Handbook of Tropical Medicine

Handbook of
Tropical Medicine

Edited by **Charline Ryler**

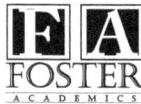

FA
FOSTER
A C A D E M I C S

New Jersey

Published by Foster Academics,
61 Van Reypen Street,
Jersey City, NJ 07306, USA
www.fosteracademics.com

Handbook of Tropical Medicine
Edited by Charline Ryler

International Standard Book Number: 978-1-63242-221-7 (Hardback)

Printed in the United States of America.

Contents

Preface

This handbook of tropical medicine includes various topics relevant in disease epidemiology, prevention and treatment. Tropical medicine has surfaced and retained its position as a significant discipline for the analysis of diseases native in the tropic, specifically those diseases which have infectious etiology. And the emergence and reemergence of several tropical pathologies have currently provoked the interest of numerous fields of the analysis of tropical medicine, inclusive of novel infectious agents. Information based on evidence along with ordered updates are required. This book provides up-to-date information on various diseases and conditions of interest in the field. It encompasses pathologies caused by helminths and protozoans. It serves as a great source of information with a broad geographical perspective as the contributions are made by veteran authors from across the globe.

After months of intensive research and writing, this book is the end result of all who devoted their time and efforts in the initiation and progress of this book. It will surely be a source of reference in enhancing the required knowledge of the new developments in the area. During the course of developing this book, certain measures such as accuracy, authenticity and research focused analytical studies were given preference in order to produce a comprehensive book in the area of study.

This book would not have been possible without the efforts of the authors and the publisher. I extend my sincere thanks to them. Secondly, I express my gratitude to my family and well-wishers. And most importantly, I thank my students for constantly expressing their willingness and curiosity in enhancing their knowledge in the field, which encourages me to take up further research projects for the advancement of the area.

Editor

Tropical Diseases Due to Protozoa and Helminths

Malaria Chemoprophylaxis for the International Traveler, Current Options and Future Possibilities

Ross Parker and Kevin Leary
Uniformed Services University of the Health Sciences
USA

1. Introduction

Malaria remains the most important parasitic disease in the world, causing approximately 250 million infections annually and one million deaths, mostly in African children. International travelers are at risk of developing malaria when visiting endemic regions, and account for an estimated 30,000 cases of malaria annually (World Health Organization, 2011). The parasite is transmitted by the female Anopheles mosquito and is caused by four protozoa of the *Plasmodium* genus *(P. falciparum, P. vivax, P. ovale* and *P. malaria). P. falciparum* causes the most significant disease burden with the highest morbidity and mortality. In addition to mosquito control and avoidance measures, chemoprophylaxis remains a critical component for preventing malaria infection in non-immune travelers.

Addressing malaria chemoprophylaxis for the international traveler can be challenging. In addition to patient-specific factors, the provider must consider a wide array of other variables, such as the predicted risk of malaria associated with the destination, type and duration of exposure during the trip as well, as the profile of the drug being prescribed. Seasonal, geographic, and climate are among the environmental variables that should be addressed to appreciate risk of malaria transmission. There can be upwards of a 200-fold difference in relative risk of contracting malaria depending on geographic variables for the international traveler, with sub-Saharan Africa conferring the greatest risk (Leder et al., 2004; Freedman, 2008). The traveler's accommodations, anticipated understanding and adherence to mosquito avoidance and control measures, chemoprophylaxis and access to appropriate medical care contribute to the risk of morbidity and mortality associated with malaria.

Patient-specific variables can also present challenges to the provider. Pregnant, nursing and pediatric travelers present unique considerations when determining the most appropriate chemoprophylactic regimen. Pregnant patients incur a much higher risk of mortality and morbidity from malaria than non-pregnant travelers, and require extensive counselling on the risks and benefits of proposed travel to areas at risk of transmission. Emerging parasite drug resistance patterns, side-effect profiles, both long and short term, contraindications and poor adherence are additional challenges that need to be considered when selecting an appropriate antimalarial chemoprophylactic agent. In addition, how to address chemoprophylaxis in long-term travelers, generally defined as travel greater than six-months in duration, can be very difficult as consensus guidelines in this population are not available (Chen et al., 2006).

It has been over ten years since the U.S. Food and Drug Administration has approved an antimalarial chemoprophylactic drug. Lack of market incentive, increasing difficulty in the design and execution of clinical trials, as well as the changing ethical environment after Declaration of Helsinki 2000 have contributed to the lag in continued development for the malaria chemoprophylaxis indication (Dow et al., 2008).

2. Education

Before travel, counseling the individual on the specific risks in the areas they may be visiting is an essential part of trip preparation. When counseling the traveler prior to visiting an endemic area, they must be made aware of the route of transmission of malaria, associated symptoms, variable incubation periods prior to symptom onset, when to seek medical aid, and the risks of contracting the disease, including death, especially in high-risk populations. They need to be aware that recent immigrants to non-malaria endemic areas returning to their home of origin to visit friends and relatives (VFR's) are at high risk for contracting malaria as acquired immunity is not long lasting (Centers for Disease Control and Prevention, 2012). Travelers should be counseled on proper personal protective measures including mosquito bite avoidance, especially during the peak transmission periods of evening and nighttime hours, mechanical and chemical barrier protection, vector control, and the appropriate use and importance of chemoprophylaxis.

Malaria can be effectively treated if suspected and recognized early and appropriate medical intervention is made within a timely manner. Time to symptom onset from initial exposure can vary, ranging as early as 7 days following a mosquito bite to several months or greater following departure from an endemic region. The diagnosis of malaria is a medical emergency since time to definitive treatment is a critical factor in determining clinical outcome. For these reasons, travelers should be counseled to seek medical care as soon as possible if they have any symptoms that may be related to malaria. The clinical presentation of malaria consists of a nonspecific, flu-like illness manifested by fever, chills, malaise, anorexia and headache. In cases of severe illness, altered mental status, seizures, respiratory disease (ARDS) and coma may be present (CDC, 2012).

Availability of medical care while traveling should be explored prior to travel. There may be rare instances where the chemoprophylaxis regimen is suboptimal or the traveler does not agree to medically advised chemoprophylaxis. In cases when the traveler develops clinical symptoms consistent with malaria and does not have timely access to medical care and definitive parasitological diagnosis, presumptive, self-administered therapy may be considered (WHO, 2010; CDC, 2012). When prescribing presumptive self-treatment, the CDC recommends a consecutive 3-day course of either atovaquone-proquanil or artemether-lumefantrine. One should never use the same drug for treatment that had been prescribed for prophylaxis. It should be stressed to the traveler that even though presumptive treatment may be available, they should seek medical care as soon as possible.

3. Personal protective measures

Several measures can be taken by the traveler while in endemic areas to reduce the risk of mosquito bites, thus reducing the risk of contracting malaria. The *Anopheles* mosquito only feeds at night, making the hours between dusk and dawn those that the traveler must be most vigilant for vector avoidance and mosquito control measures. Staying indoors, sleeping in screened-structures, and using mosquito nets during peak feeding times are all effective and relatively simple ways to reduce transmission of malaria. Other protective measures including clothing that minimizes exposed skin, eliminating mosquito breeding sites, and using appropriate repellents/insecticides on skin and clothing, should be discussed with the traveler as well (Chen et al., 2006; CDC, 2012).

A systematic literature review concluded that environmental management programs were highly effective at reducing the morbidity and mortality associated with malaria, and if educated properly travelers can reduce their risk significantly through these personal and environmental protective measures (Keiser et al., 2005).

Insecticides such as permethrin can be used as a spray to kill mosquitoes on contact, or can be used to impregnate clothes and mosquito nets for long-term protection. A 2003 randomized-controlled trial in sub-Saharan Africa showed a reduction in all-cause child mortality by 15-33% with the use of permethrin treated bed nets and curtains, and a 1995 study of permethrin impregnated uniforms in Columbian soldiers showed a decrease in incidence of malaria from 14% to 3% (Phillips-Howard & Nahlen et al., 2003; Soto & Medina et al., 1995), indicating mosquito avoidance and control measures can be highly effective in preventing malaria transmission.

Repellents prevent arthropod bites via alterations to sensorial organs. There are several different commercially available repellents including DEET (N,N-diethly-3-methyl-benzamide), picaridin (2-(2-hydroxyethyl)-1-piperidinecarboxylic acid 1-methylpropyl ester), oil of lemon eucalyptus (para-menthane-3,8-diol), and IR3535 (3-[N-butyl-N-acetyl]-aminopropionic acid, ethyl ester). The efficacy and duration of repellents vary considerably among products and species of mosquito (Zielinski-Gutierrez et al., 2012). Several studies have suggested DEET and picaridin to be the most efficacious and long lasting (Fradin & Day, 2002; Trigg, 1996; Govere et al., 2000; Badolo et al., 2004). Both DEET and picaridin demonstrate efficacy between five and seven hours after application, with variations in efficacy and duration of effectiveness related to repellent concentration, humidity, temperature, perspiration, exposure to water, and abrasion (Zielinski-Gutierrez et al., 2012). There seems to be a ceiling effect with DEET at concentrations above 50%, where higher concentrations do not offer additional benefit.

DEET, at concentrations up to 50%, can be used on children over two months of age. Children less than two months should be protected with a child carrier covered with a mosquito net. Beyond labeled precautions, the U.S. Environmental Protection Agency (EPA) and CDC do not recommend additional warnings for repellents in children > 2 months, pregnant or lactating women (Zielinski-Gutierrez et al., 2012). Like physical barriers, repellents and insecticides are only effective if used properly and consistently, thus ensuring the traveler is aware of proper use before departing is an essential part of pre-trip counseling.

4. Chemoprophylaxis

Educating travelers on the clinical indications, as well as proper use and risks of chemoprophylaxis is an important part of pre-travel counseling. Patients should be told of the options available for the area they are traveling based on CDC recommendations, and when clinically indicated, an appropriate chemoprophylaxis should be chosen and prescribed based on the patient's medical history, tolerability of side effects, compliance, and known resistance in the area (Table 1). Resistance to antimalarial drugs is growing, and is a major public health concern (WHO, 2010). Resistance of *P. falciparum* to chloroquine, the most widely available and least expensive chemoprophylaxis agent, is now widespread, except in a few limited areas of the Caribbean, Central and South America, and a few countries in the Middle East. Resistance to mefloquine is spreading and has been confirmed in areas of SE Asia including along the borders of Burma and China, Laos and Burma, Thailand and Burma, Thailand and Cambodia, and in southern Vietnam (CDC, 2012).

4.1 Chloroquine

Chloroquine is a 4-aminoquinoline oral antimalarial agent first introduced in the 1940's. It has good bioavailability, is rapidly absorbed and appreciably concentrated in tissues such as the liver, spleen, and to a lesser extent in the CNS (WHO, 2010). Its plasmodicidal activity is thought to be related to its interaction with malarial DNA, specifically haem detoxification (Castelli et al., 2010; WHO, 2010). Chloroquine is dosed once weekly and is effective against the erythrocytic stages of sensitive plasmodium species.

Chloroquine has long shown its efficacy against malaria, and was a cornerstone of treatment until growing resistance became a problem in the 1980's (Castelli et al., 2010). *P. falciparum* resistance to chloroquine is widespread, thus making it an acceptable choice only in chloroquine sensitive areas. There is some evidence of mutations making non-falciparum strains resistant, with resistance of *P. vivax* to chloroquine reported in areas of Papua New Guinea, West Papua, Guyana, Vanuatu, Myanmar, Indonesia, and India (WHO, 2010; Kain et al., 2001; Davis et al., 2003).

Chloroquine has a generally mild side effect profile with the most common events being nausea, headache, blurred vision, insomnia, and pruritis (Castelli et al., 2010). Serious side effects, although rare, include myopathy, hepatitis, hearing loss, Stevens-Johnson Syndrome, seizures, and irreversible retinopathy (WHO, 2010). Retinopathy is usually seen after 100g cumulative dose, which is equivalent to what a long-term traveler may ingest in 5-6 years of weekly dosing (Chen et al., 2006). Chloroquine-induced retinopathy is rare in patients taking malaria prophylaxis and is more frequently seen in the higher doses administered for the treatment of rheumatoid arthritis (CDC, 2012). In a large (N=2701) trial of peace corps volunteers undergoing malaria prophylaxis it was found that chloroquine was better tolerated and had fewer serious side effects than mefloquine or doxycycline, however prophylaxis in general was not tolerated well with 9% reporting severe events and 23% at some point changing their prophylactic medication (Korhonen et al., 2007).

Chloroquine is considered safe for use in children and pregnancy, however strict adherence to weight-based dosing must be adhered to for children since serious adverse events have been reported in children receiving as little as 1 gram of chloroquine (Chen et al., 2006). While chloroquine is safe for breast-feeding mothers, the infant should receive separate prophylaxis as the amount of chloroquine secreted in breast milk is not sufficient for protection.

Chloroquine is available in 500mg tablets, which is equivalent to 300mg chloroquine base. Dosing is done weekly starting 2 weeks before travel into an endemic area and for 4 weeks after leaving the area. Pediatric dosing is 5mg/kg base, never to exceed adult dosing.

While generally considered a safe and efficacious drug, the growing resistance to chloroquine is making it a choice only available in limited areas of the world. However, because it is one of two current drugs considered safe in pregnant women and children, and because it is fairly well tolerated, it will remain a viable choice for prophylaxis if resistance patterns are taken into account when prescribing.

4.2 Primaquine

Primaquine phosphate is an oral antimalarial agent first approved by the FDA in 1952. The mechanism of action is not well understood, but its plasmodicidal activity is thought to be related to disruption of the parasitic electron transport chain (Castelli et al., 2010). It has a short half-life of approximately seven hours, thus requiring daily dosing. Before the approval of primaquine, there was no available treatment of relapsing malaria because anti-malarial drugs available at the time were only effective against the erythrocytic stages of Plasmodium species (Shanks et al., 2001). Primaquine's approval was important because it is effective against both the erythrocytic and exoerythocytic stages of Plasmodium species, making it an effective choice for *P.vivax, P. ovale, or P. falciparum* (WHO, 2010; Shanks, Kain et al., 2001). However, it is only FDA-approved for the treatment of vivax malaria, but has long been used for treatment off-label for other species and is the drug of choice for terminal prophylaxis in travelers at risk for relapsing malaria (Castelli et al., 2010; Hill et al., 2006).

Multiple clinical trials have shown the efficacy of primaquine against both vivax and falciparum malaria (Shanks et al., 2001). In two placebo controlled trials on the island of New Guinea it was shown that primaquine had an efficacy of 93 - 95% against *P. falciparum* and 88 - 90% against *P. vivax* (Baird et al., 2001; Fryauff et al., 1995). In two placebo controlled trials done in Columbia good efficacy was also seen, with an overall efficacy of 89% against *P. falciparum* and 88% against *P. Vivax* (Soto et al., 1998, 1999). While good efficacy has been seen in the past, there is emerging evidence of increasing resistance to *P. Vivax* strains in some areas of Oceana, South East Asia, and South America (Baird, 2009).

Primaquine is a well-tolerated medication with the most common side effects being nausea, vomiting, and abdominal cramps (Fryauff et al., 1995). It was shown to have better tolerability than chloroquine in Irian Jaya transmigrates, and in a retrospective study of travelers to Ethiopia it had favorable tolerability compared to mefloquine and doxycycline (Schwartz & Regev-Yochay, 1999; Baird et al., 2001). Severe hemolytic anemia can occur in patients with glucose-6-phosphate dehydrogenase (G6PD) deficiency and should be avoided in any patient with this enzymopathy. All patients taking primaquine should be evaluated for G6PD deficiency prior to receiving this drug (Hill et al., 2006).

Off-label dosing recommendations are 30mg base per day for 14 days for terminal prophylaxis, and 30mg per day 1-2 days before travel and continued for 7 days after travel for prophylaxis (CDC, 2012). It should be taken with food to limit side effects. Dosing for children is 0.5 mg/kg base per day. It has been shown safe in studies up to one year with no labeled restrictions on duration of use (Fryauff et al., 1995; Chen et al., 2006). Primaquine is contraindicated in pregnant women, making prevention or treatment of malaria in areas with *P.vivax* difficult in this population. If used as a primary prophylaxis, it negates the need for terminal prophylaxis, however, if another primary chemoprophylaxis is chosen, and relapsing malaria is a concern, it makes a good choice for terminal prophylaxis.

4.3 Mefloquine

Mefloquine hydrochloride is a methanol-quinoline oral antimalarial agent whose mechanism of action is not completely understood, but is thought to be similar to quinine

(Castelli et al., 2010). It acts as a blood schizonticide, making it highly effective against the erythrocytic stages of Plasmodium species, however it does not have any exoerythrocytic activity. Mefloquine has a long half-life, with the average being 21 days, thus only requiring once-weekly dosing. Mefloquine is effective against chloroquine resistant Plasmodium species, however there are some areas in SE Asia with known mefloquine resistance. Of note, mefloquine has been found to have serious neuropsychiatric adverse events, which limit its usefulness in certain populations (Castelli et al., 2010; Croft & Garner, 2008).

Mefloquine efficacy has been shown to be greater than 90% in multiple clinical trials (Kain, Shanks et al., 2001), the longest of which was in Peace-Corps volunteers in Africa during the early 1990's. In addition, a review of mefloquine trials found that it did prevent malaria in chloroquine resistant areas (Croft & Garner, 2000). Although an effective medication, the endemic risk of malaria, current resistance patterns, the drug's side effect profile and the patient's medical and psychiatric history should be carefully considered before prescribing mefloquine (Croft & Garner, 2000).

The mefloquine label lists many side effects, the most common of which are nausea, vomiting, diarrhea, and abdominal pain. However, it also states that mefloquine can cause serious mental problems including anxiety, paranoia, hallucinations, and suicidal thoughts. These psychiatric problems may lead to prophylaxis discontinuation, and should be considered when choosing the appropriate chemoprophylactic regimen. The high rate of side effects associated with mefloquine has been shown in several clinical trials including a randomized, double blind controlled study of 623 travelers. This study found that mefloquine had the highest rate of neuropsychiatric adverse events at 37%, with the highest proportion of the events in women. A retrospective study of 4240 patients taking malaria prophylaxis completed in 2009 also showed that mefloquine had the highest incidence of neuropsychiatric events among antimalarials, and that there were 22 deaths including 5 suicides associated with normal doses of the drug (Jacquerioz & Croft, 2009). There also have been clinical trials showing that mefloquine has a higher rate of discontinuation than either placebo (3.3% for mefloquine overall) or atovaquone and proguanil (5% vs. 3.9% of atovaquone and proguanil) due to GI upset, dizziness, and neuropsychological events (Kain et al., 2001; Hogh et al., 2000). Additionally, Mefloquine has been linked with an increased risk of seizures and cardiac arrhythmias, and a 2008 FDA post marketing review associated pneumonitis and eosinophilic pneumonia with the use of mefloquine (FDA, 2008).

Mefloquine is a safe choice for children and women. It is available in 250mg tablets, with the dose being 1 pill weekly for adults and for children over 45kg. Mefloquine should be taken with food or water. Prophylactic therapy should begin ≥ 2 weeks before travel to endemic areas, and must continue four weeks after leaving the area. The effectiveness of mefloquine against resistant species of plasmodium still makes it a good choice for travelers going to chloroquine resistant regions such as Africa, and the fact that it is safe in children and pregnant women make it a much more versatile drug. However, the neuropsychiatric adverse events and other side effects should be taken into account when choosing it as a prophylactic medication.

4.4 Doxycycline

Doxycycline is a broad-spectrum antibiotic derived from oxytetracycline that acts on the 30S ribosome subunit thus disrupting protein synthesis, and has activity against not only bacteria, but several parasitic diseases as well. It has a short half-life, necessitating daily dosing and can be used as a malarial chemoprophylaxis in areas with known chloroquine and mefloquine resistance (Kain et al., 2001). It does not have activity against the exoerythorcytic stages of malaria making it a less efficacious choice for areas of the world with endemic *P. vivax* and *P. ovale*.

Several studies have shown the efficacy of prophylactic doxycycline in the prevention of malaria. In a double-blind, placebo controlled study doxycycline had 99% efficacy in the prevention of malaria in soldiers in Irian Jaya, Indonesia (Ohrt et al., 1997). In a separate trial investigating the prophylactic efficacy of azithromycin vs. doxycycline in 213 adult volunteers in a malaria endemic area it was found that daily doxycycline had an efficacy of 92.6% vs. 82.7% for daily azithromycin (Andersen et al., 1998). In addition, doxycycline was well tolerated in both of these studies.

While generally well tolerated, the most common side effects of doxycycline are primarily gastrointestinal including nausea, vomiting, diarrhea, glossitis, dysphagia, and rare instances of esophagitis and esophageal ulceration (Castelli et al., 2010). Doxycycline is a photosensitizing agent, and thus care must be taken to prevent over exposure to the sun while on this medication. Doxycycline also increases the risk for vaginal candidiasis by inhibiting the growth of natural vaginal flora. In a randomized, double-blind, placebo controlled trial of 623 non-immune travelers requiring short-term malaria chemoprophylaxis, doxycycline demonstrated a comparable side-effect profile to atovaquone/proquanal (Schlagenhauf et al., 2003). Importantly however, this study used doxycycline monohydrate, the more expensive form of the drug that has a favorable gastrointestinal side-effect profile. The findings of this study should not be extrapolated to the use of doxycycline hyclate or the non-enteric coated forms of doxycycline, where tolerability would likely be less favorable and might affect adherence to this chemoprophylactic drug.

The dosing for adults is 100mg daily. It is contraindicated in children under 8 years of age due to the risk of permanent discoloration of the teeth, and in pregnant or breast-feeding women due to the risk of toxicity to the fetus/infant (CDC, 2012). The recommended dosing for children ≥ 8 years of age is 2.2 mg/kg up to 100mg/day (CDC, 2012). Treatment should start one to two days before and last for 28 days after leaving an endemic area. Doxycycline should be taken with copious water to reduce the risk of esophagitis and may be taken with food to reduce GI side effects, although caution should be taken to avoid concomitant administration of antacids, magnesium salts, or bismuth subsalicylate as these may decrease intestinal absorption. The traveler should remain upright for at least 30 minutes following administration to reduce the risk of esophageal irritation or ulceration.

4.5 Atovaquone and proguanil hydrochloride

Atovaquone and proguanil is a combination antimalarial that works by inhibiting parasite mitochondrial electron transport and parasitic DNA synthesis by inhibiting dihydrofolate reductase. Proguanil significantly enhances the ability of atovaquone to inhibit parasitic mitochondrial electron transport (Kain et al., 2001; McKeage & Scott, 2003; Srivastava & Vaidya, 1999).

Atovaquone/proguanil is a once daily medication that is effective against both the erythrocytic and exoerythorcytic stages of malaria making this an acceptable choice not only for *P. falciprum*, but also *P. vivax and P. ovale*, both of which have hepatic life cycles. The efficacy of atovaquone as a causal prophylaxis was seen in a small volunteer challenge study in which it was shown that parasites were eliminated prior to the establishment of erythrocytic infection, thus supporting causal efficacy (Shapiro et al., 1999). Atovaquone/proquanal has demonstrated efficacy for malaria prophylaxis in areas with predominantly *P. vivax* (Soto et al., 2006).

Atovaquone/proguanil's suppressive prophylaxis effectiveness has been shown in several clinical trials, three of which were among semi-immune populations in Gabon, Kenya, and Zambia and conducted as double-blinded, randomized, and placebo controlled trials, where overall efficacy of 98% in preventing malaria was observed in this population (Lell et al., 1998; Shanks et al., 1998; Sukwa et al., 1999; Kain et al., 2001). In two other large studies, in which non-immune travelers to malaria endemic regions were randomized to receive atovaquone/proguanil, mefloquine, or chloroquine plus proguanil, none of the patients in the atovaquone/proguanil arms who completed the study developed malaria (Hogh et al., 2000; Overbosch et al., 2001). It was also shown to be 100% effective against *P. falciparum* in non-immune Columbian soldiers (Soto et al., 2006). In a study of non-immune Indonesian immigrants, atovaquone/proguanil was 93% effective at preventing *P. falciparum* and 84% effective at preventing *P.vivax* (Ling et al., 2002).

The causal prophylactic activity of atovaquone/proguanil results in required dosing for only 1-week post exposure vs. up to 4 weeks with antimalarials that only have activity against the erythrocytic stage of the parasite, which may contribute to better adherence by travelers than some other malaria prophylaxis (Kain et al., 2001). In addition, the discontinuation rate due to side effects of the medication was found to be lower in atovaquone/proguanil then either mefloquine or chloroquine/proguanil (1.2%, vs. 5.0% and 0.2% vs. 2.0%, respectively) (Hogh et al., 2000; Overbosch et al., 2001). In a randomized control study, atovaquone/proguanil had a relatively low incidence of reported side effects compared to other available chemoprophylactic agents (Schlagenhauf et al., 2003). The most serious side effects of atovaquone/proguanil, although rare, include Steven-Johnson Syndrome, and a transient elevation of liver enzymes, while the most common were headache, abdominal pain, cough, diarrhea, and myalgias (McKeage & Scott, 2003).

Atovaquone/proguanil tablets are available in two formulations, adult and pediatric with the adult tablet containing 250mg of atovaquone and 100mg of proguanil, and the pediatric tablet containing 62.5 mg and 25mg of atovaquone and proguanil, respectively. Adult dosing is 1 adult tablet daily for 1-2 days before travel into an endemic area, daily throughout the stay, and then for 7 days once out of the endemic area. Dosing in the pediatric population is the same as for adults, except the number of pediatric tablets given daily is weight based. Atovaquone is highly a lipophilic compound in which the rate and extent of absorption is increased when taken with dietary fat, thus atovaquone/proguanil should be taken with food or a milky drink. While the safety of atovaquone/proguanil in the adult and pediatric populations has been shown through clinical trials, the safety during pregnancy is unknown and is contraindicated in this population. In addition, this medication should be avoided in mother's breastfeeding infants under 5kg and should not be used in patients with severe renal impairment (creatinine clearance < 30 ml/min).

While there are some case reports of resistance, in general atovaquone/proguanil is an efficacious, well-tolerated medication that should be considered first line in chloroquine and mefloquine resistant areas. The cost is higher than with other antimalarial chemoprophylactic drugs, which may limit its use in certain circumstances. Once atovaquone/proguanil becomes generic, this drug may be a more affordable option for malaria chemoprophylaxis in the future.

	Atovaquone/	Doxycycline	Primaquine	Mefloquine	Chloroquine
Adult Dose, scheduling	250mg/150mg once daily, 1-2 days before entering endemic region and 7 days after last exposure	100 mg once daily, 1-2 days before entering endemic region and 4 weeks after last exposure	30 mg base once daily, 1-2 days before entering endemic region and 7 days after last exposure	250 mg once weekly, 2 weeks before entering endemic region and 4 weeks after last exposure	500 mg (300mg base) once weekly, begin 1-2 weeks before entering endemic region and continue 4 weeks after last exposure
Pediatric	Yes for children 5 kg, weight based dose (only FDA-approved for children 11kg (see text)	Contraindicated < 8 years of age	Yes, weight based dose	Yes, for children >5kg and > 6 months, see text for children 5 kg or younger than 6 months of age	Yes, 5mg/kg base once weekly up to adult dose
Pregnancy	Insufficient data, not recommended	Contraindicated	Contraindicated	Yes	Yes
Limits on	None	4 months	None	None	None
Advantages	Very well tolerated, convenient, good efficacy	Inexpensive, relatively well tolerated, good efficacy, available worldwide	Inexpensive, relatively well tolerated, effective against all malaria species	Inexpensive, convenient, effective against all malaria species	Inexpensive, relatively well tolerated, convenient
Disadvantages	Expensive, contraindicated for poor renal function	Photosensitivity, increased risk for vaginal yeast infections, inconvenient	G6PD testing required before administration	Growing resistance, poorly tolerated, neurotoxicity, contraindicated with active or recent depression and other psychiatric disorders	Wide spread resistance, only useful in limited areas of the world
Comments	May become more affordable once generic.	May protect against rickettsial infections and leptospirosis as well as malaria	Not US FDA approved for chemoprophylaxis, dosing based on CDC recommendations	Contraindicated in those allergic to quinine/quinidine, cardiac conduction abnormalities	May worsen psoriasis

Table 1. Malaria Prophylaxis Options

5. Special populations

Children and pregnant women are at the highest risk for severe malaria when traveling to endemic areas and increased vigilance should be taken when dealing with these populations. It should be recommend that travel to endemic areas with a risk of transmission be avoided by these populations if possible, however if patients insist, the provider should stress that the traveler or the parents of the traveler insure that both personnel protective measures and chemoprophylaxis are strictly adhered to.

5.1 Pregnancy

Contracting malaria while pregnant puts the mother at an increased risk for adverse outcomes. Malaria infection during pregnancy has been associated with premature labor, abortion and stillbirth. The traveler should be counseled that the diagnosis of malaria in pregnancy may be difficult due to relatively low parasitemia at clinical presentation. A very high degree of suspicion should be taken when a pregnant women presents with fever in an endemic area, as missing the diagnosis could have grave consequences (McGready et al., 2004). Appropriate precautions should be followed including mosquito avoidance and control measures discussed previously as well as chemoprophylaxis when clinically indicated. Reviewing label-specific information and current CDC recommendations should be adhered to. There are no published data indicating elevated risks with the use of DEET in pregnant or lactating women, and current U.S. Environmental Protection Agency and CDC sources do not advise additional precautions for using FDA-approved insect repellants in this population (Koren et al., 2003; Zielinski-Gutierrez et al., 2012). Chemoprophylaxis in pregnancy is limited, as both doxycycline and primaquine are contraindicated, and atovoquone/proguanil is not currently recommended due to lack of safety data from clinical studies. Medications considered safe during pregnancy include chloroquine and mefloquine. While data in the past have only recommended mefloquine in the last half of pregnancy, current recommendations state that there is no evidence of adverse outcome if taken in any of the three trimesters of pregnancy when no other option is available (CDC, 2012).

5.2 Children

Children are at risk of malaria and the associated complications while traveling to endemic areas, and should have the same personal protective measures as adults. DEET has been shown to be safe and effective and is recommended for use by both the CDC and the American Academy of Pediatrics (AAP) for all children over 2 months of age at concentrations between 10-30% based on duration of protection required (Koren et al., 2003; AAP, 2009, 2011; CDC, 2012). Chemoprophylaxis for children is not as restricted as for pregnant women, with contraindications including doxycyline usage in children under 8 and primaquine usage in G6PD deficient patients. Atovaquone/proguanil is FDA approved for children greater than 11kg but recommended for off-label use by the CDC and AAP for children >5 kg. Mefloquine is only FDA approved for children > 5 kg and older than 6 months of age, but when necessary recommend off-label for children < 5kg and any age (AAP, 2009; CDC, 2012). Parents of very young infants should be counseled to avoid areas endemic for malaria given the risk of severe disease in this population. Adherence to personal protective measures and chemoprophylaxis if often poor in children, and thus it must be stressed to the traveling parent the importance of these precautions.

6. Existing challenges and future possibilities

As outlined in this chapter, there are only five available options for malaria chemoprophylaxis in the United States, one of which, primaquine, is not FDA approved for this indication. Emerging resistance, traveler intolerance, non-adherence, side effects and contraindications to existing options warrant development of newer agents for future chemoprophylactic use.

Resistance to existing drugs is well documented. Wide spread chloroquine resistance has led to the use of this drug in only very limited areas of the world, and mefloquine resistance continues to emerge. Doxycycline resistance has not been established and there is no well accepted definition or validated approach to measuring primaquine resistance (Baird, 2009). Primaquine tolerant or refractory strains of *P. vivax* have been well described, notably the Chesson strain from New Guinea (Collins & Jeffery, 1996). As resistance continues to emerge among existing options for the prevention of malaria, the importance of developing new and effective chemoprophylactic drugs for the international traveler becomes critical.

There are very few candidates currently being developed for malaria chemoprophylaxis, and the last FDA approval for this indication, atovoquone/proquanil, was over ten years ago in 2000. Doxycycline and mefloquine received FDA approval for malaria chemoprophylaxis in the preceding 11 years prior to the atovoquone/proquanil approval. The current lack of development of drugs for this indication is unprecedented and is cause for great concern.

Many reasons have been postulated for the lack of candidates in the developmental pipeline for the chemoprophylaxis indication. Obvious barriers are the lack of market incentive for this indication, although it is clear that the number of international non-immune travelers visiting endemic malarious regions has increased substantially in the last few decades, with case fatality rates ranging from 1-3% for falciparum malaria (Chen & Keystone, 2005). One challenge that has been attributed to stalled development in this area is the 5th Amendment to the Declaration of Helsinki (DH2000). First adopted by the World Medical Association (WMA) in 1964, the Declaration of Helsinki was an attempt to formally identify core ethical principles and guidelines for physicians and others involved in the design, execution and oversight of clinical research (Carlson et al., 2004). Principles relating to the use of placebo in clinical trials, post-trial access to investigational drugs, and social benefit as defined in DH2000, have presented challenges to existing models and development strategies for antimalarial chemoprophylactic drugs. Strategies to address these challenges in clinical development have been proposed (Dow et al., 2008).

Azithromycin, piperaquine, and tafenoquine have all been suggested as possible future chemoprophylactic drugs (Dow et al., 2008). Azithromycin has shown some promise, however future study is needed with combination agents to clarify its role for this indication (Chen & Keystone, 2005).

Tafenoquine, an 8-aminquinolone is a synthetic analogue of primaquine. First developed by the Walter Reed Army Institute of Research as WR238605 or etaquine, tafenoquine has a very long elimination half-life of approximately 14 days allowing weekly dosing. This novel compound shows promise for causal chemoprophylaxis against *P. falciparum* and *P. vivax*, as well as radical cure of *P. vivax*. It has been shown in rhesus monkeys to have 10x higher potency than primaquine for causal prophylaxis, and has demonstrated greater activity against blood and liver-stage parasites *in vitro*. (Cooper et al., 1994; Shanks et al., 2001).

In phase I studies of tafenoquine the drug is well tolerated with single doses up to 600mg and with chronic dosing (6 months) at 200mg weekly following a load of 200mg daily for 3 days (Brueckner et al., 1998; Leary et al., 2009) with no dose-limiting adverse events. The most common side effects observed are gastrointestinal, including heartburn, nausea and gas, usually associated with higher (>200mg) dosing. The most significant toxicity associated with tafenoquine is the potential to induce hemolysis in G6PD deficient individuals and methemoglobinemia (Crockett & Kain, 2007). GlaxoSmithKline, in partnership with Medicines for Malaria Venture, are undertaking an ascending-dose safety study of tafenoquine in G6PD heterozygous patients to identify the maximum safe dose in this population (MMV, 2011).

There have been several placebo-controlled trials evaluating tafenoquine as a causal antimalarial chemoprophylactic drug. In a study of non and semi-immune Thai soldiers, tafenoquine was administered monthly at 400mg, following a 1200mg loading dose (given as 400mg/day for 3 days) for a total of 6 months and demonstrated a protective efficacy 96% for *P. vivax* and 100% for multidrug-resistant *P. falciparum* (Walsh et al., 2004).

In a dose ranging prophylactic trial of tafenoquine to prevent *P. falciparum* in Gabon semi-immunes, which included children, doses of 25mg, 50mg, 100mg or 200mg/day for three consecutive days were tested. Tafenoquine was given one week following treatment with halofantrine. Subjects were actively followed for positive blood smears at day 56 and day 77 following tafenoquine dosing. Notwithstanding the 25mg dose, which uniformly failed, tafenoquine demonstrated 100% protective efficacy (PE) at all doses of 50mg or greater at day 56 and had PE of 80%, 93% and 100% at day 77 for doses of 50mg, 100mg and 200mg, respectively (Lell et al., 2000).

In a 13-week prophylactic trial in Kenyan semi-immune adults, tafenoquine was evaluated at weekly doses of 200mg and 400mg followed by a 600mg and 1200mg 3-day load, respectively. A third group consisted of a loading dose (1200mg load), followed by weekly placebo and a fourth group received placebo only throughout the 13-week period. The 200mg and 400mg weekly doses demonstrated PE of 91% and 93%, respectively. The loading dose only group had a PE of 80% (Shanks et al., 2001).

A large randomized, non-placebo controlled trial of non-immune Australian soldiers evaluated tafenoquine, dosed at 200mg weekly for 6 months following a loading dose (200mg/day for 3 days) while deployed to East Timor. Study participants were randomized 3:1 to receive either tafenoquine (n=492) or mefloquine (n=162) throughout their deployment. Although treatment-emergent adverse events were similar between the two groups and tafenoquine was well-tolerated during the study, there were no cases of malaria in any group. Exposure to malaria could not be assessed and therefore efficacy was not established (Nasveld et al., 2010).

In a subset of subjects (n=74) in the East Timor study who received tafenoquine, detailed safety assessments were conducted which detected vortex keratopathy. This finding had no effect on visual acuity and was fully resolved within one year following cessation of therapy (Nasveld et al., 2010). More extensive clinical ophthalmic evaluation of tafenoquine in a subsequent phase 1 safety trial further supports the vortex keratopathy seen with tafenoquine is not clinically significant (Leary et al., 2009).

Tafenoquine shows promise as a causal prophylactic drug and is currently being developed for a radical cure indication for *P. vivax* through a joint collaboration between GlaxoSmithKline and Medicines for Malaria Venture (MMV, 2011).

7. Conclusion

Addressing malaria chemoprophylaxis for the international traveler can be challenging and should be done within the context of a comprehensive medical evaluation well before visiting the endemic region. Malaria is a life-threatening illness and requires a multidimensional, individually tailored approach to ensure the most appropriate measures, including non-drug strategies, are taken to prevent infection if the traveler is exposed. Existing chemoprophylactic drugs offer effective options for the international traveler, however emerging resistance, side effect profiles and contraindications limit use in many circumstances. Future effort is needed to identify and develop new effective and safe options for malaria chemoprophylaxis.

The views expressed in this chapter are those of the authors and do not necessarily reflect the official policy or position of the Department of the Navy, Army or Air Force, the Department of Defense, nor the U.S. Government

8. References

AAP (2009). American Academy of Pediatrics Red Book.

AAP. (2011). "American Academy of Pediatrics." Retrieved July 10, 2011, 2011, from http://www.aap.org/.

Andersen, S. L., A. J. Oloo, et al. (1998). "Successful double-blinded, randomized, placebo-controlled field trial of azithromycin and doxycycline as prophylaxis for malaria in western Kenya." Clin Infect Dis 26(1): 146-150.

Badolo, A., E. Ilboudo-Sanogo, et al. (2004). "Evaluation of the sensitivity of Aedes aegypti and Anopheles gambiae complex mosquitoes to two insect repellents: DEET and KBR 3023." Trop Med Int Health 9(3): 330-334.

Baird, J. K. (2009). "Resistance to Therapies for Infection by *Plasmodium vivax*." Clinical Microbiology Reviews 22(3): 508-534.

Baird, J. K., M. D. Lacy, et al. (2001). "Randomized, parallel placebo-controlled trial of primaquine for malaria prophylaxis in Papua, Indonesia." Clin Infect Dis 33(12): 1990-1997.

Brueckner, R. P., K. C. Lasseter, et al. (1998). "First-Time-In-Humans Safety and Pharmacokinetics of WR 238605, a New Antimalarial." American Journal of Tropical Medicine and Hygiene 58(5): 645-649.

Carlson, R. V., K. M. Boyd, et al. (2004). "The revision of the Declaration of Helsinki: past, present and future." British Journal of Clinical Pharmacology 57(6): 695-713.

Castelli, F., S. Odolini, et al. (2010). "Malaria prophylaxis: A comprehensive review." Pharmaceuticals 3(10): 3212-3239.

CDC (2012). Infectious Disease Related to Travel, Malaria. Atlanta, U.S. Department of Health and Human Services, Public Health Service.

Chen, L. H. and J. S. Keystone (2005). "New Strategies for the Prevention of Malaria in Travelers." Infectious Disease Clinics of North America 19: 185-210.

Chen, L. H., M. E. Wilson, et al. (2006). "Prevention of malaria in long-term travelers." Journal of the American Medical Association 296(18): 2234-2244.

Collins, W. E. and G. M. Jeffery (1996). "Primaquine Resistance in *Plasmodium Vivax*." American Journal of Tropical Medicine and Hygiene 55(3): 243-249.

Cooper, R. D., W. K. Milhous, et al. (1994). "The efficacy of WR238605 against the blood stages of a chloroquine resistant strain of Plasmodium vivax." Trans R Soc Trop Med Hyg 88(6): 691-692.

Crockett, M. and K. C. Kain (2007). "Tafenoquine: a promising new antimalarial agent." Expert Opininion on Investigational Drugs 16(5): 705-715.

Croft, A. M. and P. Garner (2000). "Mefloquine for preventing malaria in non-immune adult travellers." Cochrane Database Syst Rev(2): CD000138.

Croft, A. M. and P. Garner (2008). "WITHDRAWN: Mefloquine for preventing malaria in non-immune adult travellers." Cochrane Database Syst Rev(1): CD000138.

Davis, T. M., D. A. Syed, et al. (2003). "Toxicity related to chloroquine treatment of resistant vivax malaria." Ann Pharmacother 37(4): 526-529.

Dow, G. S., A. J. Magill, et al. (2008). "Clinical development of new prophylactic antimalarial drugs after the 5th Amendment to the Declaration of Helsinki." Ther Clin Risk Manag 4(4): 803-819.

FDA. (2008). "Postmarketing Reviews - Volume 1, Number 4, Summer 2008." Retrieved June 25th, 2011, from http://www.fda.gov/Drugs/DrugSafety/DrugSafetyNewsletter/ucm120613.htm.

Fradin, M. S. and J. F. Day (2002). "Comparative efficacy of insect repellents against mosquito bites." N Engl J Med 347(1): 13-18.

Freedman, D. O. (2008). "Clinical practice. Malaria prevention in short-term travelers." N Engl J Med 359(6): 603-612.

Fryauff, D. J., J. K. Baird, et al. (1995). "Randomised placebo-controlled trial of primaquine for prophylaxis of falciparum and vivax malaria." Lancet 346(8984): 1190-1193.

Govere, J., D. N. Durrheim, et al. (2000). "Efficacy of three insect repellents against the malaria vector Anopheles arabiensis." Med Vet Entomol 14(4): 441-444.

Hill, D. R., J. K. Baird, et al. (2006). "Primaquine: report from CDC expert meeting on malaria chemoprophylaxis I." Am J Trop Med Hyg 75(3): 402-415.

Hogh, B., P. D. Clarke, et al. (2000). "Atovaquone-proguanil versus chloroquine-proguanil for malaria prophylaxis in non-immune travellers: a randomised, double-blind study. Malarone International Study Team." Lancet 356(9245): 1888-1894.

Jacquerioz, F. A. and A. M. Croft (2009). "Drugs for preventing malaria in travellers." Cochrane Database Syst Rev(4): CD006491.

Kain, K. C., G. D. Shanks, et al. (2001). "Malaria chemoprophylaxis in the age of drug resistance. I. Currently recommended drug regimens." Clin Infect Dis 33(2): 226-234.

Keiser, J., B. H. Singer, et al. (2005). "Reducing the burden of malaria in different eco-epidemiological settings with environmental management: a systematic review." Lancet Infect Dis 5(11): 695-708.

Koren, G., D. Matsui, et al. (2003). "DEET-based insect repellents: safety implications for children and pregnant and lactating women." CMAJ 169(3): 209-212.

Korhonen, C., K. Peterson, et al. (2007). "Self-reported adverse events associated with antimalarial chemoprophylaxis in peace corps volunteers." Am J Prev Med 33(3): 194-199.

Leary, K. J., M. A. Riel, et al. (2009). "A Randomized, Double-Blind, Safety and Tolerability Study to Assess the Ophthalmic and Renal Effects of Tafenoquine 200mg Weekly versus Placebo for 6 Months in Healthy Volunteers." American Journal of Tropical Medicine and Hygiene 81(2): 356-362.

Leder, K., J. Black, et al. (2004). "Malaria in Travelers: A Review of the GeoSentinel Surveillance Network." Clin Infect Dis 39: 1104-1112.

Lell, B., J. F. Faucher, et al. (2000). "Malaria chemoprophylaxis with tafenoquine: a randomised study." Lancet 355: 2041-2045.

Lell, B., D. Luckner, et al. (1998). "Randomised placebo-controlled study of atovaquone plus proguanil for malaria prophylaxis in children." Lancet 351(9104): 709-713.

Ling, J., J. K. Baird, et al. (2002). "Randomized, placebo-controlled trial of atovaquone/proguanil for the prevention of Plasmodium falciparum or Plasmodium vivax malaria among migrants to Papua, Indonesia." Clin Infect Dis 35(7): 825-833.

McGready, R., E. A. Ashley, et al. (2004). "Malaria and the pregnant traveller." Travel Med Infect Dis 2(3-4): 127-142.

McKeage, K. and L. Scott (2003). "Atovaquone/proguanil: a review of its use for the prophylaxis of Plasmodium falciparum malaria." Drugs 63(6): 597-623.

MMV. (2011). "MMV Interactive Science Portfolio: Tafenoquine." Retrieved July 5th, 2011, 2011, from www.mmv.org/research-development/science-portfolio.

Nasveld, P. E., M. D. Edstein, et al. (2010). "Randomized, Double-Blind Study of the Safety, Tolerability, and Efficacy of Tafenoquine versus Mefloquine for Malaria Prophylaxis in Nonimmune Subjects." Antimicrob Agents Chemother 54(2): 792-798.

Ohrt, C., T. L. Richie, et al. (1997). "Mefloquine compared with doxycycline for the prophylaxis of malaria in Indonesian soldiers. A randomized, double-blind, placebo-controlled trial." Ann Intern Med 126(12): 963-972.

Overbosch, D., H. Schilthuis, et al. (2001). "Atovaquone-proguanil versus mefloquine for malaria prophylaxis in nonimmune travelers: results from a randomized, double-blind study." Clin Infect Dis 33(7): 1015-1021.

Phillips-Howard, P. A., B. L. Nahlen, et al. (2003). "The efficacy of permethrin-treated bed nets on child mortality and morbidity in western Kenya I. Development of infrastructure and description of study site." Am J Trop Med Hyg 68(4 Suppl): 3-9.

Schlagenhauf, P., A. Tschopp, et al. (2003). "Tolerability of malaria chemoprophylaxis in non-immune travellers to sub-Saharan Africa: multicentre, randomised, double blind, four arm study." BMJ 327(7423): 1078.

Schwartz, E. and G. Regev-Yochay (1999). "Primaquine as prophylaxis for malaria for nonimmune travelers: A comparison with mefloquine and doxycycline." Clin Infect Dis 29(6): 1502-1506.

Shanks, G. D., D. M. Gordon, et al. (1998). "Efficacy and safety of atovaquone/proguanil as suppressive prophylaxis for Plasmodium falciparum malaria." Clin Infect Dis 27(3): 494-499.

Shanks, G. D., K. C. Kain, et al. (2001). "Malaria chemoprophylaxis in the age of drug resistance. II. Drugs that may be available in the future." Clin Infect Dis 33(3): 381-385.

Shanks, G. D., A. J. Oloo, et al. (2001). "A New Primaquine Analogue, Tafenoquine (WR 238605), for Prophylaxis against Plasmodium falciparum Malaria." Clin Infect Dis 33: 1968-1974.

Shapiro, T. A., C. D. Ranasinha, et al. (1999). "Prophylactic activity of atovaquone against Plasmodium falciparum in humans." Am J Trop Med Hyg 60(5): 831-836.

Soto, J., F. Medina, et al. (1995). "Efficacy of permethrin-impregnated uniforms in the prevention of malaria and leishmaniasis in Colombian soldiers." Clin Infect Dis 21(3): 599-602.

Soto, J., J. Toledo, et al. (2006). "Randomized, double-blind, placebo-controlled study of Malarone for malaria prophylaxis in non-immune Colombian soldiers." Am J Trop Med Hyg 75(3): 430-433.

Soto, J., J. Toledo, et al. (1998). "Primaquine prophylaxis against malaria in nonimmune Colombian soldiers: efficacy and toxicity. A randomized, double-blind, placebo-controlled trial." Ann Intern Med 129(3): 241-244.

Soto, J., J. Toledo, et al. (1999). "Double-blind, randomized, placebo-controlled assessment of chloroquine/primaquine prophylaxis for malaria in nonimmune Colombian soldiers." Clin Infect Dis 29(1): 199-201.

Srivastava, I. K. and A. B. Vaidya (1999). "A mechanism for the synergistic antimalarial action of atovaquone and proguanil." Antimicrob Agents Chemother 43(6): 1334-1339.

Sukwa, T. Y., M. Mulenga, et al. (1999). "A randomized, double-blind, placebo-controlled field trial to determine the efficacy and safety of Malarone (atovaquone/proguanil) for the prophylaxis of malaria in Zambia." Am J Trop Med Hyg 60(4): 521-525.

Trigg, J. K. (1996). "Evaluation of a eucalyptus-based repellent against Anopheles spp. in Tanzania." J Am Mosq Control Assoc 12(2 Pt 1): 243-246.

Walsh, D. S., C. Eamsila, et al. (2004). "Efficacy of Monthly Tafenoquine for Prophylaxis of Plasmodium vivax and Multidrug-Resistant P. falciparum Malaria." The Journal of Infectious Diseases 190: 1456-1463.

WHO (2010). Guidelines for the treatment of malaria. Geneva, Switzerland, World Health Organization.

WHO. (2011). "World Health Organization Website." Retrieved July 13th, 2011, from http://www.who.int/malaria/en/.

Zielinski-Gutierrez, E., R. A. Wirtz, et al. (2012). Protection against Mosquitoes, Ticks, & Other Insects & Arthropods (Chapter 2, The Pre-Travel Consultation). The Yellow Book: CDC Health Information for International Travel 2012.

Effects of Irrigated Rice Fields and Seasonality on *Plasmodium* Transmission in West Africa, Particularly in Central Côte d'Ivoire

Benjamin G. Koudou[1,2,3], Marcel Tanner[4,5] and Juerg Utzinger[4,5]

[1]*Vector Group, Liverpool School of Tropical Medicine, Pembroke Place, Liverpool*
[2]*Centre Suisse de Recherches Scientifiques, Abidjan,*
[3]*University of Abobo-Adjame´, Abidjan,*
[4]*Department of Epidemiology and Public Health,*
Swiss Tropical and Public Health Institute, Basel,
[5]*University of Basel, Basel,*
[1]*UK*
[2,3]*Côte d'Ivoire*
[4,5]*Switzerland*

1. Introduction

The transmission of the parasites that cause human malaria is influenced by myriad environmental factors, including changes in agricultural practices, deforestation, and water-resources development and management (Ijumba and Lindsay, 2001; Ijumba et al., 2002; Keiser et al., 2005; Guerra et al., 2006), climatic factors such as rainfall, humidity and temperature (Reiter, 2008), and various cultural, economic, political and social factors, including health-seeking behaviour, urbanization, armed conflict and war (Esse et al., 2008; Baragatti et al., 2009). Drug resistance in the causative parasites and insecticide resistance in the mosquito vectors are also important factors that now influence malaria transmission (Reiter, 2008). Each year, in many parts of Africa, the local populations of anopheline mosquitoes build up rapidly and peak shortly after the onset of the rainy season (Mbogo et al., 1995). In two studies on the relationships between mosquito abundance, malaria transmission and rainfall in West Africa, 70%–90% of the children investigated were found infected with *Plasmodium spp.* after the rainy season (Bonnet et al., 2002; Koudou et al., 2009). It is particularly during and at the end of the rainy season that malaria becomes one of the leading causes of mortality and health-seeking at dispensaries and hospitals in this region (Rey et al., 1987). Not only season but also changing patterns of agriculture, particularly irrigated rice farming, influence malaria transmission in Africa (Ijumba & Lindsay, 2001; Diuk-Wasser et al., 2007; Sogoba et al., 2007).

Additionally, malaria transmission, *Plasmodium* prevalence rates, the proportion of presumptive and clinically-confirmed malaria episodes have been studied in two villages of central Côte d'Ivoire: one with irrigated rice farming (Zatta) and one without (Tiémélékro) (Koudou et al., 2009). Due to a farmers' conflict over land and socio-political issues, irrigated rice farming was interrupted in Zatta in 2003. The goal of this contribution to a book chapter is to evaluate the relationship between *Plasmodium* transmission, seasonality and agriculture practices.

2. Methods

2.1 Study sites
The study described here was carried out in the villages of Tiemelekro (geographical coordinates: 6°500 N, -4°170 W) and Zatta (6°880 N, -5°390 W), located in central Côte d'Ivoire (Figure 1). A detailed description of Tiemelekro, including climatic conditions, current health care delivery structures and key demographic and socioeconomic indicators, has been presented recently (Girardin et al., 2004). Zatta is located 7 km north-west of Yamoussoukro, the capital city of Côte d'Ivoire. The mean annual temperature in this village is 26.5°C and the mean annual precipitation is 1280 mm. There is a long rainy season between April and July and a shorter one in October/November. A dispensary, run by two local nurses, is located in Zatta and also covers nearby settlements. Two small dams were constructed in this village in the mid-1970s. Since 1997, a very large irrigated rice field has been cultivated on an estimated surface area of 36 ha, in close proximity to human habitations. However, due to unstable socio-political conditions and a farmers' conflict over land, rice irrigation was interrupted in 2000 and again in 2003/2004.

Living conditions and several of the investigated household characteristics are comparable between the two study villages. For example, similar proportions of houses utilized iron-corrugated sheets as roofing material (93.8% in Tiemelekro vs. 92.9% in Zatta), and had running water at home (74.1% vs. 65.4%). On the other hand, improved sanitation facilities were less prominent in Tiemelekro than in Zatta (17.0% vs. 47.6%). With regard to personal protective measures against mosquito bites, the proportion of people sleeping under a bednet was similarly low in both villages (8.4–11.2%), whereas use of fumigating coils was much more pronounced in Zatta (47.3%) when compared to Tiemelekro (9.1%).

2.1.1 Rainfall data collection
The Ivorian "Societe d'Exploitation et de Developpement Aeroportuaire et Meteorologique" (SODEXAM) holds rainfall data for the study area, from 1971 onwards. For the present study, monthly rainfall data from 2002 to 2005 were extracted from the society's records.

2.1.2 Adult mosquitos' collection
Overall, 13 entomological surveys were carried out: seven in the long rainy seasons (in the April and June of 2002, the April, May, June and July of 2003, and the May of 2005), and six in dry seasons (in the February and August of 2002, 2003 and 2005). Adult mosquitoes were collected by means of human-bait night catches. The surveys in 2002 and 2005 were each conducted between 18.00 and 06.00 hours, both inside and outside sentinel houses. Each of the six surveys carried out in 2003, however, covered shorter time periods (from 22:00 to 06:00 hours) and the collectors were only stationed inside the sentinel house because of the unstable socio–political situation at the time. Overall, 96, 48 and 32 night catches were carried out in 2002, 2003 and 2005, respectively. No surveys could be undertaken in 2004, as it was then considered too dangerous to reach the study villages.

2.1.3 Laboratory procedures
Adult mosquitoes were brought to a laboratory and processed. Firstly, the physiological age of each female *Anopheles* and the corresponding parity rate (i.e. the proportion of female mosquitoes that had laid eggs at least once) were determined by dissection of ovaries and

Effects of Irrigated Rice Fields and Seasonality on Plasmodium Transmission in West Africa, Particularly in Central Côte d'Ivoire

21

examination of tracheoles (Detinova, 1962). For quality control, a random sample of 10% of the mosquitoes investigated were re-examined by a senior technician. Secondly, a proportion of *An. gambiae* female having laid eggs at least once was checked for *P. falciparum* infection, in an ELISA for detecting the parasite's circumsporozoite protein (Beier et al.,

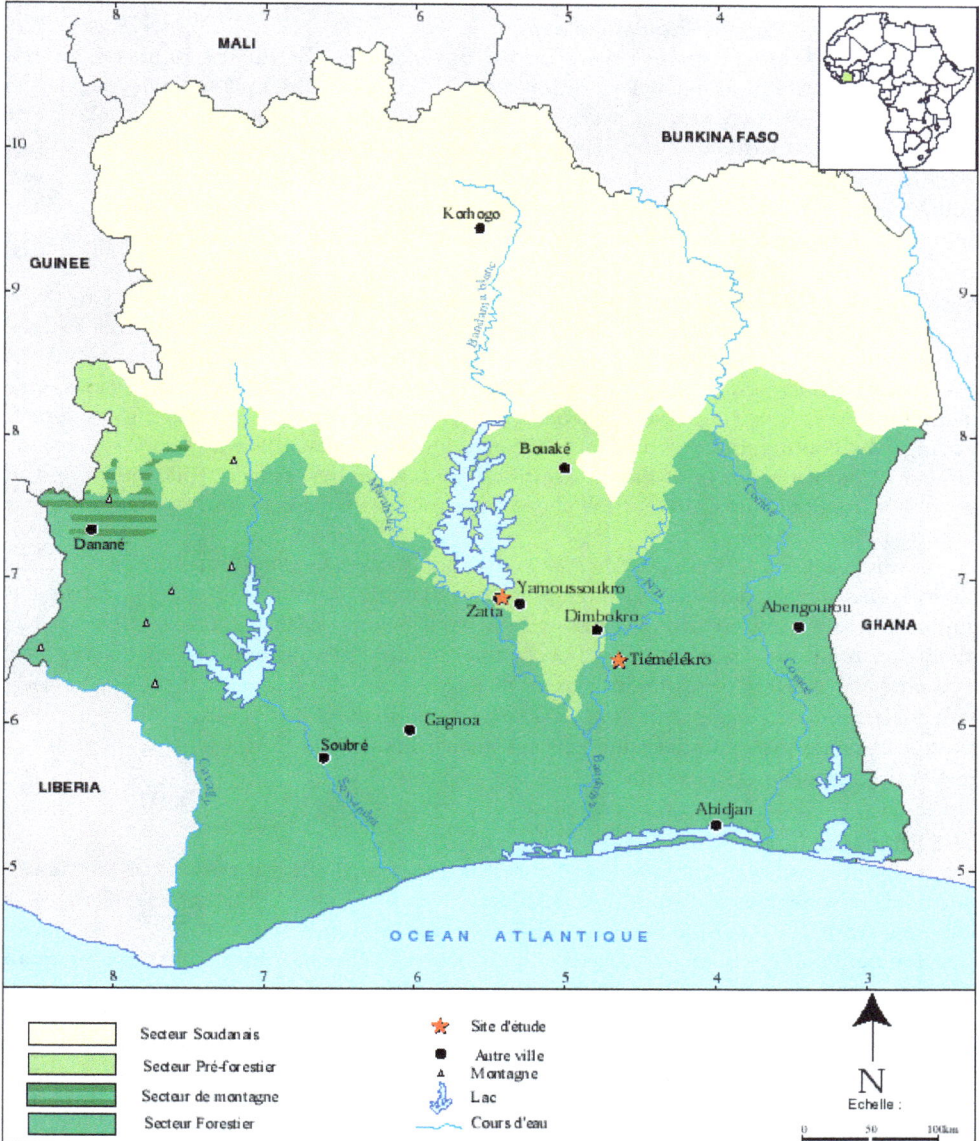

Fig. 1. Vegetation mapping of Côte-d'Ivoire presenting both study sites (Zatta and Tiemelekro) located in the central part of the country.

1988). Thirdly, some of the females belonging to the *An. gambiae* complex were identified to species level, in a PCR-based assay (Scott et al., 1993). Finally, some of the mosquitoes belonging to the *An. funestus* group were further identified using an assay based on a multiplex PCR (Koekemoer et al., 2002; Cohuet et al., 2003).

2.1.4 Clinical and Parasitological surveys

Repeated cross-sectional surveys were carried out in the study villages to assess malaria parasitaemia and clinical malaria in children aged ≤15 years. The first survey was done in June 2002. In 2003, two surveys were carried out in Zatta and three in Tiémélékro. The research team first worked in the primary schools and all children aged between 7 and 15 years from randomly selected classes were invited for a finger prick blood sample. Next, mothers and caregivers of under 7-year-old children were invited to accompany their children to a designated community location where a blood sample was taken from each child.

Thick and thin blood films were prepared on microscope slides. The slides were air-dried prior to transfer to a nearby laboratory where they were stained with Giemsa for 45 min. The slides were examined by the same experienced laboratory technician throughout the study under a microscope at high magnification. *Plasmodium* species and gametocytes were identified and counted against 200 leucocytes. When less than 10 parasites were found, reading was continued for a total of 500 leucocytes. Parasitaemia was expressed by the number of parasites per µl of blood, assuming for a standard count of 8000 leucocytes/µl blood. For quality control, 10% of the slides were randomly selected and re-examined by a second senior technician.

In our study, fever was defined when an individual had an axillary temperature >37.5 ∘C. Clinical malariawas defined as fever plus parasitaemia (Smith et al., 1994). Particular emphasis was placed on clinical cases with a parasitaemia >5000 parasites/_l blood. The latter threshold has been chosen after comparing the proportions of fever cases and asymptomatic carriers for different classes of parasite density (Gaye et al., 1989). Subjects with malaria-related symptoms (e.g. headache) plus axillary temperature >37.5 ∘C were given artesunate plus amodiaquine (the respective first-line antimalarial treatment at the time of the study) and paracetamole.

2.1.5 Ethical issues

The study protocol was approved by the institutional research commission of the Centre Suisse de Recherches Scientifiques (Abidjan, Côte d'Ivoire). Ethical clearance was obtained from the Ivorian Ministry of Public Health and National Malaria Control Programme. People who acted as bait and collectors in the mosquito collections were all volunteers and signed informed consent forms. During the study, Patients with malaria-related symptoms who presented at the dispensaries and mosquitoes' collectors were treated and protected for free against malaria by artesunate–amodiaquine chemoprophylaxis (artesunate–amodiaquine being the recommended, first-line treatment for malaria in Côte d'Ivoire at the time of the present study) and all mosquitoes' collectors were immunized against yellow fever. The heads of household in both study sites were informed and the parents or legal guardians of participating children signed a written informed consent sheet.

Effects of Irrigated Rice Fields and Seasonality on Plasmodium Transmission in West Africa, Particularly in Central Côte d'Ivoire

23

3. Results

3.1 Species composition of *An. gambiae* complex and *An. funestus* group

A total of 110 mosquitoes were identified to species level by PCR: 60 from Tiémélékro and 50 from Zatta. Within *Anopheles* spp. morphologically identified as *An. gambiae* complex, 100% were *An. gambiae s. s.* With regard to the *An. funestus* group, it consisted of 100% *An. funestus s. s.*

3.2 Effects of agricultural practices (irrigated rice fields & vegetable farming) on *Plasmodium* transmission

Comparison between years revealed that the biting rate of *An. gambiae s.l.* in Zatta decreased several-fold from 49.3 bites per person per night (b/p/n) in 2002 to 7.9 b/p/n in 2003 (likelihood ratio test (LRT=1072.66; P<0.001). In Tiemelekro, the biting rates recorded in 2002 and 2003 remained fairly constant. These observations were paralleled by a marked decrease in the infective rate of *An. gambiae s.l.* in Zatta (4.6–1.2%), and an increase in Tiemelekro (3.1–7.6%). Meanwhile, the entomological inoculation rate (EIR) of *An. gambiae s.l.* decreased 21-fold in Zatta, from 789 to 38 infective bites per person per year (ib/p/y), whereas it remained high in Tiemelekro (233 vs. 342 ib/p/y). In Zatta, the return to irrigated rice farming in January 2005 was paralleled by a significant increase of the EIR ranging from 38 infective bites per person per year (ib/p/y) in 2003 to 295 ib/p/y in 2005. In Tiémélékro high EIRs were found in 2003 (342 ib/p/y) and 2005 (572 ib/p/y).

3.3 Effects of agricultural practices (irrigated rice fields & vegetable farming) on *Plasmodium* prevalence and clinical malaria cases

3.3.1 Irrigated rice fields and *Plasmodium* prevalence

In both villages, the peak prevalence of *P. falciparum* was generally observed in children aged 3-6 years. There were three exceptions: in Tiémélékro, the peak prevalence of *P. falciparum* during the May 2005 survey was found in the youngest age group ($\leq$ 2 years), whereas in Zatta, the highest prevalence in the baseline survey (June 2002) and the second last survey (May 2005) was observed in children aged 7-15 years.

In June 2002, similarly high *P. falciparum* prevalence rates were observed in Zatta (85.4%) and Tiémélékro (86.1%). In Zatta, a significant decrease in the mean *P. falciparum* prevalence rate occurred from 2002 to 2003 (58.4%; χ^2 = 42.33, degree of freedom (df) = 1; P < 0.001). There was a significant increase from 2003 to 2005 (66.0%; χ^2 = 14.78, df = 1, P = 0.012). In Tiémélékro, the *P. falciparum* prevalence rate in June 2003 (78.2%) was significantly lower than during the June 2002 survey (χ^2 = 4.92, df = 1; P = 0.027). The annual *P. falciparum* prevalence rate decreased significantly from 2003 (70.7%) to 2005 (60.4%; χ^2 = 17.27, df = 1; P < 0.001).

3.3.2 Fever cases and asymptomatic carriers, stratified by parasite density

Table 1 shows how many of the children examined with parasitaemia in the 2003 surveys were either asymptomatic carriers or presented with a fever. There was a strong seasonal variation in the proportion of fever cases among individuals with parasitaemia. In Zatta, for example, the proportion of fever cases among *Plasmodium*-positive individuals was significantly higher towards the end of the rainy season (August) when compared to the dry season (March) (22.1% **versus** 9.9%; χ^2 = 9.90, df = 1; P = 0.002). In Tiémélékro, considerably higher frequencies of fever cases among *Plasmodium*-positive individuals were recorded during the peak rainy season in June (27.3%) and towards the end of the rainy season in August (25.5%) when compared to the dry season in March (15.9%; $P < 0.05$ for both comparisons).

In Zatta, all individuals with a high level of parasitaemia ($\geq$ 5000 parasites/μl blood) presented with fever, accounting for a highly significant difference between the proportion of asymptomatic carriers and fever cases in this parasitaemia class ($P < 0.001$). Similarly, there was a highly significant association between the fever cases and high parasitaemia in the three surveys carried out in 2003 in Tiémélékro ($P < 0.05$). No statistically significant difference was found in children with lower parasitaemias (1000-5000 parasites/μl of blood), neither in Zatta (March: $\chi^2 = 1.53$; df = 1; $P = 0.068$ and August: $\chi^2 = 0.116$; df = 1; $P = 0.733$) nor in Tiémélékro (March: $\chi^2 = 0.18$; df = 1; $P = 0.671$, June: $\chi^2 = 2.23$; df = 1; $P = 0.135$ and August: $\chi^2 = 0.001$; df = 1; $P = 0.973$).

3.3.3 Annual variation of presumptive cases and malaria transmission

In Zatta, 966, 812, 693 and 884 presumptive cases were recorded in 2002, 2003, 2004 and 2005, respectively. The annual number of presumptive malaria cases decreased significantly by 15.1% and 14.7%, respectively, from 2002 to 2003 (IRR = 0.841, $P < 0.001$) and from 2003 to 2004 (IRR = 0.853, $P = 0.002$). An opposite trend was observed from 2004 to 2005; the number of presumptive malaria cases increased significantly by 27.5% (IRR = 1.276, $P < 0.001$). The monthly number of presumptive cases was not related to the monthly number of infective bites per person (IRR = 0.994, $P = 0.827$).

Date of survey	P. falciparum parasitaemia (parasites/μl blood)	Tiémélékro		Zatta	
		No. (%) of asymptomatic carriers	No. (%) of children with fever	No. (%) of asymptomatic carriers	No. (%) of children with fever
March 2003	< 1000	69 (54.8%)	13 (10.3%)	135 (73.4%)	9 (4.2%)
	1000-5000	37 (29.4%)	6 (4.8%)	57 (26.8%)	9 (4.2%)
	$\geq$ 5000	0 (0)	1 (0.8%)	0 (0)	3 (1.4%)
	Total	106 (84.1%)	20 (15.9%)	192 (90.1%)	21 (9.9%)
June 2003[a]	< 1000	86 (52.1%)	34 (20.6%)	n.a.	n.a.
	1000-5000	32 (19.4%)	7 (4.2%)	n.a.	n.a.
	$\geq$ 5000	2 (1.2%)	4 (2.4%)	n.a.	n.a.
	Total	120 (72.7%)	45 (27.3%)	n.a.	n.a.
August 2003	< 1000	99 (50.5%)	22 (11.2%)	78 (57.4%)	12 (8.8%)
	1000-5000	46 (23.5%)	16 (8.2%)	28 (20.6%)	7 (5.1%)
	$\geq$ 5000	1 (0.5%)	12 (6.1%)	0 (0)	11 (8.1%)
	Total	146 (74.5%)	50 (25.5%)	106 (77.9%)	30 (22.1%)
Overall 2003 (number of positive children/ number of total children)		54.0% (372/689)	16.7% (115/689)	49.8% (298/598)	8.5% (51/598)

n.a.: not assessed

[a] No survey carried out in June 2003 in Zatta due to unstable sociopolitical situation

Table 1. Number (%) of children infected with P. falciparum who were asymptomatic carriers or presented with fever, stratified by different levels of parasitaemia, in the two study villages of Tiémélékro and Zatta, central Côte d'Ivoire.

Effects of Irrigated Rice Fields and Seasonality on Plasmodium Transmission in West Africa, Particularly
in Central Côte d'Ivoire

25

In Tiémélékro, the yearly numbers of presumptive malaria cases were 2089, 1858, 1655 and 1541. Thus, we observed significant decreases in the yearly number of presumptive cases by 11.1% from 2002 to 2003 (IRR = 0.889, P < 0.001), 9.0% from 2003 to 2004 (IRR = 0.910, P = 0.005) and 8.9% from 2004 to 2005 (IRR = 0.911, P = 0.008).

As in the case of Zatta, the monthly number of presumptive cases was not related to the monthly number of infective bites per person (IRR = 1.007; P = 0.776).

3.4 Effects of seasonality on *Plasmodium* Transmission
Tables 2 and 3 summarise the mean biting rate, infection rate and the entomological inoculation rate (EIR) of *An. gambiae* and *An. funestus* in the two study villages in 2002, 2003 and 2005.

3.4.1 Relationship between season and biting and infection rates
In Zatta, significantly higher *An. gambiae s. s.* biting rates were recorded in the dry seasons of 2002 and 2005 when irrigated rice farming was practiced, compared to the dry season of 2003 when irrigated rice farming was interrupted (LRT comparing 2002 with 2003: 13.79, LRT comparing 2005 with 2003: 20.50; both P <0.001). In 2003, there was no seasonal difference in the biting rate of *An. gambiae s. s.* (LRT = 0.13; P = 0.900) and *An. funestus s. s.* (LRT = 0.17, P = 0.879). In Tiémélékro, in 2002 (LRT = 1.84; P = 0.069) and 2005 (LRT = 0.56; P = 0.455), there were no significant differences in *An. gambiae s. s.* biting rates between the dry and the rainy season. In 2003, the biting rate was significantly higher in the long rainy season (LRT = 3.87, P <0.001). Regarding *An. funestus s. s.* biting rates, those recorded in the dry season of 2002 (LRT = 6.15) and 2003 (LRT = 4.50) were significantly higher than those recorded in the rainy season (both P <0.001). The difference in the biting rates between the dry and rainy season in 2005 also showed statistical significance (LRT = 3.26; P = 0.031).

3.4.2 Relationship between season and *Plasmodium* transmission
In both villages, higher EIRs of *An. gambiae s. s.* were usually recorded in the rainy season. For example, in Zatta, the EIR of *An. gambiae s. s.* recorded in the rainy seasons of 2002 and 2005 were 458 and 365 infective bites per person per season (ib/p/s), respectively. In 2003, when irrigated rice farming was interrupted in Zatta, *P. falciparum* transmission by *An. gambiae s. s.* and *An. funestus s. s.* only occurred during the rainy season. In Tiémélékro, in the rainy seasons of 2003 and 2005, the number of infective bites recorded for *An. gambiae s. s.* (357 and 208 ib/p/s, respectively) were 3-14 times higher than in the dry seasons (25 and 77 ib/p/s in the respective years). In 2002, in contrast, the EIR of *An. gambiae s. s.* recorded in the dry season was 2.5 times higher than the one recorded in the rainy season.

The highest EIRs of *An. funestus s. s.* were usually noted during the dry season. In Tiémélékro, this species was the primary *P. falciparum* transmitter during the dry season of 2005 when 207 ib/p/s were recorded. With regard to infection rates, with the exception of the 2005 infection rate of *An. funestus s. s.* recorded in Tiémélékro (χ^2 = 4.47, P = 0.035), no significant differences were observed between seasons, neither for *An. gambiae s. s.* nor for *An. funestus s. s.* in any village.

Malaria vector	Entomological parameter	Dry season		Rainy season		χ² or LRT	P value
		Mean (n)	95% CI	Mean (n)	95% CI		
An. gambiae							
2002[a]	Biting rate	38.7	36.3-41.1	59.9	56.9-68.2	3.79	<0.001
	Infection rate	4.8 (1,120)	3.6-6.1	4.2 (978)	3.0-5.5	0.33	0.564
	Parity rate	40.4 (673)	36.7-44.1	31.1 (1,157)	28.4-33.8	16.28	<0.001
	Total EIR	338	-	458	-		
2003[b]	Biting rate	7.1	5.4-9.3	8.3	5.0-11.6	0.13	0.900
	Infection rate	0.0 (65)	0.0-0.2	1.7 (176)	0.0-3.6	1.12	0.290
	Parity rate	61.9 (63)	49.8-74.2	36.7 (139)	28.6-44.8	11.16	<0.001
	Total EIR	0	-	26	-		
2005[c]	Biting rate	18.3	11.8-24.7	58.6	23.8-93.4	20.50	<0.001
	Infection rate	2.3 (127)	0.2-5.8	3.4 (136)	1.7-5.2	0.37	0.542
	Parity rate	52.9 (194)	45.2-60.6	46.2 (199)	40.6-52.0	1.71	0.191
	Total EIR	77		365			
An. funestus							
2002[a]	Biting rate	0.0	0.0-0.2	0.0	0.0	0	0
	Infection rate	0.0 (0)	0.0	0.0 (0)	0.0	0	0
	Parity rate	0.0 (0)	0.0	0.0 (0)	0.0	0	0
	Total EIR	0		0			
2003[b]	Biting rate	1.4	0.7-2.4	1.2	0.6-2.1	0.17	0.879
	Infection rate	0.0 (18)	0.0-0.2	2.3 (44)	0.0-6.8	0.42	0.519
	Parity rate	0.0 (9)	0.0-0.2	58.3 (12)	25.6-91.1	7.88	0.005
	Total EIR	0	-	5	-		
2005[c]	Biting rate	2.7	1.1-4.4	0.6	0.0-1.5	0.61	0.435
	Infection rate	8.3 (8)	0.0-28.4	0.0 (3)	0.0	0.87	0.824
	Parity rate	70.9	24.3-84.3	60.0	0.0-100.0	0.58	0.216
	Total EIR	41		0			0

In brackets are the number of malaria vectors analyzed; LRT (likelihood ratio test)
[a]Irrigated rice farming performed in a synchronized manner
[b]Interruption of rice cultivation
[c]Irrigated rice farming performed in a synchronized manner

Table 2. Monthly average biting rate, infection rate, parity rate and entomological inoculation rate (EIR) of *An. gambiae* and *An. funestus* during the dry season and the rainy season in 2002, 2003 and 2005 in Zatta, central Côte d'Ivoire

Malaria vector	Entomological parameter	Dry season		Rainy season		χ^2 or LRT	P value
		Mean (n)	95% CI	Mean (n)	95% CI		
An. gambiae							
2002*	Biting rate	19.6	18.1-21.1	12.6	11.2-14.1	1.84	0.069
	Infection rate	4.1 (268)	1.7-6.5	2.6 (531)	1.3-4.0	1.27	0.260
	Parity rate	72.5 (240)	66.8-78.2	52.4 (597)	48.4-56.4	28.34	<0.001
	Total EIR	146	-	60	-		
2003**	Biting rate	5.2	3.8-7.0	24.7	21.6-28.3	3.87	<0.001
	Infection rate	2.6 (35)	0.0-8.7	7.9 (467)	5.4-10.4	1.19	0.274
	Parity rate	59.0 (39)	42.8-75.1	58.6 (449)	54.0-63.1	0.002	0.961
	Total EIR	25	-	357	-		
2005**	Biting rate	3.9	2.1-5.7	16.7	9.1-24.4	10.56	<0.001
	Infection rate	10.9 (52)	3.7-17.3	6.8 (163)	2.6-10.6	1.47	0.226
	Parity rate	48.3 (103)	33.3-63.4	81.1 (201)	75.5-86.7	30.19	<0.001
	Total EIR	77	-	208	-		
An. funestus							
2002	Biting rate	5.0	4.1-5.9	0.7	0.4-1.1	6.15	<0.001
	Infection rate	3.1 (97)	0.0-6.6	7.7 (26)	0.0-18.7	1.11	0.292
	Parity rate	65.4 (185)	58.5-72.3	50.0 (22)	27.3-72.7	2.02	0.155
	Total EIR	28	-	9	-		
2003	Biting rate	8.4	6.6-10.5	4.0	2.9-5.4	4.50	<0.001
	Infection rate	3.6 (55)	0.0-8.7	9.1 (66)	1.9-16.2	1.45	0.229
	Parity rate	75.0 (60)	63.7-86.3	69.0 (42)	54.4-83.6	0.44	0.507
	Total EIR	55	-	67	-		
2005	Biting rate	29.9	20.9-38.9	1.0	0.6-1.9	3.26	0.031
	Infection rate	3.8 (131)	1.2-5.6	17.6 (11)	0.0-37.8	4.47	0.035
	Parity rate	65.1 (203)	50.6-73.2	91.7 (12)	73.3-100.0	3.61	0.057
	Total EIR	207	-	32	-		

In brackets are the number of malaria vectors analyzed; LRT (likelihood ratio test)
*Vegetable farming is performed intensively with 2 production cycles per year
**Vegetable farming is performed intensively with 1 production cycle per year

Table 3. Monthly average biting rate, infection rate, parity rate and entomological inoculation rate (EIR) of *An. gambiae* and *An. funestus* during the dry season and the rainy season in 2002, 2003 and 2005 in Tiémélékro, central Côte d'Ivoire

4. Discussion

The interruption of irrigated rice farming due to a farmers' dispute over land property rights, coupled with an unstable socio-political situation in the face of the 2002-2004 armed conflict (Betsi et al., 2006; Fürst et al., 2009) offered a unique opportunity to study the dynamics of malaria transmission. Our analyses complement previous publications

(Girardin et al., 2004; Koudou et al., 2005, 2007, 2009), now with an explicit focus on the effect of seasonality on malaria transmission under changing agro-ecological conditions. The following points are offered for discussion.

Firstly, biting rates of *An. gambiae* in both villages were usually significantly higher in the rainy season than in the dry season. When irrigated rice farming was interrupted in Zatta in 2003, much lower biting rates were observed than in the preceding year and in 2005, but there were no seasonal differences. Hence, the interruption of irrigated rice farming appeared to have hidden the effect of season on *An. gambiae* biting rate. These findings are in agreement with previous investigations in the humid savannah of Côte d'Ivoire: in an area characterised by intensive agriculture, the biting rate of *An. gambiae* increased significantly a few weeks after the beginning of the rainy season, whereas it decreased and became lowest towards the end of the dry season (Doannio et al., 2006). Moreover, the blunting of seasonal differences in biting rates due to changing patterns in irrigated rice farming has been documented previously for the savannahs of Senegal (Faye et al., 1993) and Mali (Dolo et al., 2004). In contrast to *An. gambiae* with the highest biting rates usually observed in the rainy season, the highest biting rates of *An. funestus* were consistently recorded in the dry season regardless of the prevailing agricultural activity. Moreover, interruption of irrigated rice farming in Zatta showed no effect.

Secondly, with the only exception of a significantly higher infection rate of *An. funesuts* in Tiémélékro in the rainy season compared to the dry season of 2005, infection rates of both *An. gambiae* and *An. funestus* showed no clear seasonal patterns. Different results were reported from Dielmo, a holoendemic area in Senegal, where the infection rate of malaria vectors showed considerable seasonal variation (Fontenille et al., 1997). The observations made in Senegal corroborated previous findings obtained in the savannah area in the north of Côte d'Ivoire (Dossou-Yovo et al., 1995), and other findings documenting a high infection rate of *An. funestus* at the beginning of the dry season in an irrigated rice area compared to a non-irrigated rice farming area (Dossou-Yovo, 2000). It should be noted, however that the mean annual infection rate of *An. gambiae* in Zatta was significantly higher when irrigated rice farming was in place (in 2002 and 2005) compared to a year with interrupted irrigated rice farming (Koudou et al., 2005).

Thirdly, the influence of changing patterns of irrigated rice farming on the *An. gambiae*-specific EIR in Zatta has been discussed elsewhere (Koudou et al., 2005, 2007). In brief, interruption of irrigated rice farming resulted in several-fold lower EIRs compared to normal years. Here, we now document that seasonal patterns of transmission remained. Indeed, considerably higher EIRs were observed for *An. gambiae* in the rainy season compared to the dry season. Of note, the EIR of *An. gambia* in the dry season of 2003 in Zatta dropped to zero. In Tiémélékro, high EIRs were recorded throughout the study period for *An. gambiae* and, in general, EIRs were higher in the rainy season compared to the dry season. *An. funestus* seemed to play an important role in the transmission of malaria, particularly in the dry season. Our results therefore confirm previous observations made elsewhere in the northern savannah of Côte d'Ivoire (Dossou-Yovo, 2000) and in southern Cameroon (Bonnet et al., 2002). Whilst *An. gambiae* was the key *P. falciparum* transmitter mainly during the rainy season, *An. funestus* was the main vector species during the dry season. It is interesting to note that a previous study focusing on climatic models for suitable malaria transmission in Africa, based on monthly rainfall and temperature data, concluded that an average of 80 mm rainfall per month, for at least 3-5 months, is a minimum to ascertain stable malaria transmission (Craig et al., 1999). Usually, a rapid rise in the

An. gambiae population at the beginning of the short rainy season was followed by an increase in the EIR (Bonnet *et al.*, 2002).

With regard to *An. funestus*, the highest EIRs were usually observed during the dry season. Indeed, *An. funestus* is often abundant and has high EIR during dry season compared to the rainy season (Fontenille et al., 1997; Manga et al., 1997). *An. funestus* was identified as the main malaria vector in the Guinean climatic region, in East Africa and Madagascar (Robert et al., 1985; Severini et al., 1990). As shown in our study, despite the presence of irrigated rice field, there is a great variability in the annual EIR values and seasonality would seem to play a key role (Mabaso et al., 2007).

Finally, an important finding of our study is that in Zatta, where irrigated rice farming was interrupted in 2003/2004, *Plasmodium* prevalence rates and the number of presumptive malaria cases decreased. This observation is corroborated by a significant decrease in the EIR from 2002 to 2003 (Koudou et al., 2005) and a significant increase from 2003 to 2005 (Koudou et al., 2007). This study demonstrated also that irrigated rice cultivation is associated with elevated malaria prevalence rates, as well as high numbers of presumptive malaria cases, as seen in Burundi (Coosemans, 1985), Kenya (Githeko et al., 1993) and Madagascar (Marrama et al., 1995). However, research carried out in Tanzania showed that irrigated rice farming was not associated with a higher risk of malaria. One important reason for this observation is that farmers engaged in irrigated rice have the opportunity to gain some extra money, part of which is spent for protective measures against malaria. A reduced risk of malaria despite enhanced rice production has been termed 'paddies paradox' (Ijumba & Lindsay, 2001).

5. Conclusion

In conclusion, analyses of our entomological data revealed that malaria transmission in two different agro-ecological settings of central Côte d'Ivoire is very high, but there are clear seasonal patterns. Whilst the interruption of irrigated rice farming in one of the two study villages resulted in a highly significant reduction in the EIR, seasonal patterns of transmission remained. Hence, even in intensive agriculture areas, the effect of season on malaria transmission must be taken into consideration for the design of integrated interventions and their monitoring.

Additionally, in Zatta, from 2002 to 2003, the highly significant reduction in the annual EIR was paralleled by a significant reduction in the *Plasmodium* prevalence rate, and the proportions of presumptive and clinically-confirmed malaria cases. Once irrigated rice farming was resumed, there was an increase in entomological and parasitological parameters of malaria. In Tiémélékro, despite the significant increase in the EIR from the year 2002 to 2005 (Koudou et al., 2005, 2007), malaria prevalence rates, and the presumptive and clinical malaria cases decreased. Hence, the reduction of malaria transmission in endemic areas does not necessary reduce the incidence of clinical malaria episodes (Charlwood et al., 1998), highlighting the complex relationship between these parameters.

6. Acknowledgements

Our thanks are addressed to the local authorities and villagers of Tiémélékro and Zatta, and the district health officers of Dimbokro and Yamoussoukro, for their commitment in the present study. This investigation received financial support from the 'Fonds Ivoiro Suisse de

Développement Economique et Sociale' (FISDES) and the Swiss Federal Commission for Fellowships for Foreign Students (CFBEE). While the field works were ongoing Profs Benjamin Koudou and Marcel Tanner were partially supported by the National Centre of Competence in Research (NCCR) North-South, integrated programme #4 (IP4) entitled "Health and Well-being". JU acknowledges financial support from the Swiss National Science Foundation (project no. PPOOB--102883 and PPOOB--119129).

7. References

Baragatti, M., Fournet, F., Henry, M. C., Assi, S., Ouedraogo, H., Rogier, C. & Salem, G. (2009). Social and environmental malaria risk factors in urban areas of Ouagadougou, Burkina Faso. *Malaria Journal*, 8, 13.

Betsi, N. A., Koudou, B. G., Cissé, G., Tschannen, A. B., Pignol, A. M., Ouattara, Y., Madougou, Z., Tanner, M. & Utzinger, J. (2006). Effect of an armed conflict on human resources and health systems in Côte d'Ivoire: prevention of and care for people with HIV/AIDS. *AIDS Care*, 18, 356-365.

Beier, M. S., Schwartz, I. K., Beier, J. C., Perkins, P. V., Onyango, F., Koros J. K., Campbell, G. H., Andrysiak, P.M. & Brandling-Bennet, A. D. (1988). Identification of malaria species by ELISA in sporozoite and oocyst infected *Anopheles* from western Kenya. *American Journal of Tropical Medicine and Hygiene*, 39, 323-327.

Bonnet, S., Paul, R. E. I., Gouagna, C, Safeukui, I., Meunier, J. Y., Gounoue, R. & Boudin, C. (2002). Level and dynamics of malaria transmission and morbidity in an equatorial area of South Cameroon. *Tropical Medicine and International Health*, 7, 249-256.

Charlwood, J.D., Smith, T., Lyimo, A., Kitua, Y., Masanja, H., Booth, M., Alonso, P.L. & Tanner, M. (1998). Incidence of Plasmodium falciparum infection in infants in relation to exposure to sporozoïte-infected Anophelines. Am. J. Trop. Med. Hyg. 59, 243-251.

Cohuet, A., Simard, F., Toto, F., J. C., Kengne, P., Coetzee, M. & Fontenille D. (2003). Species identification within the *Anopheles funestus* group of malaria vectors in Cameroon and evidence for a new species. *American Journal of Tropical Medicine and Hygiene*, 69, 200-205.

Coosemans, M.H. (1985). Comparison of malarial endemicity in a rice-growing area and a cotton-growing area of the Rusizi Plain, Burundi. Ann. Soc. Belge Med. Trop. 65, 187-200.

Craig, M. H., Snow, R. W. & le Sueur, D. (1999). African climatic model of malaria transmission based on monthly rainfall and temperature. *Parasitology Today*, 15, 105-111.

Detinova, T. S. (1962). Age-grouping methods in Diptera of medical importance, with special reference to some vectors of malaria. World Health Organization, Geneva, 220p.

Diuk-Wasser, M. A., Touré, M. B., Dolo, G., Bagayoko, M., Sogoba, N., Sissoko, I., Traoré, S. F. & Taylor, C. E. (2007). Effect of rice cultivation patterns on malaria vector abundance in rice-growing villages in Mali. *American Journal of Tropical Medicine and Hygiene*, 76, 869-874.

Doannio, J. M. C., Dossou-Yovo, J., Diarrassouba, S., Rakotondraibe, M. E., Chauvancy, G. & Rivière, F. (2006). Comparaison de la composition spécifique et de la dynamique des populations de moustiques dans deux villages du centre de la Côte d'Ivoire, avec et sans périmetre de riziculture irriguée. *Bulletin de la Société de Pathologie Exotique*, 99, 1-3.

Dolo, G., Briët, O. J. T., Dao, A., Traoré, S. F., Bouaré, M., Sogoba, N., Niaré, O., Bagayogo, M., Sangaré, D., Teuscher, T. & Touré, Y. T. (2004). Malaria transmission in relation to rice cultivation in the irrigated Sahel of Mali. *Acta Tropica*, 89, 147-159.

Dossou-Yovo, J. (2000). Etude éthologique des moustiques vecteurs du paludisme en rapport avec les aspects parasitologiques de la transmission du *Plasmodium* dans la région de Bouaké. Thèse de doctorat d'Etat en entomologie médicale. Université de Cocody, Abidjan, Côte d'Ivoire.

Dossou-Yovo, J., Doannio, J., Rivière, F. & Chauvancy, G. (1995). Malaria in Côte d'Ivoire wet Savannah region: the entomological inputs. *Tropical Medicine and Parasitology*, 46, 263-269.

Essé, C., Utzinger, J., Tschannen, A. B., Raso, G, Pfeiffer, C., Granado, S., Koudou, B. G., N'Goran, E. K., Cissé, G., Girardin, O, Tanner, M. & Obrist, B. (2008). Social and cultural aspects of 'malaria' and its control in central Côte d'Ivoire. *Malaria Journal*, 7, 224.

Faye, O., Fontenille, D., Hervé, J. P., Diack, P. A., Diallo, S. & Mouchet, J. (1993). Malaria in the sahelian region of Senegal. 1. Entomological transmission findings. *Annales de la Société Belge de Médecine Tropicale*, 73, 21-30.

Fontenille, D., Lochouarn, L., Diagne, N., Sockhna, C., Lemasson, J. J., Diatta, M., Konaté, L., Faye, F., Rogier, C. & Trape, J. F. (1997). High annual and seasonal variations in malaria transmission by anophelines and vector species composition in Dielmo, a holoendemic area in Senegal. *American Journal of Tropical Medicine and Hygiene*, 56, 247-253.

Fürst, T., Raso, G., Acka, C. A., Tschannen, A. B., N'Goran, E. K. & Utzinger, J. (2009). Dynamics of socioeconomic risk factors for neglected tropical diseases and malaria in an armed conflict. *PLoS Neglected Tropical Diseases*, 3, e513.

Gaye, O., Bah, L., Faye, F. & Baudon, C. (1989). Une étude de la morbidité palustre en milieu rural et urbain au Sénégal. *Med. Trop.* 49, 59-62.

Girardin, O., Dao, D., Koudou, B. G., Essé, C., Cissé, G., Yao, T., N'Goran, E. K., Tschannen, A. B., Bordmann, G., Lehmann, B., Nsabiman, C., Keiser J., Killeen, G. F., Singer, B. H, Tanner, M. & Utzinger, J. (2004). Opportunities and limiting factors of intensive vegetable farming in malaria endemic Côte d'Ivoire. *Acta Tropica* 89, 109-123.

Githeko, A.K., Service, M.W., MBogo, C.M., Atieli, F.K. & Jumao, F.O. (1993). Plasmodium falciparum sporozoite and entomological inoculation rates at Ahero rice irrigation scheme and the Miwani sugar-belt in Western Kenya. Ann. Trop. Med. Parasitol. 87, 379-391.

Guerra, C. A., Snow, R. W. & Hay, S. I. (2006). A global assessment of closed forests, deforestation and malaria risk. *Annals of Tropical Medicine and Parasitology*, 100, 189-204.

Ijumba, J. N. & Lindsay, S. W. (2001). Impact of irrigation on malaria in Africa: paddies paradox. *Medical and Veterinary Entomology*, 15, 1-11.

Ijumba, J. N., Mosha, F. W. & Lindsay, S. W. (2002). Malaria transmission risk variations derived from different agricultural practices in an irrigated area of northern Tanzania. *Medical and Veterinary Entomology*, 16, 28-38.

Keiser, J., Castro, M. C., Maltese, M. F., Bos, R., Tanner, M., Singer, B. H. & Utzinger, J. (2005). Effect of irrigation and large dams on the burden of malaria on a global and regional scale. *American Journal of Tropical Medicine and Hygiene*, 72, 392-406.

Koekemoer, L. L., Kamau, L, Hunt, R. H. & Coetzee, M. (2002). A cocktail polymerase chain reaction assay to identify members of the *Anopheles funestus* (Diptera: Culicidae) group. *American Journal of Tropical Medicine and Hygiene*, 66, 804-811.

Koudou, B. G., Adja, A. M., Matthys, B., Cissé, G, Koné, M., Tanner, M. & Utzinger, J. (2007). Pratiques agricoles et dynamique de la transmission du paludisme dans deux différentes zones eco-épidemiologiques, au centre de la Côte d'Ivoire. *Bulletin de la Société de Pathologie Exotiques*, 100, 124-126.

Koudou, B. G., Tano, Y., Doumbia, M., Nsanzabana, C., Cissé, G., Girardin, O., Dao, D., N'Goran, E. K., Vounatsou, P., Bordmann, G., Keiser, J., Tanner, M. & Utzinger, J. (2005). Malaria transmission dynamics in central Côte d'Ivoire: the influence of changing patterns of irrigated rice agriculture. *Medical and Veterinary Entomology* 19, 27-37.

Koudou, B. G., Tano, Y., Keiser, J., Vounatsou, P., Girardin, O., Klero, K., Koné, M., N'Goran, E. K., Cissé, G., Tanner, M. & Utzinger, J. (2009). Effect of agricultural activities on prevalence rates, and clinical and presumptive malaria episodes in central Côte d'Ivoire. *Acta Tropica*, 111, 268-274.

Mabaso, M. L., Craig, M., Ross, A., Smith, T. (2007). Environmental predictors of the seasonality of malaria transmission in Africa: the challenge. *American Journal of Tropical Medicine and Hygiene*, 76, 33-38.

Manga, L., Toto, J. C., Le Goff, G. & Brunhes, J. (1997). The bionomics of *Anopheles funestus* and its role in malaria transmission in a forest area of southern Cameroon. *Transactions of the Royal Society of Tropical Medicine and Hygiene*, 91, 232-233.

Marrama, L., Rajaonarivelo, E., Laventure, S. & Rabison, P. (1995). Anopheles funestus et la riziculture sur les plateaux de Madagascar. *Cahiers Santé*, 5, 415-419.

Mbogo, C. N. M., Snow, R. W., Khamala, C. P. M, Kabiru, E. W., Ouma, J. H., Githure, J. L., Marsh, K. & Beier, J. C. (1995). Relationships between *Plasmodium falciparum* transmission by vector populations and the incidence of severe disease at nine sites on the Kenyan coast. *American Journal of Tropical Medicine and Hygiene*, 52, 201-206.

Reiter, P. (2008). Climate change and mosquito-borne disease: knowing the horse before hitching the cart. *Revue Scientifique et Technique*, 27, 383-398.

Robert, V., Gazin, P., Boudin, C., Molez, J. F., Ouédraogo, V. & Carnevale, P. (1985). La transmission du paludisme en zone de savane arborée et en zone rizicole des environs de Bobo-Dioulasso, Burkina Faso. *Annales de la Société Belge de Médecine Tropicale*, 65 (Suppl. 2), 201-214.

Scott, J. A., Brogdon, W. G. & Collins, F. H. (1993). Identification of single specimens of the *Anopheles gambiae* complex by the polymerase chain reaction. *American Journal of Tropical Medicine and Hygiene*, 49, 520-529.

Severini, C., Fontenille, D. & Ramiakajato, M. R. (1990). Importance d'*An. funestus* dans la transmission du paludisme au hameau de Mahitsy, à Tananarive, Madagascar. *Bulletin de la Société Pathologie Exotique*, 83, 114-116.

Smith, T., Armstrong-Schellenberg, J. & Hayes, R. (1994). Attributable fraction estimates and case definitions for malaria in endemic areas. *Stat. Med.* 13, 2345-2358.

Sogoba, N., Doumbia, S., Vounatsou, P., Bagayoko, M. M., Dolo, G., Traoré, S. F., Maïga, H. M., Touré, Y. T. & Smith, T. (2007). Malaria transmission dynamics in Niono, Mali: the effect of the irrigation systems. *Acta Tropica*, 101, 232-240.

3

Amoebiasis in the Tropics: Epidemiology and Pathogenesis

A. Samie[1], A. ElBakri[2] and Ra'ed AbuOdeh[2]

[1]Molecular Parasitology and Opportunistic Infection Program, Department of Microbiology, University of Venda, Private Bag X5050 Thohoyandou 0950
[2]Medical Laboratory Technology Department, College of Health Sciences, University of Sharjah, Sharjah,
[1]South Africa
[2]United Arab Emirates

1. Introduction

Entamoeba histolytica is a protozoan parasite that causes amebic dysentery and liver abscess. The disease is common in tropical regions of the world where hygiene and sanitation is often approximate. The epidemiology of *E. histolytica* has been studied around the world. However, there is a dearth of comprehensive literature on the epidemiology of this pathogen as well as its pathogenicity in the tropical and underdeveloped regions of the world where the disease is actually more common. Epidemiological figures in many endemic tropical countries are often overestimated because of inaccurate identification. Accurate data on the prevalence of the pathogenic strain(s) of *E. histolytica* in those regions will allow for the effective cure of patients with anti-amoebic drugs thus preventing the development of resistant types and reducing management costs.

With the advents of HIV and AIDS, several organisms have been identified as potential opportunistic pathogens. However, it is not clear whether amoebiasis is an opportunistic infection or not. Up to date, very little data has been published on the occurrence of *E. histolytica* in relation to HIV and AIDS. In developed countries amebiasis tends to be more common in older patients and occurs mostly among men who have sex with men or in institutions. However, in tropical regions, the epidemiology of amoebiasis is completely different and is more common among the general population and particularly among patients attending health care centers with diarrhea. Therefore, it is important to understand the epidemiology of this pathogen in tropical areas where it is responsible for most morbidity and mortality.

The recent reclassification of *E. histolytica* into different species now including the pathogenic *Entamoeba histolytica* and the non pathogenic *Entamoeba dispar* and *Entamoeba moshkovskii* has further added to the complexity of the epidemiology of amoebiasis since these three species cannot be differentiated by microscopy that is the most commonly used diagnostic method particularly in tropical countries where resources are limited, but can only be differentiated by the use of molecular methods such as the polymerase chain reaction based methodologies. Recent development of simpler but more sensitive methods such as the Loop-Mediated Isothermal Amplification (LAMP) should improve the understanding of the epidemiology of this disease.

Over the past few years we have studied the epidemiology of E. histolytica in African countries (Cameroon, Zimbabwe, and South Africa). In the present chapter, we review these and other studies conducted in the African continent as well as other tropical regions in the light of new and more specific and sensitive molecular methods. The pathogenesis mechanism of amoebiasis is still not clear and recently differences in population levels of E. histolytica strains isolated from asymptomatic and symptomatic individuals have been shown to exist. One of the factors believed to be the determinant of the various clinical presentations of the disease is the organism's virulence. The different methodologies used for the detection and epidemiology of amoebiasis will be reviewed as well as the role of E. histolytica in HIV disease. Recent advances on the pathogenesis and control of amoebiasis will also be reviewed.

Amoebiasis caused by the protozoan parasite E. histolytica was first recognized as a deadly disease by Hippocrates who described a patient with fever and dysentery (460 to 377 B.C.). With the application of a number of new molecular biology-based techniques, tremendous advances have been made in our knowledge of the diagnosis, natural history, and epidemiology of amoebiasis. Amoebiasis remains an important health problem in tropical countries where sanitation infrastructure and health are often inadequate (Ximénez et al., 2009). Clinical features of amoebiasis range from asymptomatic colonization to amoebic colitis (dysentery or diarrhea) and invasive extraintestinal amoebiasis, which is manifested most commonly in the form of liver abscesses (Fotedar et al., 2007). Current WHO estimates of 40-50 million cases of amoebic colitis and amoebic liver abscess (ALA) and up to 100,000 deaths annually, place amoebiasis second only to malaria in mortality (Stanley 2003; Ravdin 2005; WHO/PAHO/UNESCO 1997). Global statistics on the prevalence of E. histolytica infection indicates that 90% of individuals remain asymptomatic while the other 10% develop clinically overt disease (Jackson et al, 1985; Haque et al., 1999). Although all the deaths could be due to invasive E. histolytica infections, the value for the prevalence of E. histolytica is an overestimate since it dates from before the separation of the pathogen E. histolytica from the non-pathogen E. dispar (Diamond & Clark, 1993). Recently however, Entamoeba moshkovskii, a morphologically identical species, has been detected in individuals inhabiting endemic areas of amoebiasis (Ali et al., 2003, Fotedar et al., 2008, Khairnar et al., 2007, Parija & Khairnar, 2005) and could be contributing to the prevalence figures. Thus, the reclassification of E. histolytica into the three morphologically identical yet genetically different species has further added to the complexity of the epidemiology of amoebiasis since they cannot be differentiated by microscopy that is the most commonly used diagnostic method particularly in tropical countries where resources are limited. Furthermore, the worldwide prevalence of these species has not been specifically estimated. Thus, obtaining accurate species prevalence data remains a priority as there are gaps in our knowledge for many geographic regions of the tropics.

Although only a minority of E. histolytica infections - one in every four asymptomatic intestinally infected individuals - progress to development of clinical symptoms (Gathiram and Jackson, 1987; Blessmann et al., 2003; Haque et al., 2006), the exact basis for this difference remains mostly unsolved. This might be partly due to the differences in the pathogenic potential of the infecting strains (Burch et al., 1991) and/or the parasite genotype

(Ali et al., 2007) or due to the variability of the host immune response against amoebic invasion (Mortimer and Chadee, 2010).

The disease mechanism and the exact prevalence and incidence of infection caused by *E. histolytica* are still unknown. The epidemiological data available for endemic countries however, albeit sporadic, is based mostly on the microscopic identification of the *E. histolytica/E. dispar/E. moshkovskii* complex, often inaccurately reported as "*E. histolytica*". To date many highly sensitive and specific techniques such as enzyme-linked immuno-sorbent assays (ELISA) and polymerase chain reaction (PCR) have been developed for the accurate identification and detection of *E. histolytica* in various clinical samples (Ackers, 2002). It is anticipated that these molecular tools will allow us to reconstruct a more reliable picture of the true epidemiology of the disease mainly in endemic regions of the world and to better our understanding of the role of the parasite and/or host factors that determine the disease outcome.

2. Biology of *Entamoeba histolytica*

Entamoeba histolytica trophozoites (Figure 1) live and multiply indefinitely within the mucosa of the large intestine feeding normally on starches and mucous secretions and interacting metabolically with the host's gut bacteria. However, such trophozoites commonly initiate tissue invasion when they hydrolyze mucosal cells and absorb the predigested products in order to meet their dietary provisions. Filopodia (tiny cytoplasmic extensions) that form from the surface of their trophozoites are believed to play a role in the pathogenicity of certain strains. Examples of functions related to pathogenesis include: endocytosis and/or pinocytosis, exocytosis, tissue penetration, cytotoxic substances release or contact cytolysis of host cells. Other host factors that may also influence the invasiveness of *E. histolytica* are the oxidation-reduction potential and gut contents pH both of which are largely influenced by the overall nutritional state of the host.

Once the parasites invade the intestinal wall, they reach the submucosa and the underlying blood vessels. From there, trophozoites travel in the blood to sites such as the liver, lungs or skin. These parasite forms are now considered to be dead-end course since they cannot leave the host and cause infection in others. Encystation occurs in the intestinal lumen, and cyst formation is complete when four nuclei are present. These infective cysts are passed into the environment in human feces and are resistant to a variety of physical conditions. On occasions, trophozoites may exit in the stool, but they cannot survive outside the human host. The signals leading to encystations or excystation are poorly understood, but findings in the reptilian parasite *Entamoeba invadens* suggest that ligation of a surface galactose-binding lectin on the surface of the parasite might be the one trigger for encystations (Stanley, 2003; Eichinger, 2001). Also, several previous proteomic and transcriptomic studies have shown that a few dozens of Rab genes/proteins are involved in important biological processes, such as stress response, virulence, and pathogenesis, and stage conversion (Picazarri et al., 2008; Chatterjee et al., 2009; Novick and Zerial, 1997; Stenmark, 2009; Nozaki and Nakada-Tsukui, 2006). EhRab11A was reported to be recruited to the cell surface by iron or serum starvation, and was suggested to be involved in encystation (McGugan and Temesvari, 2003). In contrast, EhRab11B is involved in cysteine protease secretion, and its overexpression enhanced the secretion of cysteine protease (Mitra et al., 2007; Nozaki and Nakada-Tsukuia, 2006).

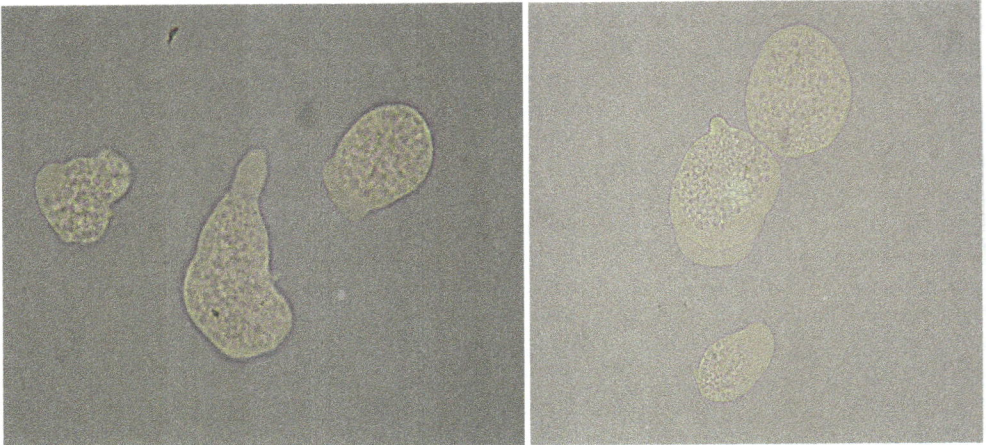

Fig. 1. *Entamoeba histolytica* trophozoites observed under the microscope stain with methylene blue (Observe that the cells did not accept the stain since they were still alive at the time the picture was taken) (Photos by Samie A)

The life cycle of *E. histolytica* is simple and consists of an infective cyst stage (10 to 15 µm in diameter) and a multiplying trophozoite stage (10 to 60 µm in diameter). Like other protozoa, *E. histolytica* appears incapable of de novo purine synthesis. Biochemical analysis has indicated that glutathione is not present. For this reason, *E. histolytica* is different from higher eukaryotes. It also uses pyrophosphate instead of ATP (McLaughlin and Aley, 1985). Mature cysts in the large intestine leave the host in large numbers and remain viable and infective in a moist, cool environment for at least 12 days. In water, cysts can live for up to 30 days. Nonetheless, they are rapidly killed by desiccation, and temperatures below 5°C and above 40°C. Mature cysts are also resistant to chlorine levels normally used to disinfect water. When swallowed, cysts pass through the stomach unharmed. In the small intestine, where conditions are alkaline and as a result of nuclear division, eight motile trophozoites are produced. These motile trophozoites then settle in the large intestine lumen, where they divide by binary fission and feed on host cells, bacteria and food particle (Figure 2). This is the first chance of the parasite making contact with the mucosa.

The organisms' biochemistry and metabolism have been reviewed by McLaughlin and Aley (1985). It has many hydrolytic enzymes, including phosphatases, glycosidases, proteinases, and an RNAse. Major metabolic end products are carbon dioxide, ethanol and acetate. *E. histolytica* is more of a metabolic opportunist which is able to exploit oxygen when it is present in the environment. Glucose is metabolized via the Embden-Meyerhof pathway exclusively, and fructose phosphate is phosphorylated, prior to lysis, by enzymatic reactions unique to *Entamoeba* spp. Pyruvate is converted mostly to ethanol, even in the presence of oxygen, via coenzyme-A, and pyruvate oxidase. Terminal electron transfers are accomplished with ferredoxinlike iron-sulphur proteins, a trait that may contribute to the efficacy of metronidazole in treatment. Similar metabolic traits in *Trichomonas vaginalis* and *Giardia lamblia* also are metronidazole targets. Mitogen Activated Protein Kinases (MAPK) – a group of proline directed serine/threonine kinases

(Bardwell, 2006) - regulate a number of different cellular processes such as proliferation, and response to a variety of environmental stresses like osmotic stress, heat shock and hypoxia (Junttila, 2008). The existence of MAPK homologues has been documented in certain parasitic protozoa. For instance ERK1 and ERK2 homologues of *Giardia lamblia* have been shown to play a critical role in trophozoite differentiation into cysts (Ellis et al., 2003), Pfmap2, a MAPK homologue in *Plasmodium falciparum* is essential for the completion of the asexual phase of the parasite lifecycle (Dorin-Semblat et al., 2006) and *Leishmania major* MAPK homologues exhibit an increased phosphotransferase activity in response to pH and temperature shift (Morales et al., 2007). On the other hand, *E. histolytica* has been shown to possess a single homologue of a typical MAPK gene (EhMAPK). Activation of EhMAPK in *E. histolytica* has been found to be associated with stress survival such as heat shock and oxidative stress response (Ghosh et al, 2010).

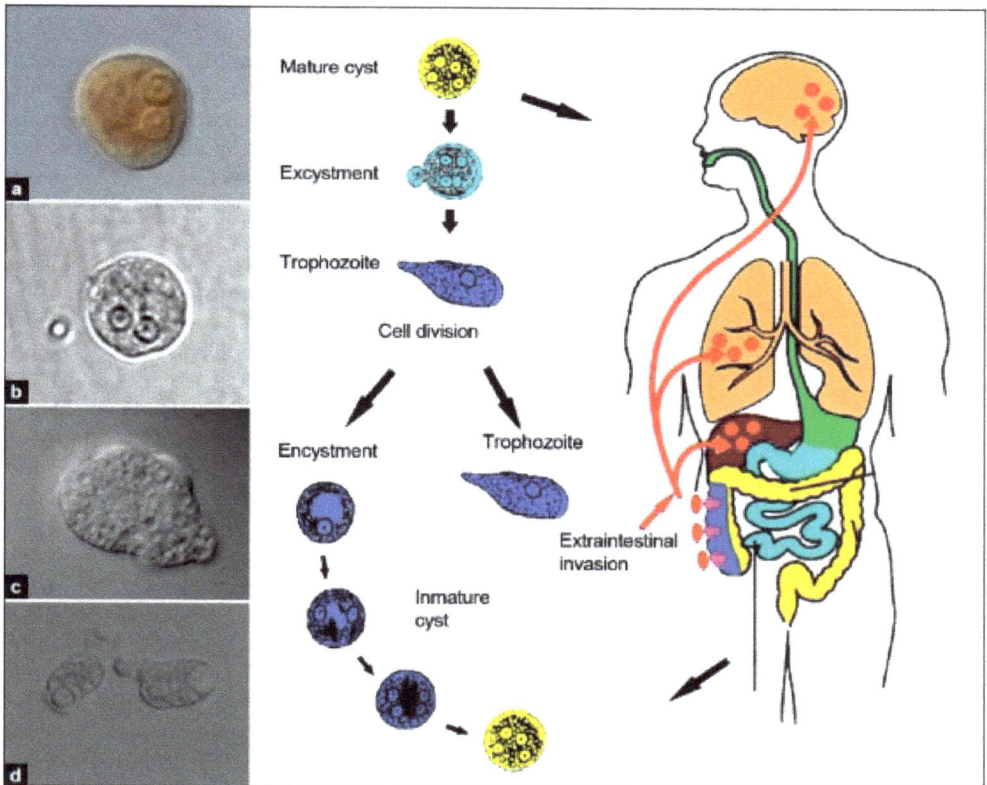

Fig. 2. Life cycle of *E. histolytica/ E. dispar*. a) Mature cyst stained with 4% Lugol solution (100× magnification). b) Mature cyst without staining (100×). c) Trophozoite observed with differential interference contrast (DIC) (100×). d) Trophozoites of *E. histolytica* species with phagocyted erythrocytes (DIC 40×). Obtained with permission from Ximenez et al (2011).

3. Epidemiology of amoebiasis and its occurrence in the era of HIV and AIDS

The epidemiology of amoebiasis around the world is complicated by the existence of three different forms that are morphological identical but genetically distinct and include *E. histolytica* which is a known pathogen, *E. dispar* and *E. moshkovskii* which are non pathogens (Ali et al., 2008). This is particularly relevant to the African continent as well as many other developing countries in the world, including Latin American and Asian countries, where there is lack of specific diagnostic tools. According to some studies conducted in some African countries (Alonzo et al., 1993; Molback et al., 1994; Njoya et al., 1999; Roche et al., 1999) from 6% to 75% of the population carry the parasite. These studies were conducted using microscopic examination giving a general idea on the distribution of the disease in the population. Such results require confirmation by techniques that clearly differentiate *E. histolytica* from *E. dispar*, which is not pathogenic. Countries in Central and Latin America where the parasite displays endemic behavior include Mexico, Brazil, and Ecuador. In Mexico for example, the incidence rate of intestinal amoebiasis from 1995 to 2000 was reported to be between 1000 and 5000 cases/100,000 inhabitants annually. Incidence values from 2002 to 2006 were 1128.8 to 615.85/100,000 inhabitants per year. As in other developing countries, those under 15 years of age were the most frequently affected group, with a notable increase in children aged 5–9 (Ximenez, 2009). In Aracaju, Brazil, Lawson et al (2004) demonstrated *E. histolytica* in 1% of cases whereas *E. dispar* was found in 13% of the cases. Whilst in Pernambuco state, northeastern Brazil *E. dispar* was found in 74.19% of culture positive samples using the PCR method, no *E. histolytica* was reported (Pinheiro *et al.*, 2004). In a remote area of Ecuador, Gatti et al (2002) using isoenzyme analysis reported an 18.9% infection rate with *E. histolytica* while 70.3% were infected with *E. dispar*. In the Indian subcontinent, the prevalence of intestinal amoebiasis among hospitalized patients was found to be around 11.7% using microscopy. However, using molecular biology tools such as PCR, *E. histolytica* was shown to be in 3.5% of those infected (Khairnar et al., 2007). In another endemic country such as Bangladesh and using ELISA antigen detection kits, *E. histolytica* prevalence was found to be 4.2% among children living in the urban slums of Dhaka (Haque et al. 2006). Many studies have been conducted in different parts of the world, (Ghosh et al., 2000) but the region most concerned by this problem (Africa) remains unexplored. Thus, the epidemiology of amoebiasis still remains very uncertain particularly in this part of the world.

Following the HIV/AIDS pandemic, numerous studies demonstrated that intestinal parasites such as *Cryptosporidium* sp, Microsporidia sp, *Isospora belli*, and *Cyclospora cayetenensis* were frequently associated with episodes of severe and often fatal diarrhea in both industrialized and poor countries. There have been controversies around the impact of HIV on the occurrence of amebiasis. However, recent data have shown an increase in the occurrence of *E. histolytica* among HIV patients in countries such as Japan, Mexico, Taiwan, and South Africa (Moran et al., 2005; Hung et al., 2008; Samie et al., 2009; Watanabe et al., 2011). With the hall mark of HIV infection being the depletion of CD4+ T cells count (below 200 cells/µl) and the progressive decline of the mucosal immunologic defense mechanisms, HIV/AIDS patients become prone to life-threatening gastrointestinal manifestations such as diarrhea (Stark et al., 2009). Table 1 provides a summary of the prevalence studies reporting *E. histolytica* and/or *E. histolytica / E. dispar* infections in HIV positive individuals in different countries. The association of *E. histolytica* infections with HIV positive individuals in some studies is not clear-cut. In a Mexican study no clear association between *E. histolytica* and

HIV has been noted. In this study, the prevalence of *E. histolytica* in HIV/AIDS patients was 25.3% compared to 18.4% in a control HIV-group (Moran et al., 2005). Other studies in South American countries have shown no obvious association. However, a significant association between high levels of serum anti-*E. histolytica* antibodies and the presence of *E. histolytica* in the stool has been noted in studies from both Vietnam (Blessman et al., 2006) and Africa (Stauffer et al., 2006). In a South African study in the Vhembe district in the northern part of the country, a positive association between *E. histolytica* infection and HIV-positive individuals has been indicated. Among the HIV-positive individuals, those with CD4+ count less than 200 cells/µl, were relatively more likely to be seropositive for *E. histolytica* (Samie et al., 2010). In a Chinese study, a higher seroprevalence of *E. histolytica* infections was also found in HIV-infected patients (Chen et al, 2007). Furthermore, two studies conducted in Taiwan revealed a positive association as well (Hung et al., 2005; Tsai et al., 2006).

Country	Prevalence of *Entamoeba species*	Reference
Cuba	1.5% (*E. histolytica/dispar*)	Escobedo, A. A. 1999
Bogota, Colombia	13% (*E. histolytica*)	Florez et al., 2003
San Pedro Sula, Honduras	5.8% (*E. histolytica*)	Lindo et al., 1998
Venezuela (Zulia state)	10.8% (*E. histolytica*)	Rivero et al., 2009
Brazil	3.3% and 1% (*E. histolytica/ dispar* before and after HAART)	Bachur et al., 2008
Mexico	25.3% in HIV+ and 18.5% in HIV-contacts (*E. histolytica*)	Moran et al., 2005
Tajikistan	25.9% (*E. histolytica/dispar* non HIV)	Matthys et al., 2011
Northern India	7.7% (*E. histolytica*)	Prasad et al., 2000
Taiwan	5.8% (*E. histolytica* in HIV patients)	Hung et al., 2008
Bangladesh	2.1% vs. 1.4% in diarrhea and control (*E. histolytica*)	Haque et al., 2009
India (Kolkata)	3.6% (*E. histolytica*)	Mukherjee et al., 2010
Sydney, Australia	3.2% (*E. histolytica/ E. dispar*)	Stark et al., 2007
Mazandaran province, Iran	1.6% (*E. histolytica*)	Daryani et al., 2009
Uganda	1.4% (*E. histolytica*)	Brink et al., 2002
Ethiopia	10.3% (*E. histolytica*)	Hailemariam et al., 2004
Dakar, Senegal	5.1% (*E. histolytica*)	Gassama et al., 2001
South Africa	12.4% (*E. histolytica*)	Samie et al., 2006

Table 1. Global prevalence of *E. histolytica* in HIV-infected and non-infected persons.

Over the past decade, there has been an increasingly reported risk of amebiasis in East Asian countries like Japan, Taiwan and South Korea particularly among men who have sex with men (MSM) probably due to oral-anal sexual contact (Hung et al., 2008; Watanabe et al., 2011). In Japan, *E. histolytica* often occur in institutions of mentally retarded individuals where outbreaks of amebiasis have been described with the prevalence rate and positive serology rate as high as 38.2% and 67.1%, respectively (Nishise et al., 2010) and has been occurring more often in HIV positive patients (Watanabe et al., 2011). In addition to HIV/AIDS, the increasing use of organ transplants and other immunosuppressed conditions such as neutropenia have been considered important risk factor for invasive amoebiasis in many countries. In Colombia for example, a study of organ transplant patients revealed that about 24.7% had detectable antiamoebic antibodies (Reyes et al., 2006) whereas in another study 14.3% neutropenic patients were found to have antiamoebic antibodies (Cardona et al., 2004).

Certain risk behaviors, such as homosexual relations and practicing oro-anal sex, can exacerbate the possibility of acquiring *E. histolytica* infections as well as other intestinal parasites such as *Cryptosporidium* spp., where the symptomatic pictures are more severe than those of immunocompetent individuals (Tatiana et al., 2008; Hung 2008). A recent study in Vietnam had indicated that socio-economic and personal hygiene factors determined infection with *E. histolytica*, rather than exposure to human and animal excreta in agricultural activities (Pham duc et al., 2011). In a study in Bangladesh, it was shown that wet environment is not the only factor that affects the detection curve of *E. histolytica*, but anti-Carbohydrate Recognition Domain IgA level in the gut is another determining factor for its occurrence in a closed population (Haque et al., 2006). Although, numerous seroprevalence studies suggest that HIV/AIDS individuals are at a higher risk of *E. histolytica* infections and are therefore more likely to develop symptomatic infections or severe forms of the disease, modest data exist to support these findings and further research is needed to confirm this hypothesis.

4. Diagnosis of amoebiasis

Amoebiasis diagnosis rests on the demonstration of *E. histolytica* trophozoites or cysts in stool or colonic mucosa of patients. For many years a direct smear examined either as a wet mount or fixed and stained was done by microscopic examination of stool. Repeated stool sample examinations (at least three) may be needed. The presence of haematophagous amoebic trophozoites in a stool sample has always suggested *E. histolytica* infections (Gonzalez-Ruiz, A. et al 1994). Nonetheless, the specificity of this finding was further reduced when it was demonstrated that in some patients *E. dispar* also contains RBCs (Fotedar et al., 2007). Also, in view of the high frequency of *E. dispar* in many areas, dysentery due to entities such as shigellosis and campylobacter will probably be misdiagnosed as amoebic colitis if microscopy is the sole diagnostic criteria (Stanley 2003). However, in the absence of haematophagous trophozoites, the sensitivity of microscopy is limited by its ability to distinguish between samples infected with *E. histolytica* and the morphologically identical *E. dispar* and *E. moshkovskii*. Confusion between *E. histolytica*, other non-pathogenic amoeba and white blood cells such as macrophages and polymorphonuclear cells in feces frequently result in the overdiagnosis of amoebiasis. Delays in the processing of stool samples affect the sensitivity of light microscopy, which under the best circumstances is only 60% of that of the stool culture method followed by isoenzyme analysis (Krogstad et al., 1978).

Stool culture technique followed by isoenzyme analysis has been considered as the "gold standard" for many years. This method has been used to distinguish between *E. histolytica* and *E. dispar*. For more details on the culture technique the reader is advised to consult reference (Clark and Diamond, 2002). Culture of *E. histolytica* can be performed from fecal specimens, rectal biopsy specimens, or liver abscess aspirates. However, the process usually takes between 1-4 weeks to perform and requires sophisticated laboratory equipment making it not feasible as a routine procedure especially in the developing world where *E. histolytica* is rampant. The rate of success of *E. histolytica* culture in reference laboratories has been reported to be between 50 and 70%. Moreover, isoenzyme (zymodeme) analysis is labor intensive, costly and often produces false-negative results for many microscopy positive stool specimens (Strachan et al., 1988).

Serological methods may be useful diagnostically to detect infections with *E. histolytica* in developed countries where infections are not as common as in endemic developing nations (Ohnishi et al., 1997). In developing countries individuals are constantly exposed to *E. histolytica* making serological tests unable to definitively distinguish past from current infections (Caballero et al., 1994). Amoebic serology is highly sensitive and specific for the diagnosis of ALA (Zengzhu et al., 1999). Conversely, a study of asymptomatic individuals living in an *E. histolytica* endemic area of Vietnam revealed that about 83% of those infected had detectable anti-amoebic antibodies (Blessmann et al., 2002). Several assays for the detection of antibodies to *E. histolytica* infections have been developed (Table 2). These include: indirect hemagglutination (IHA), latex agglutination, immunoelectrophoresis, counterimmunoelectrophoresis (CIE), the amebic gel diffusion test, immunodiffusion, complement fixation, indirect immunofluorescence assay (IFA), and enzyme-linked immunosorbent assay (ELISA). With the exception of ELISA, all the other tests have been either costly to perform (Complement fixation), less sensitive and nonspecific (IHA and Latex agglutination test), time consuming (immunodiffusion) or requires skills in culture and antigen preparation (IFA) (Fotedar et al., 2007).

Serological Assay	Sensitivity (%)	Specificity (%)	Reference(s)
IHA	100[a], 99	90.9-100[a] , 99.8	Pillai et al., 1999; Hira et al., 2001
Novagnost *Entamoeba* IgG	>95	>95	Manufacturer's recommendation
I.H.A. Amoebiasis	93	97.5	Robert et al., 1990
Amebiasis Serology microplate ELISA	95	97	Manufacturer's recommendation
RIDASCREEN *Entamoeba* (IgG detection)	100, 97.7-100 (100)	95.6, 97.4 (100)	Manufacturer's recommendation; Knappik et al., 2005

Table 2. List of some of the commercially available antibody assays used for the diagnosis of amoebiasis.

ELISA is a reliable, easy to perform and rapid method for the diagnosis of *E. histolytica* infections especially in developing countries. It has been used widely for the study of the epidemiology and diagnosis of symptomatic amoebiasis (intestinal and/or extraintestinal). An ELISA to detect antibodies to *E. histolytica* has been shown to be 97.9% sensitive and 94.8% specific for detection of *E. histolytica* antibodies in ALA patients in a non endemic country (Hira et al., 2001). Unlike IgG, immunoglobulin M (IgM) is short lived and does not remain in the serum for longer periods making it a very useful marker for the detection of present or current *E. histolytica* infections. An ELISA for the detection of serum IgM antibodies to the amoebic Gal or GalNAc-inhibitable adherence lectin has been reported. In this study, conducted in Egypt, anti-lectin IgM antibodies in the serum were detected in 45% of patients who had been suffering from acute colitis for <1 week (Abd-Alla et al., 1998). Since there is no cross-reaction with other non-*E. histolytica* parasites (Goncalves et al., 2004), the use of ELISA thus seems to be an excellent choice for the routine laboratory diagnosis as well as the surveillance and control of amoebiasis in the developing world.

The newer methods available to distinguish between *E. dispar* and *E. histolytica* have thrown into question the commonly accepted figure of 500 million infections worldwide suggesting that the actual number may be closer to 50 million. PCR and monoclonal antibody techniques are now available to distinguish between these three species in fresh and preserved stool samples, including those with mixed infections. Several investigators have developed ELISAs that detect antigens in fresh stool samples with sensitivity closer to that of stool culture methods and PCR. These ELISAs are usually easy and rapid to perform. Copro-antigen based ELISA kits specific for *E. histolytica* exploit monoclonal antibodies against the Gal/GalNAc-specific lectin of *E. histolytica* (*E. histolytica* II; TechLab, Blacksburg, VA) or against serine-rich antigen of *E. histolytica* (Optimum S kit; Merlin Diagnostika, Bornheim-Hersel, Germany). Other ELISA kits include the Entamoeba CELISA PATH kit (Cellabs, Brookvale, Australia) and the ProSpecT EIA (Remel Inc.; previously manufactured by Alexon-Trend, Inc., Sunnyvale, CA) (Fotedar et al., 2007). The early nineties of the 20th century have witnessed the introduction by TechLab of an ELISA kit for the specific detection of *E. histolytica* in feces. This antigen detection test captures and detects the parasite's Gal/GalNAc lectin in stool samples. It can also be used for the detection of the lectin antigen in the serum and liver abscesses in patients with invasive intestinal amoebiasis and ALA (Haque et al., 2000). However, the diagnosis of ALA normally relies on the identification of liver lesions and positive anti-*E. histolytica* serology. Yet neither provides conclusive results for ALA. The Gal/GalNAc lectin is conserved and highly immunogenic, and because of the epitopic differences in the lectins of *E. histolytica* and *E. dispar*, the test enables specific identification *E. histolytica* (Haque et al., 1993; Mirelman 1997). Because of some disadvantages observed with the TechLab ELISA kit, a newer more sensitive and specific version, TechLab *E. histolytica* II kit, was produced. This second – generation *E. histolytica* II kit has demonstrated good sensitivities and specificities when compared to real-time PCR (71 to 79% and 96 to 100%, respectively) (Roy et al., 2005; Visser et al., 2006). Other studies however, have reported a lesser sensitivity (14.3%) and specificity (98.4%) in comparison to stool culture and isoenzyme analysis (Gatti et al., 2002). Cross reactivity is another concern with the use of the assay, since it seems that *E. dispar* positive samples by means of PCR may sometimes give false-positive outcomes (Furrows et al., 2004). Accordingly, accurate detection of *E. histolytica*, *E. dispar* and *E. moshkovskii* could be helpful for diagnostic and epidemiological studies in places where it is impractical and expensive to use molecular assays and where amoebiasis is most prevalent, such as in the developing countries. An antigen detection kit for the specific identification of *E. dispar* and *E. moshkovskii* is yet to be developed.

Several PCR-based techniques that amplify and detect *E. histolytica* DNA are currently used for the clinical and epidemiological studies in non-endemic rich countries (Acuna-Soto et al.,

1993; Katzwinkel-Wladarsch et al., 1994; Calderaro et al., 2006; Hamzah et al., 2006). The sensitivity and specificity of PCR-based methods for the diagnosis of *E. histolytica* infection approach those of stool culture followed by isoenzyme analysis. PCR methods can be used to detect *E. histolytica* in stool, tissues and liver lesion aspirates. Of all the different gene targets used to identify *E. histolytica*, the small-subunit rRNA gene (18SrDNA) is believed to be more sensitive than the best antigen detection method used and performs equally well compared to stool culture (Mirelman et al., 1997).

Several groups have developed a variety of excellent conventional PCR assays, targeting different genes, for the direct detection and differentiation of *E. histolytica*, *E. dispar*, and *E. moshkovskii* DNA in clinical specimens such as stool and liver abscess samples (Tanyuksel and Petri Jr., 2003; Paul et al., 2007). Of all the targeted genes, assays amplifying the 18SrDNA genes are the ones in wide use as they are present in multiple copies on extrachromosomal plasmids thus making them easily detectable than single copy genes (Battacharya et al., 1989). Other gene targets used in PCR to study the epidemiology of *E. histolytica* include: the serine-rich *E. histolytica* protein (SREPH) gene (Stanley et al., 1990), cysteine proteinases gene and actin genes (Freitas et al., 2004). The SREHP is also used to study the genotypes of *E. histolytica* in human populations. However, it is now being replaced by the use of PCR amplification of tRNA gene-linked short tandem repeats which in addition to providing details of the epidemiology of *E. histolytica*, it also provides a tool to predict the outcome of the infection (Ali et al., 2005).

A nested multiplex PCR was developed by many groups. This method has the added advantage of increasing the sensitivity and specificity of the test whilst simultaneously detecting and differentiating *E. histolytica* and *E. dispar* from DNA extracted from microscopy-positive stool specimens (Evangelopoulos et al., 2000; Hung et al., 2005; Nunez et al., 2001). A nested PCR method for the identification of *E. moshkovskii* in fecal samples was developed as a nested 18S rDNA PCR followed by restriction endonuclease digestion (Ali et al., 2003). The method exhibited a high sensitivity and specificity (100%).

Real time PCR is another type of PCR which is more sensitive than the conventional PCR. It is faster than the conventional PCR and characterized by the elimination of gel analysis and other post-PCR analysis, thus reducing the risk of contamination and cost (Klein 2002). However, its application in developing countries is limited to research only. Real-time PCR allows specific detection of the PCR product by binding to one or two fluorescence-labeled probes during PCR, thereby enabling continuous monitoring of the PCR product formation throughout the reaction. Furthermore, real-time PCR is a quantitative method and allows the determination of the number of parasites in various samples (Fotedar et al., 2007). Despite being used for the successful identification of *E. histolytica*, *E. dispar* and *E. moshkovskii*, the various PCR methods use is still confined to research institutes in the developing world where amoebiasis is endemic. PCR-based methods application in routine clinical diagnostic laboratories in low income societies is hindered by difficulties such as cost, and time to perform the test.

A new platform for the detection of pathogens has been developed known as loop-mediated isothermal amplification (LAMP) and was developed in 2000 by Notomi and colleagues. This method uses a set of two specifically designed inner primers and two outer primers that recognize six distinct regions of the targeted DNA. The reaction is performed under isothermal conditions and simple incubators, such as a water bath or heat block, are adequate for the specific amplification of the desired genetic material. Considering these advantages, the LAMP assay could be a useful and valuable diagnostic tool particularly in developing countries where most of the infections are common as well as in hospital laboratories. Recently this method was developed specifically for the detection of *E. histolytica* (Liang et al., 2009). The efficiency of the developed method was compared to that of existing PCR methodology and was similar in terms of sensitivity and specificity. This method needs further evaluations to be used in local conditions in Africa in order to improve the understanding of amebiasis in the continent as well as elsewhere.

5. Pathogenicity of amoebiasis

E. histolytica causes intestinal and extraintestinal amoebiasis based on the site of infection. Though most infections do not harm the host (asymptomatic infections), establishment in the colonic mucosa via the Galactose/N-acetyl Galactosamine inhibitable lectin (Gal-lectin) is a pre-requisite for the disease (Chadee et al., 1987). Pathogenic forms of the parasite are known to secrete enzymes that facilitate their invasion into the mucosa and sub-mucosa causing deep-flask shaped ulcers (Figure 3), and in some cases entering the circulation and reaching internal organs like the liver, lungs, skin, etc. The disease in the colon is the most common with acute diarrhoea and dysentery accounting for 90% of the clinical amoebiasis cases (Espinosa-Cantellano and Martínez-Palomo, 2000) and only 1% involve the liver (Haque et al., 2003) (Figure 4).

5.1 Asymptomatic colonization
Asymptomatic infections are characterized by the parasite living in perfect harmony within the host. *E. histolytica* trophozoites have developed elusive tactics to prevent them from being purged from the host.. By modulating signals by intestinal epithelial cells (IEC), trophozoites direct anti-inflammatory host responses leading to a tolerogenic/hyporesponsive immune state favourable to their survival (Kammanadiminti and Chadee, 2006). Furthermore, products secreted by non-pathogenic *E. histolytica* strains normally disrupt and suppress NFκB signaling and as a result diminish pro-inflammatory responses normally detrimental to the parasite (Artis, 2008). Interleukin 10 (IL-10), an anti-inflammatory cytokine, has been shown to play a significant role in maintaining this hyporesponsive state. On the other hand, a deficiency of IL-10 more often than not predisposes the host to develop the clinical amoebiasis (Hamano et al., 2006)

5.2 Intestinal amoebiasis
After an incubation period of 1-4 weeks, the parasite invade the colonic mucosa, producing characteristic ulcerative lesions and a profuse bloody diarrhea (amoebic dysentery). Amoebic invasion through the mucosa and into the submucosa is the hallmark of amoebic colitis. Contact of the trophozoites via the Gal/GalNAc lectin triggers a signaling cascade initiating the death of the host cell through different mechanisms such as phagocytosis, cytotoxicity and caspase activation instigating the invasive (intestinal and/or extra-intestinal) stages of the disease. Other molecules involved in the disease process include: a serine-rich *E. histolytica* protein (SREHP), amoebapores, and cysteine proteases (Boettner at al., 2002; Mortimer and Chadee, 2010). Activation of damaging inflammatory and non-

inflammatory responses following contact of the trophozoites to the gut wall induces a massive neutrophil infiltration across the epithelium into the underlying tissues resulting in weakening of epithelial cells and the mucous layer and allowing trophozoites to invade the intestinal epithelium and disseminating to other bodily sites (Ackers and Mirelman, 2006). The ulcers formed may be generalized involving the whole length of the large intestine or they may be localized in the ileo-caecal or sigmoido-rectal regions. Ulcers are normally disconnected with sizes varying from pin-head size to more than 2.5 cm in diameter. They may be deep or superficial. Base of the deep ulcers is generally formed by the muscularis layer. Nonetheless, superficial ulcers do not extend beyond the muscularis layer. A large number of fatalities results from perforated colons with concomitant peritonitis. *E. histolytica* also causes amoebomas. These are pseudotumoural lesions, whose formation is associated with necrosis, inflammation and oedema of the mucosa and submucosa of the colon. These granulomatous masses may obstruct the bowel.

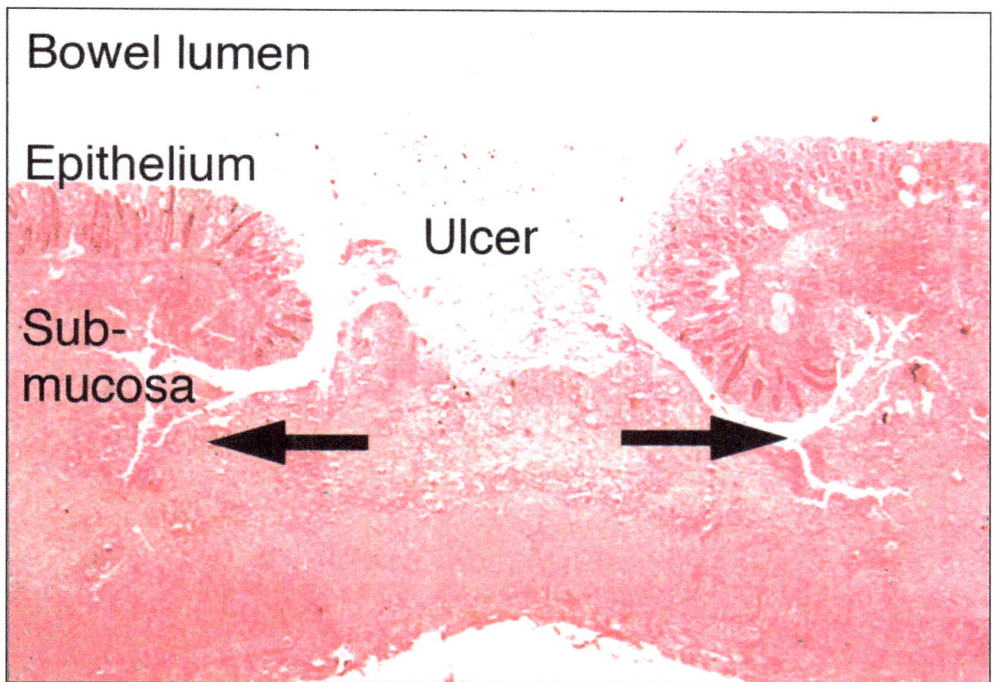

Fig. 3. "Flask-shaped" ulcer of invasive intestinal amebiasis (hematoxylin-eosin, original magnification ×50). Source: **Pritt B S , Clark C G Mayo Clin Proc. 2008;83:1154-1160: Mayo Clinic Proceedings**

While the serine rich *E. histolytica* protein (SREHP) have been shown to promote adhesion of the trophozoites to host cells, cysteine proteases (CP), are known for their virulence in other protozoa as well as in tumour metastasis. Five *E. histolytica* proteins (EhCP1, 2, 3, 5 and 112) have been identified. All are alleged to play a role in the destruction of host cells, phagocytosis, together with the recruitment of neutrophils and macrophages and the induction of intestinal inflammation (Mortimer and Chadee, 2010). Moreover, EhCP5 has also been shown to perform a variety of functions such as evasion of the host complement and immune system by preventing the activation of the classical complement system via the inactivation of IgG and the degradation of IgA (Laughlin and Temesvari, 2005).

Equally important in the pathogenesis and virulence of *E. histolytica* is the role of the phagosome-associated proteins. Many have been identified and their function in endocytosis and pathogenesis has been established. Examples include: EhRacA, EhRacG, EhPAK, actin and several Rab7-related GTPases (Laughlin and Temesvari, 2005). Cytokines such as IL-1β, IL-1α, IL-8 and TNF-α are suspected of aggravating the disease process and driving the immunopathogenesis mechanism (Kammanadiminti et al., 2003). Although neutrophils are known to cause intestinal tissue damage they are nevertheless critical for controlling the infection. Nonetheless, host and/or parasite factors normally play a role in determining whether the parasite is cleared or the disease becomes established (Asgharpour et al., 2005).

Although most intestinal invasions heal following an acute inflammatory response, *E. histolytica* evades destruction in a modest number of individuals and a chronic state is established. This chronic state is associated with the development of a non-protective adaptive immune response. Human data, in vitro and in vivo models support a paradigm that Th1 responses in the gut clear *E. histolytica*, while Th2 responses through the production of IL-4 are anti-protective, likely through suppressing IFN-γ. It is not yet clear what signals drive an anti-protective Th2 immune response instead of an effective protective Th1 response towards the infection. Evidence suggesting that genetics, the MHC restriction, nutrition and bacterial flora might play a role in directing the immune response towards *E. histolytica* infection exists. For example, the MHC class II allele DQBl*0601 was reported to be associated with resistance to *E. histolytica* (Mortimer and Chadee, 2010). Susceptibility to ALA has been found to be associated with HLA-DR3 and complotype SC01 in some Mexican populations; this association is not seen for amoebic colitis or asymptomatic colonization with *E. histolytica* (Stanley, 2003).

5.3 Extraintestinal amoebiasis

About 5% individuals with intestinal amoebiasis, 1-3 months after the disappearance of the dysenteric attack, develop extraintestinal amoebiasis. Once in the blood, the parasite uses many different strategies to avoid elimination by the host and reaches other sites in the body (such as the liver, lungs, brain, etc). The most common extraintestinal site affected by the parasite is the liver and an Amoebic liver abscess (ALA) is its most common manifestation, predominantly seen in adult males. This chronic stage of ALA is characterized by defective cell-mediated immunity and the suppression of T cells and their defective proliferative responses (Campbell et al., 1999). *E. histolytica* trophozoites reaching the liver create their unique abscesses, which are well circumscribed regions of cytolysed liver cells, liquefied cells, and cellular debris. The lesions are surrounded by connective tissue enclosing few inflammatory cells and trophozoites. Parenchymal cells adjacent to the lesion are often unaffected. However, lysis of neutrophils by *E. histolytica* trophozoites might release mediators that lead to the death of liver cells, and extend damage to hepatocytes not in direct contact with the parasite. Studies have shown that in ALA in mice, most hepatocytes die from apoptosis, but necrosis is also present. In ALA from humans, the small numbers of amoebas relative to the size of the abscess suggests that *E. histolytica* can kill hepatocytes without direct contact (Stanley 2003). From the liver, *E. histolytica* trophozoites may enter into the general circulation and reach other organs (Figure 4).

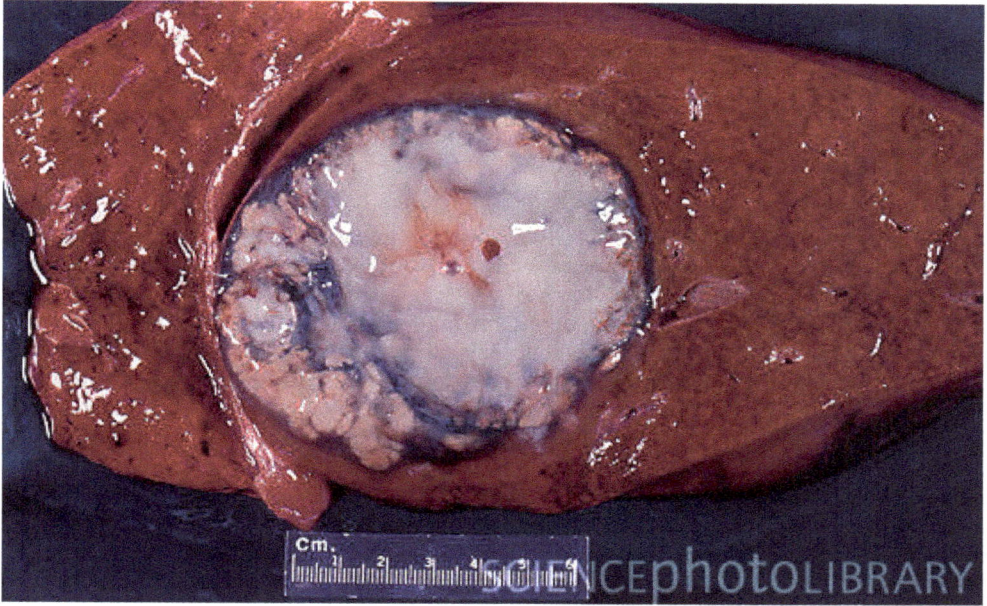

Fig. 4. Amoebic Liver abscess. Gross specimen of liver tissue with an abscess (white) that formed due to infection of the organ with *Entamoeba histolytica*. Source: http://www.sciencephoto.com/media/250248/enlarge

6. Role of genetic characteristics of the infecting strains in the pathogenesis of amoebiasis

The outcome of an infection may depend on several factors among which the genetic characteristics of the specific pathogen have been identified as an important one. Few polymorphic genetic loci have been identified and targeted to aid in the study of the population structure of *E. histolytica* strains and their possible relationships with the parasite's virulence and disease outcome (Clark, 2006; Paul et al., 2007). Examples of these genetic markers include protein coding genes (serine – rich *E. histolytica* protein, [SREHP] and Chitinase) and non-coding DNA (Strain Specific Gene and tRNA gene linked short tandem repeats [STR]) of PCR-amplified genes (Haghighi et al., 2003; Samie et al., 2008). In a study in Bangladesh, the tRNA-linked STR genotyping system has provided evidence that the parasite genome does influence the outcome of infection. tRNA-linked STR genotyping was also behind the recent observation of differences between parasite genotypes in the intestine and the liver abscess of same patients (Ali et al., 2007). Few studies, albeit inconclusive, using the polymorphic SREHP marker have indicated that certain SREHP profiles might be responsible for the presentation of intestinal amoebic symptoms (Ayeh-kumi et al., 2001; Samie et al., 2008). Yet, all studies with SREHP marker did support previous findings of extensive genetic diversity among *E. histolytica* isolates from the same geographic origin (Ayeh-kumi et al., 2001; Simonishvili et al., 2005; Samie et al., 2008; Tanyuksel et al., 2008). Thus, it seems that the parasite genotype does play a role in the outcome of infection in humans thus linking parasite diversity and virulence. Other approaches, such as SNP identification coupled with microarray-based analysis of gene expression or proteomic comparisons among parasites will be needed to identify the actual genes responsible for these results and to help us understand the mechanism of parasite virulence and pathogenesis (Ali et al., 2008).

7. Conclusions

Up to date, there are still large gaps in our knowledge of species prevalence rates in different regions of the world particularly in the African continent where very few studies are being conducted using molecular methods. In order to address this limitation, there is need to implement species-specific diagnosis of E. histolytica, E. dispar and E. moshkovskii, particularly in countries where these organisms are endemic.   Based on the limited information available to date it appears that molecular and genomic studies are still needed combined to molecular epidemiology studies in order to advance our understanding of amoebiasis. The currently available genome sequence is very useful in better understanding the biology of the parasite, however, E. histolytica strains from Africa still need to have the genome sequenced. Comparative genomics will probably allow the understanding of the pathogenicity of some strains of E. histolytica compared to non-pathogenic strains as well as better understanding of E. dispar in relation to E. histolytica. Further collaborations between scientists from developed countries and those from developing countries is essential in answering questions on the epidemiology, pathogenesis and biochemistry of E. histolytica which is the causing agent of amoebiasis.

8. References

Abd-Alla MD, and Ravdin JI (2002). Diagnosis of amebic colitis by antigen capture ELISA in patients presenting with acute amebic diarrhea in Cairo Egypt. Trop Med Int Health 7: 365--370.

Abd-Alla MD, Jackson TG and Ravdin JI (1998). Serum IgM antibody response to the galactose-inhibitable   adherence lectin of Entameoba histolytica. Am J Trop Med Hyg 59: 431-434.

Ackers JP (2000). The diagnostic implications of the separation of Entamoeba histolytica and Entamoeba dispar. J Biosci 27: 573-578.

Acuna-Soto R, Samuelson J, De Girolami P, Zarate L, Millan-Velasco F, Schoolnick G, Wirth D (1993) Application of the polymerase chain reaction to the epidemiology of pathogenic and nonpathogenic Entamoeba histolytica. Am J Trop Med Hyg 48: 58-70.

Ali IKM, Hossain MB, Roy S, Ayeh-Kumi PF, Petri WA, Jr, Haque R, Clark CG (2003). Entamoeba moshkovskii infections in children, Bangladesh. Emerg Infect Dis 9:580–584.

Ali IKM, Mondal U, Roy S, Haque R, Petri WA, Jr, Clark CG (2007). Evidence for a link between parasite genotype and outcome of infection with Entamoeba histolytica. J Clin Microbiol 45: 285–289.

Ali IK, Zaki M and ClarkCG (2005). Use of PCR amplification of tRNA gene-linked short tandem repeats for genotyping *Entamoeba histolytica*. J Clin Microbiol 43: 5842-5847.

Ali IK, Clark CG, Petri Jr. WA (2008). Molecular epidemiology of amoebiasis. Infect Genet Evol 8: 698-707.

Ali IK, Mondal U, Roy S, Haque R, Petri Jr.WA, Clark CG (2007). Evidence for a link between parasite genotype and outcome of infection with *Entamoeba histolytica*. J Clin Microbiol 45: 285-289.

Ali IK, Solaymani-Mohammadi S, Akhter J, Roy S, Gorrini C, Calderaro A, Parker SK, Haque R, Petri Jr.WA, Clark CG (2008). Tissue invasion by *Entamoeba histolytica*: evidence of genetic selection and/or DNA reorganization events in organ tropism. PLoS Negl Trop Dis 2: e219.

Alonzo E, Alonzo V, Forino D, Ioli A (1993). Parasitological research conducted between 1982 and 1991 in a sample of Zinvie (Benin) residents. Med Trop 53(3):331-335.

Artis D (2008). Epithelial-cell recognition of commensal bacteria and maintenance of immune homeostasis in the gut. Nat Rev Immunol 8:411–420.

Asgharpour A, Gilchrist C, Baba D, Hamano S, Houpt E (2005). Resistance to intestinal *Entamoeba histolytica* infection is conferred by innate immunity and Gr-1+ Cells. Infect Immun 73: 4522–4529.

Ayeh-Kumi PF, Ali IM, Lockhart LA, Gilchrist CA, Petri Jr, WA, Haque R (2001). *Entamoeba histolytica*: genetic diversity of clinical isolates from Bangladesh as demonstrated by polymorphisms in the serine-rich gene. Exp Parasitol 99(2):80-88.

Bachur TP, Vale JM, Coêlho IC, Queiroz TR, Chaves Cde S (2008). Enteric parasitic infections in HIV/AIDS patients before and after the highly active antiretroviral therapy. Braz J Infect Dis. 12(2):115-122.

Bardwell L (2006) Mechanisms of MAPK signalling specificity. Biochem Soc Trans 34: 837–841.

Bhattacharya S, Bhattacharya A, Diamond LS and Soldo AT(1989). Circular DNA of Entamoeba histolytica encodes ribosomal RNA. J Protozool 36:455-458.

Blessman J, Le Van A, and Tannich E (2006). Epidemiology and treatment of amoebiasis in Hue, Vietnam. Arch Med Res 37: 270-272.

Blessmann J, Ali IKM, Nu PA, Dinh BT, Viet TQ, Van AL, Clark CG, Tannich E (2003). Longitudinal study of intestinal *Entamoeba histolytica* infections in asymptomatic adult carriers. J Clin Microbiol. 41:4745–50.

Blessmann J, Buss H, Nu PA, Dinh BT, Ngo QT, Van AL, Alla MD, Jackson TF, Ravdin JI, and Tannich E (2002). Real-time PCR for detection and differentiation of *Entamoeba histolytica* and *Entamoeba dispar* in fecal samples. J Clin Microbiol 40:4413-4417.

Blessmann J, Van Linh P, Nu PA, Thi HD, Muller-Myhsok B, Buss H, and Tannich E (2002). Epidemiology of amebiasis in a region of high incidence of amebic liver abscess in central Vietnam. Am J Trop Med Hyg 66:578-583.

Boettner DR, Hutson C, Petri Jr. WA (2002). Galactose/N-acetylgalactoseamine lectin: the coordinator of host cell killing. J Bio 6(Suppl.3):553-557.

Brink AK, Mahe C, Watera C, Lugada E, Gilks C, Whitworth J, and French N (2002). Diarrhoea, CD4 counts and enteric infections in a community-based cohort of HIV-infected adults in Uganda. J Infect 45:99-106.

Burch DJ, Li E, Reed S, Jackson TF, Stanley SL Jr (1991). Isolation of strain-specific Entamoeba histolytica cDNA clone. J Clin Microbiol 29(4):696-701.

Caballero-Salcedo A, Viveros-RogelM, Salvatierra B, Tapia-Conyer R, Sepulveda-Amor J, Gutierrez G, and Ortiz-Ortiz L (1994). Seroepidemiology of amebiasis in Mexico. Am J Trop Med Hyg 50:412-419.

Calderaro A, Gorrini C, Bommezzadri S, Piccolo G, Dettori G, and Chezzi C (2006). *Entamoeba histolytica* and *Entamoeba dispar*: comparison of two PCR assays for diagnosis in a non-endemic setting. Trans R Soc Trop Med Hyg 100:450-457.

Campbell D, Gaucher D, Chadee K (1999). Serum from *Entamoeba histolytica*-infected gerbils selectively suppresses T cell proliferation by inhibiting Interleukin-2 production. J Infect Dis 179:1495–1501.

Cardona AF, Cambariza JF, Reveiz L, Ospina EG, Poveda CM, Ruiz CA, Ramos P, Aponte DM (2004). Caracteristicas clinicas y microbiologicas de la colitis neutropenica en adultos con neoplasias hematologicas del Instituto Nacional de Cancerologia de Bogota, D.C. (Colombia). Enferm Infecc Microbiol Clin 22: 462–466.

Chadee K, Petri WA Jr, Innes DJ, Ravdin JI (1987). Rat and human colonic mucins bind to and inhibit adherence lectin of *Entamoeba histolytica*. J Clin Invest 80(5):1245-54.

Chatterjee A, Ghosh SK, Jang K, Bullitt E, Moore L, Robbins PW and Samuelson J (2009). Evidence for a "wattle and daub" model of the cyst wall of *Entamoeba*. PLoS Pathogens 5 : e1000498.

Chen Y, Zhang Y, Yang B, Qi T, Lu H, Cheng X, and Tachibana H (2007). Seroprevalence of *Entamoeba histolytica* infection in HIV-infected patients in China. Am J Trop Med Hyg 77: 825-828.

Clark CG and Diamond LS (2002). Methods for the cultivation of luminal parasitic protists of clinical importance. Clin Microbiol Rev 15:329-341.

Clark CG (2006). Methods for the investigation of diversity in *Entamoeba histolytica*. Arch Med Res 37(2):258-262.

Daryani A, Sharif M, Meigouni M, Mahmoudi FB, Rafiei A, Gholami Sh, Khalilian A, Gohardehi Sh, Mirabi AM (2009). Prevalence of intestinal parasites and profile of CD4+ counts in HIV+/AIDS people in north of Iran. Pak J Biol Sci. 12(18):1277-1281.

Diamond LS, Clark CG (1993). A redescription of *Entamoeba histolytica* Schaudinn, 1903 (Emended Walker, 1911) separating it from Entamoeba dispar Brumpt, 1925. J Eukaryot Microbiol 40:340–344.

Dorin-Semblat D, Quashie N, Halbert J, Sicard A, Doerig C, Peat E, Ranford-Cartwright L, Doerig C (2007) Functional characterization of both MAP kinases of the human malaria parasite *Plasmodium falciparum* by reverse genetics. Mol Microbiol 65: 1170–1180.

Eichinger D (2001). A role for a galactose lectin and its ligands during encystment of *Entamoeba*. J Eukaryot Microbiol 48: 17-21.

Ellis JG, Davila M, Chakrabarti R (2003). Potential involvement of extracellular signal-regulated kinase 1 and 2 in encystation of a primitive eukaryote, *Giardia lamblia*. Stage-specific activation and intracellular localization. J Biol Chem 278: 1936–1945.

Escobedo AA and Nunez FA (1999). Prevalence of intestinal parasites in Cuban acquired immunodeficiency syndrome (AIDS) patients. Acta Trop 72:125-130.

Espinosa-Cantellano M, Martínez-Palomo A (2000). Pathogenesis of Intestinal Amebiasis: From Molecules to Disease. Clin Microbiol Rev 13(2): 318-331.

Evangelopoulos A, Spanakos G, Patsoula E and Vakalis N (2000). A nested, multiplex, PCR assay for the simultaneous detection and differentiation of *Entamoeba histolytica* and *Entamoeba dispar* in faeces. Ann. Trop. Med. Parasitol. 94:233-240.

Evangelopoulos A, Spanakos G, Patsoula E, Vakalis N, and Legakis NA (2000). A nested, multiplex, PCR assay for the simultaneous detection and differentiation of *Entamoeba histolytica* and Entamoeba dispar in faeces. Ann Trop Med Parasitol 94:233-240.

Florez AC, Garcia DA, Moncada L, Beltran M (2003). Prevalence of Microsporidia and other intestinal parasites in patients with HIV infection, Bogota, 2001. Biomedica 23(3):274-82.

Fotedar R, Stark D, Beebe N, Marriott D, Ellis J, Harkness J (2007). Laboratory diagnostic techniques for *Entamoeba* species. Clin Microbiol Rev. 20(3):511-32.

Fotedar R, Stark D, Marriott D, Ellis J, Harkness J (2008). *Entamoeba moshkovskii* infections in Sydney, Australia. Eur J Clin Microbiol Infect Dis. 27:133–7.

Freitas MA, Vianna EN, Martins ES, Silva EF, Pesquero JL and Gomes MA (2004). A single step duplex PCR to distinguish *Entamoeba histolytica* from *Entamoeba dispar*. Parasitology 128:625-628.

Fujishima T, Nishise S, Ichihara M, Kobayashi S, Takeuchi T (2010). Difficulties in the treatment of intestinal amoebiasis in mentally disabled individuals at a rehabilitation institution for the intellectually impaired in Japan. Chemotherapy. 56(4):348-52.

Furrows SJ, Moody AH and Chiodini PL (2004). Comparison of PCR and antigen detection methods for diagnosis of Entamoeba histolytica infection. J Clin Pathol 57:264-266.

Gassama A, Sow PS, Fall F, Camara P, Gueye-N'diaye A, Seng R, Samb B, M'Boup S, Aidara-Kane A (2001). Ordinary and opportunistic enteropathogens associated with diarrhea in Senegalese adults in relation to human immunodeficiency virus serostatus. Int J Infect Dis 5(4):192-8.

Gathiram V, Jackson TFHG (1987). A longitudinal study of asymptomatic carriers of pathogenic zymodemes of *Entamoeba histolytica*. S Afr Med J 72:669–72.

Gatti S, Swierczynski G, Robinson F, Anselmi M, Corrales J, Moreira J, Montalvo G, Bruno A, Maserati R, Bisoffi Z, and Scaglia M (2002). Amebic infections due to the Entamoeba histolytica-Entamoeba dispar complex: a study of the incidence in a remote rural area of Ecuador. Am J Trop Med Hyg 67:123-127.

Ghosh S, Frisardi m, Rminez-Avila L, Descoteaux S, sturm-Ramirez K, Newton-Sanchez OC, Santos-precado JI, Ganguly C, Lohia A, Reed S, and Samuelson J (2000). Molecular epidemiology of *Entamoeba* spp.: Evidence of a bottleneck (Demographic Sweep) and Transcontinental Spread of Diploid Parasites.J Clin Microbiol 38(10) : 3815-3821.

Goncalves ML, da Silva VL, de Andrade CM, Reinhard K, da Rocha GC, Le Bailly M, Bouchet F, FerreiraLF, and Araujo A (2004). Amoebiasis distribution in the past: first steps using an immunoassay technique. Trans R Soc Trop Med Hyg 98:88-91.

González-Ruiz A, Haque R, Aguirre A, Castañón G, Hall A, Guhl F, Ruiz-Palacios G, Miles MA, Warhurst DC (1994). Value of microscopy in the diagnosis of dysentery associated with invasive Entamoeba histolytica. J Clin Pathol 47: 236-239.

Haghighi A, Kobayashi S, Takeuchi T, Thammapalerd N, Nozaki T (2003). Geographic diversity among genotypes of *Entamoeba histolytica* field isolates. J Clin Microbiol 41(8): 3748-56.

Haileeyesus A and Beyene P (2009). Intstinal protozoan infections amonh HIV positive persons with and without antiretroviral treatment (ART) in selected ART centres in Adama, Afar and Dire-Dawa, Ethiopia. Ethiop. J Health Dev 23(2): 133-140.

Hailemariam G, Kassu A, Abebe G, Abate E, Damte D, Mekonnen E and Ota F (2004). Intestinal parasitic infections in HIV/AIDS and HIV seronegative individuals in a teaching hospital, Ethiopia. Jpn J Infect Dis 57:41-43.

Hamano S, Asgharpour A, Stroup SE, Wynn TA, Leiter EH, Houpt E (2006). Resistance of C57BL/6 mice to amoebiasis is mediated by nonhemopoietic cells but requires hemopoietic IL-10 production. J Immunol 177: 1208–1213.

Hamzah Z, Petmitr S, Mungthin M, Leelayoova S and Chavalitshewinkoon-Petmitr P (2006). Differential detection of *Entamoeba histolytica*, *Entamoeba dispar*, and *Entamoeba moshkovskii* by a single-round PCR assay. J Clin Microbiol 44:3196-3200.

Haque R, Mondal D, Duggal P, Kabir M, Roy S, Farr BM, Sack RB, Petri WA., Jr (2006). *Entamoeba histolytica* infection in children and protection from subsequent amebiasis. Infect Immun 74:904–9.

Haque R, Mondal D, Duggal P, Kabir M, Roy S, Farr BM, Sack RB, Petri WA Jr (2006). *Entamoeba histolytica* Infection in Children and Protection from Subsequent Amebiasis. Infect Immunity 74 (2): 904-909.

Haque R, Mondal D, Karim A, Molla IH, Rahim A, Faruque AS, Ahmad N, Kirkpatrick BD, Houpt E, Snider C, Petri WA Jr (2009). Prospective case-control study of the association between common enteric protozoal parasites and diarrhea in Bangladesh. Clin Infect Dis 48(9):1191-7.

Haque R, Mondal D, Duggal P, Kabir M, Roy S, Farr BM, Sack RB, Petri WA Jr (2006). *Entamoeba histolytica* infection in children and protection from subsequent amebiasis. Infect Immun. 74(2):904-9.

Haque R, Hutson CD, Hughes M, Houpt E, Petri Jr WA (2003). Amoebiasis. N Engl J Med 348: 1565-1573.

Haque R, Ali IKM, and Petri, Jr WA (1999). Prevalence and immune response of *Entamoeba histolytica* infection in preschool children in Bangladesh. Am J Trop Med Hyg 60:1031-1034.

Haque R, Kress K, Wood S, Jackson TFGH, Lyerly D, Wilkins T, and Petri, Jr.WA (1993). Diagnosis of pathogenic *Entamoeba histolytica* infection using a stool ELISA based on monoclonal antibodies to the galactose specific adhesin. J Infect Dis 167:247-249.

Haque R, Mollah NU, Ali IKM, Alam K, Eubank A, Lyerly D, and Petri Jr.WA (2000). Diagnosis of amebic liver abscess and intestinal infection with the TechLab *Entamoeba histolytica* II antigen detection and antibody tests. J Clin Microbiol 38:3235-3239.

Hira PR, Iqbal J, Al-Ali F, Philip R, Grover S, D'Almeida E and Al-Eneizi AA (2001). Invasive amebiasis: challenges in diagnosis in a non-endemic country (Kuwait). Am J Trop Med Hyg 65:341-345.

Hung CC, Ji DD, Sun HY, Lee YT, Hsu SY, Chang SY, Wu CH, Chan YH, Hsiao CF, Liu WC, Colebunders R (2008). Increased risk for *Entamoeba histolytica* infection and invasive amebiasis in HIV seropositive men who have sex with men in Taiwan. PLoS Negl Trop Dis 2(2):e175.

Hung CC, Ji DD, Sun HY, Lee YT, Hsu SY, Ya TL, Shui YH, Sui YC, Cheng HW, Yun HC, Chin FH, Wen CL, Robert C (2008). Increased risk for *Entamoeba histolytica* infection and invasive amoebiasis in HIV seropositive men who have sex with men in Taiwan. PLOS Negl Trop Dis 2(2):e175.

Hung CC, Deng HI, Hsiao WH, Hsieh SM, Hsiao CF, Chen MY, Chang SC and Su KE (2005) Invasive amoebiasis is an emerging parasitic infection in patients with HIV infection. Archives of Internal Medicine, 165: 409-415.

Jackson TF, Gathiram V, Simjee AE (1985). Seroepidemiological study of antibody responses to the zymodemes of *Entamoeba histolytica*. Lancet. 1(8431):716-9.

Junttila MR, Li SP, Westermarck J (2008). Phosphatase-mediated crosstalk between MAPK signaling pathways in the regulation of cell survival. Faseb J 22: 954–965.

Kammanadiminti SJ, Mann BJ, Dutil L, Chadee K (2003). Regulation of toll-like receptor-2 expression by the Gal-lectin of *Entamoeba histolytica*. The FASEB 8: 155-7.

Kammanadiminti SJ, Chadee K (2006). Suppression of NF-κB Activation by *Entamoeba histolytica* in intestinal epithelial cells is mediated by heat shock protein 27. J Biol Chem 281:26112–26120.

Katzwinkel-Wladarsch S, Loscher T and Rinder H (1994). Direct amplification and differentiation of pathogenic and nonpathogenic *Entamoeba histolytica* DNA from stool specimens. Am J Trop Med Hyg 51: 115-118.

Khairnar K, Parija SC, Palaniappan R (2007). Diagnosis of intestinal amoebiasis by using nested polymerase chain reaction-restriction fragment length polymorphism assay. J Gastroenterol 42:631–640.

Klein D (2002). Quantification using real-time PCR technology: applications and limitations. Trends Mol Med 8:257-260.

Knappik M, Borner U, and Jelinek T (2005). Sensitivity and specificity of a new commercial enzyme-linked immunoassay kit for detecting Entamoeba histolytica IgG antibodies in serum samples. Eur J Clin Microbiol Infect Dis 24:701-703.

Krogstad DJ, Spencer HC Jr, Healy GR, Gleason NN, Sexton DJ, Herron CA (1978) Amoebiasis: epidemiologic studies in the United States, 1971-1974. Ann Intern Med 88: 89-97.

Kumiko Nakada-Tsukuia, Yumiko Saito-Nakanoa, Afzal Husaina and Tomoyoshi Nozaki T (2010). Conservation and function of Rab small GTPases in *Entamoeba*: Annotation of *E. invadens* Rab and its use for the understanding of *Entamoeba* biology. Exp Parasitol 126(3): 337-347.

Laughlin RC, Temesvari LA (2005). Cellular and molecular mechanisms that underlie *Entamoeba histolytica* pathogenesis: prospects for intervention. Expert Reviews in Molecular Medicine 7: 1-19.

Lawson LL, Bailey JW, Beeching NJ, Gurgel RG and Cuevas LE (2004). The stool examination reports amoeba cysts: should you treat in the face of over diagnosis and lack of specificity of light microscopy? Trop Doctor 34(1):28-30

Liang SY, Chan YH, Hsia KT, Lee JL, Kuo MC, Hwa KY, Chan CW, Chiang TY, Chen JS, Wu FT, Ji DD (2009). Development of loop-mediated isothermal amplification assay for detection of *Entamoeba histolytica*. J Clin Microbiol 47(6):1892-5.

Lindo JF, Dubon JM, Ager AL, De Gourville EM, Solo-Gabriele H, Klaskala WI, Baum VK, and Palmer CJ (1998). Intestinal parasitic infections in human immunodeficiency virus (HIV)-positive and HIV-negative individuals in San Pedro Sula, Honduras. Am J Trop Med Hyg 58:431-435.

Matthys B, Bobieva M, Karimova G, Mengliboeva Z, Jean-Richard V, Hoimnazarova M, Kurbonova M, Lohourignon LK, Utzinger J, Wyss K (2011). Prevalence and risk factors of helminths and intestinal protozoa infections among children from primary schools in western Tajikistan. Parasit Vectors 4(1):195.

McGugan Jr GC and Temesvari LA (2003). Characterization of a Rab11-like GTPase, EhRab11, of *Entamoeba histolytica*. Mol Biochem Parasitol 129 : 137–146.

McLaughlin J, and Aley S (1985). The biochemistry and functional morphology of the Entamoeba. J Protozool 32:221-240.

Mirelman D, Nuchamowitz Y, and Stolarsky T (1997). Comparison of use of enzyme-linked immunosorbent assay-based kits and PCR amplification of rRNA genes for simultaneous detection of *Entamoeba histolytica* and *E. dispar*. J Clin Microbiol 35:2405-2407.

Mitra BN, Saito-Nakano Y, Nakada-Tsukui K, Sato D and Nozaki T (2007). Rab11B small GTPase regulates secretion of cysteine proteases in the enteric protozoan parasite *Entamoeba histolytica*, Cell Microbiol 9 :2112–2125.

Molbak K, Wested N, Hojlyng N, Scheutz F, Gottschau A, Aaby P, da Silva AP (1994). The etiology of early childhood diarrhea : a community study from Guinea-Bissau.J Infect Dis 169 (3) :581-7.

Morales MA, Renaud O, Faigle W, Shorte SL, Spath GF (2007). Over-expression of Leishmania major MAP kinases reveals stage-specific induction of phosphotransferase activity. Int J Parasitol 37: 1187–1199.

Moran P, Ramos F, Ramiro M, Curiel O, González E, Valadez A, Gómez A, García G, Melendro EI, Ximénez C (2005). *Entamoeba histolytica* and/or *Entamoeba dispar*: infection frequency in HIV+/AIDS patients in Mexico City. Exp Parasitol 110(3):331-4.

Moran P, Ramos F, Ramiro M, Curiel O, Gonzalez E, Valadez A, Gomez A, Garcia G, Melendro EI and Ximenez C (2005). Infection by human immunodeficiency virus-1 is not a risk factor for amoebiasis. American Journal of Tropical Medicine and Hygiene, 73: 296-300.

Mortimer L, Chadee K (2010). The immunopathogenesis of *Entamoeba histolytica*. Exp Parasitol 126(3):336-80.

Mortimer L, Chadee K (2010). The immunopathogenesis of *Entamoeba histolytica*. Exp Parasitol 126 (3): 366-80.

Mukherjee AK, Das K, Bhattacharya MK, Nozaki T, Ganguly S (2010). Trend of *Entamoeba histolytica* infestation in Kolkata. Gut Pathog. 2(1):12.

Nishise S, Fujishima T, Kobayashi S, Otani K, Nishise Y, Takeda H, Kawata S (2010). Mass infection with *Entamoeba histolytica* in a Japanese institution for individuals with mental retardation: epidemiology and control measures. Ann Trop Med Parasitol. 104(5):383-90.

Njoya O, Njitoyap Ndam EC, Ngoue V, Ngonde Sende C (1999). Amoebic liver abscesses in Yaounde. Cahiers sante. 9(2):119-22.

Notomi T, Okayama H, Masubuchi H, Yonekawa T, Watanabe K, Amino N and Hase (2000). Loop-mediated isothermal amplification of DNA. Nucleic Acids Res. 28E63.

Novick and M. Zerial (1997). The diversity of Rab proteins in vesicle transport, Current Opinion in Cell Biology 9 (1997), pp. 496–504.

Nozaki and Nakada-Tsukui (2006). Nozaki T and Nakada-Tsukui K (2006). Membrane trafficking as a virulence mechanism of the enteric protozoan parasite *Entamoeba histolytica*, Parasitology Research 98: 179–183.

Nunez YO, Fernandez MA, Torres-Nunez D, Silva JA, Montano I, Maestre JL, and Fonte L (2001). Multiplex polymerase chain reaction amplification and differentiation of *Entamoeba histolytica* and *Entamoeba dispar* DNA from stool samples. Am J Trop Med Hyg 64:293-297.

Ohnishi K, and Murata M (1997). Present characteristics of symptomatic amebiasis due to *Entamoeba histolytica* in the east-southeast area of Tokyo. Epidemiol. Infect. 119:363-367.

Parija SC, Khairnar K (2005). *Entamoeba moshkovskii* and *Entamoeba dispar*-associated infections in Pondicherry, India. J Health Popul Nutr 23:292–295.

Paul J, Srivastava S, Bhattacharya S (2007). Molecular methods for diagnosis of *Entamoeba histolytica* in a clinical setting: An overview. Exp Parasitol 116: 35-43.

Pham Duc P, Nguyen-Viet H, Hattendorf J, Zinsstag J, Dac Cam P, Odermatt P (2011). Risk factors for *Entamoeba histolytica* infection in an agricultural community in Hanam province, Vietnam. Parasit Vectors. 4:102.

Picazarri K, Nakada-Tsukui K and Nozaki T (2008). Autophagy during proliferation and encystation in the protozoan parasite *Entamoeba invadens*, Infect Immun 76: 278–288.

Pillai DR, Keystone JS, Sheppard DC, MacLean JD, MacPherson DW, and Kain KC (1999). *Entamoeba histolytica* and *Entamoeba dispar*: epidemiology and comparison of diagnostic methods in a setting of non endemicity. Clin Infect Dis 29:1315-1318.

Pinheiro SM, Carneiro RM, Aca IS, Irmao JI, Morais MAJr, Coimbra MR and Carvalho LB Jr 2(004). Determination of the prevalence of *Entamoeba histolytica* and *E. dispar* in the pernambuco state of northeastern Brazil by a polymerase chain reaction. AmJ Trop Med Hyg 70(2):221-4.

Prasad KN, Nag VL, Dhole TN, and Ayyagari A (2000). Identification of enteric pathogens in HIV-positive patients with diarrhoea in northern India. J Health Popul Nutr 18:23-26.

Ravdin JI, Stauffer WM (2005). *Entamoeba histolytica* (amoebiasis). In: Mandell GL, Bennett JE, Dolin R, eds. Principles and Practice of Infectious Diseases, vol. 2. Ed., Phiadelphia: Churchill Livingstone; 2005: 3097-3111.

Reyes P, Cortes JA, Potdevin G, Urdaneta AM, Rosales J, Cuervo SI, Bermudez D, Arroyo PA (2006). Infecciones en pacientes con trasplante de me´dula o´ sea en el tro´ pico. Infection 10: 101.

Rivero Z, Bracho A, Calchi M, Díaz I, Acurero E, Maldonado A, Chourio G, Arráiz N, Corzo G (2009). [Detection and differentiation of *Entamoeba histolytica* and *Entamoeba dispar* by polymerase chain reaction in a community in Zulia State, Venezuela]. Cad Saude Publica. 25(1):151-9.

Robert R, Mahaza C, Bernard C, Buffard C, and Senet JM (1990). Evaluation of a new bicolored latex agglutination test for immunological diagnosis of hepatic amoebiasis. J Clin Microbiol 28:1422-1424.

Roche J, Benito A (1999). Prevalence of intestinal parasite infections with special reference to *Entamoeba histolytica* on the island of Bioko (Equatorial Guinea). Am J Trop Med Hyg 60(2):257-62.

Roy S, Kabir M, Mondal D, Ali IK, Petri Jr. WA and Haque R (2005). Real-time-PCR assay for diagnosis of *Entamoeba histolytica* infection. Clin. Microbiol. 43:2168-2172.

Samie A, Barrett LJ, Bessong PO, Ramalivhana JN, Mavhandu LG, Njayou M, and Gurreant RL (2010). Seroprevalence of *Entamoeba histolytica* in the context of HIV and AIDS: the case of the Vhembe district, in South Africa's Limpopo province. Ann Trop Med Parasitol 104 (1): 55-63.

Samie A, Obi CL, Bessong PO, Houpt E, Stroup S, Njayou M, Sabeta C, Mduluza T, Guerrant RL (2008). *Entamoeba histolytica*: genetic diversity of African strains based on the polymorphism of the serine-rich protein gene. Exp Parasitol 118(3): 354-61.

Sardar Ghosh A, Ray D, Dutta S, Raha S (2010). EhMAPK, the Mitogen-Activated Protein Kinase from Entamoeba histolytica Is Associated with Cell Survival. PLoS ONE 5(10): e13291. doi:10.1371/journal.pone.0013291.

Simonishvili S, Tsanava S, Sanadze K, Chlikadze R, Miskalishvili A, Lomkatsi N, Imnadze P, Petri Jr.WA, Trapaidze N (2005). *Entamoeba histolytica*: the serine-rich gene polymorphism-based genetic variability of clinical isolates from Georgia. Exp Parasitol 110(3):313-7.

Stanley SL Jr (2003). Amoebiasis. Lancet. 361(9362):1025-1034.

Stanley S LJr., Becker A, Kunz-Jenkins C, Foster L and Li E (1990). Cloning and expression of a membrane antigen of *Entamoeba histolytica* possessing multiple tandem repeats. Proc Natl Acad Sci USA 87:4976-4980.

Stanley SL (2003). Amoebiasis. Lancet 361, 1025-34.

Stark D, Barratt JLN, van Hal S, Marriott D, Harkness J, and Ellis JT (2009). Clinical significance of enteric protozoa in the immunosuppressed human population. Clin Microbiol Rev 22(4): 634-650.

Stark D, Fotedar R, van Hal S, Beebe N, Marriott D, Ellis TG and Harkness J (2007). Prevalence of enteric protozoa in human immunodeficiency virus (HIV)-positive and HIV-negative men who have sex with men from Sydney, Australia. Am J Trop Med Hyg 76:549-552.

Stauffer W, Abd-Alla M and Ravdin JI (2006). Prevalence and incidence of Entamoeba histolytica in South Africa and Egypt. Arch Med Res 37: 266-269.

Stenmark H (2009). Rab GTPases as coordinators of vesicle traffic, Nature Reviews Molecular Cell Biology 10:513–525.

Strachan WD, Chiodini PL, Spice WM, Moody AH and Ackers JP (1988). Immunological differentiation of pathogenic and nonpathogenic isolates of E. histolytica. Lancet i:561-563.

Tanyuksel M., Petri Jr.WA (2003). Laboratory diagnosis of amoebiasis. Clin Microbiol Rev 16: 713-729.

Tanyuksel M, Ulukanligil M, Yilmaz H, Guclu Z, Araz RE, Mert G, Koru O, Petri Jr WA. (2008). Genetic variability of the serine-rich gene of the *Entamoeba histolytica* in clinical isolates from Turkey. Turk J Med Scdi 38(3): 239-244.

Bachur TP, Vale JM, Coêlho IC, Queiroz TR, Chaves Cde S (2008). Enteric parasitic infections in HIV/AIDS patients before and after the highly active antiretroviral therapy. Braz J Infect Dis 12(2):115-122.

Tsai JJ, Sun HY, Tsai KS, Chang SY, Hsieh SM, Hsiao CF, Yen JH, Hung CC, Chang SC (2006). Higher seroprevalence of Entamoeba histolytica infection is associated with human immunodeficiency virus type 1 infection in Taiwan. Am J Trop Med Hyg 74(6):1016-9.

Visser LG, Verweij JJ, Van Esbroeck M, Edeling WM, Clerinx J, Polderman AM (2006). Diagnostic methods for differentiation of Entamoeba histolytica and Entamoeba dispar in carriers: performance and clinical implications in a non-endemic setting. Int J Med Microbiol 296:397-403.

WHO (1997). "WHO/PAHO/UNESCO report. A consultation with experts on amoebiasis. Mexico City, Mexico 28-29 January 1997. Epidemiological Bulletin 18 (1): 13-14.

Ximénez C, Morán P, Rojas L, Valadez A, Gómez A, Ramiro M, Cerritos R, González E, Hernández E, and Oswaldo P (2011). Novelties on Amoebiasis: A Neglected Tropical Disease. J Glob Infect Dis 3(2): 166–174.

Ximénez C, Morán P, Rojas L, Valadez A, Gómez A (2009). Reassessment of the epidemiology of amebiasis: state of the art. Infect Genet Evol 9(6):1023-32.

Zengzhu G, Bracha R, Nuchamowitz Y, Cheng W and Mirelman D (1999). Analysis by enzyme-linked immunosorbent assay and PCR of human liver abscess aspirates from patients in China for *Entamoeba histolytica*. J Clin Microbiol 37:3034-3036.

4

Retrospective Analysis of Leishmaniasis in Central Tunisia: An Update on Emerging Epidemiological Trends

Akila Fathallah Mili[1,3], Fatma Saghrouni[1], Zeineb BenSaid[2],
Yusr Saadi- BenAoun[3], Ikram Guizani[3] and Moncef BenSaid[1]
[1]Laboratory of Parasitology, Farhat Hached Hospital, Sousse
[2]Service of Dermatology, Farhat Hached Hospital, Sousse
[3]Laboratory of Parasitic Epidemiology and Ecology (LEEP) - LR00SP04,
Institut Pasteur, Tunis
Tunisia

1. Introduction

This study aimed at describing the spatio-temporal distribution of leishmaniasis in patients who have sought diagnosis in the laboratory of Parasitology of Farhat Hached hospital, Sousse, Tunisia, across the 1986-2010 period in order to: **i)** highlight important features and trends of leishmaniasis and its epidemiology; **ii)** and to assess whether the activity of the unit reflects the situation of the disease at the national level and whether it could constitute an indicator of public health relevance.

2. Current situation of leishmaniasis in Tunisia

Tunisia is located in Northern Africa, bordering the Mediterranean sea between Algeria and Libya. Its climate is of the hot temperate Mediterranean type. Bioclimatic zones range from humid in the north to saharian in the extreme south (Figure 1).
The country is divided into 24 governorates, each composed of a variable number of "delegations"; and each delegation is subdivided into localities also named "imadas" (Figure 2). Four forms of leishmaniasis are known to occur in Tunisia: i) the sporadic cutaneous leishmaniasis (SCL); ii) the chronic cutaneous leishmaniasis (CCL); iii) the zoonotic cutaneous leishmaniasis (ZCL); iv) the visceral leishmaniasis (VL).

2.1 The sporadic cutaneous leishmaniasis (SCL)

This form is caused by dermotropic zymodemes of *Leishmania infantum*, mainly the zymodeme MON 24 and to a lesser extent MON 1 (Aoun et al., 2000, 2008; Ben Ismail et al, 1986, 1992; Gramiccia et al., 1991; Haouas et al., 2007; Kallel et al., 2005, 2008b). The dog is supposed to be the reservoir as it is the case for the viscerotropic zymodemes and *Phlebotomus perfiliewi* as the phletotomine vector. But other vectors can not be excluded; following an outbreak of SCL in the locality of Oued Souani, le Kef governorate, *P. langeroni* was found infected by *L. infantum* (Guerbouj et al., 2007).

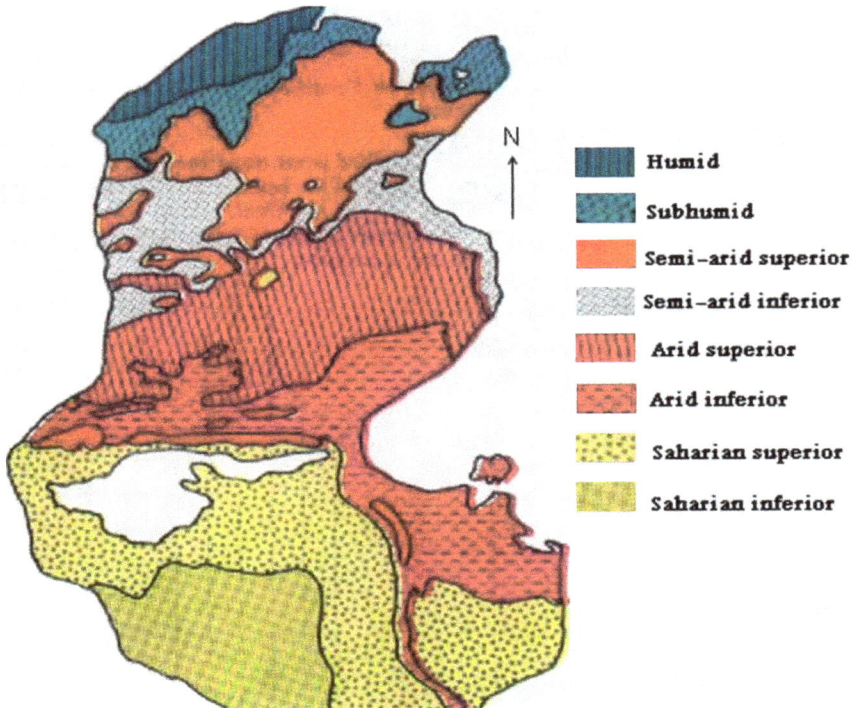

Legend:
- Humid
- Subhumid
- Semi-arid superior
- Semi-arid inferior
- Arid superior
- Arid inferior
- Saharian superior
- Saharian inferior

Fig. 1. Map of Tunisia showing the distribution of bioclimatic zones.

SCL was first described in 1917 in a patient from Sakiet Sidi Youssef (Le Kef governorate) located next to the Algerian frontier (Nicolle & Blanc, 1917), and again in 1945 (Chadli et al., 1968; Vermeil, 1956). Since 1945, the disease has sporadically been reported with, however, an incidence that gradually increased from a median of one case /year between 1945 and 1955 to 22 cases /year in the 1990s and 59 cases/year in the 2000s (Table 1; Anonymous ; Ben Abda et al., 2009; Ben Said et al., 2006; Ben Ismail & Ben Rachid, 1989; Ben Rachid et al., 1983, 1992; Chadli et al., 1968 ; Chaffai et al., 1988; Ladjimi & Lakhoua, 1955 ; Vermeil, 1956). SCL has long been supposed to be confined to the humid and subhumid bioclimatic areas north to the "dorsale" or "tunisian Ridge" (the eastern extension of the Atlas mountains), in rural areas where its distribution overlaps with that of VL (Ben Ismail et al., 1989; Ben Rachid et al., 1983; Ben Rachid & Ben Ismail, 1989; Chadli et al., 1986 ; Vermeil, 1956). However, over the last three decades, many cases originating from central Tunisia governorates (Monastir, Sousse, Mahdia and Kairouan) and referred to our laboratory were found to be very suggestive of SCL on the basis of epidemiological, clinical and parasitological criteria. Typed strains obtained from some of these patients proved indeed to be *L. infantum* (Ben Said et al., 2006). These data were very indicative of SCL spread towards the south of the country. These findings were further confirmed by additional reports (Aoun et al, 2000, 2008; Ben Abda et al., 2009; Kallel et al., 2008a, 2008b). The revised SCL distribution is shown in figure 3. SCL usually occurs sporadically within no particular season. However, over the last few years, local outbreaks were reported like that of Sidi Bourouis in Siliana governorate, which involved more than 30 patients over a short period (Bel Hadj et al., 2003).

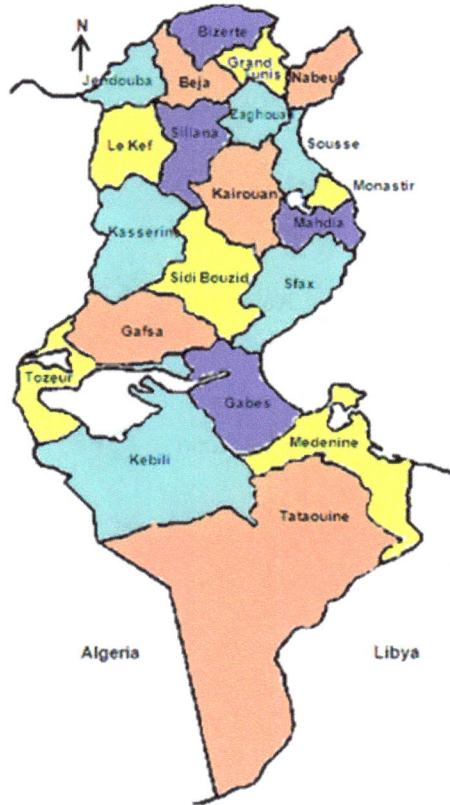

Fig. 2. Map of Tunisia showing its subdivision into 24 governorates (Grand Tunis is composed of 4 governorates).

Years	Nb of cases	Median
1945-55	10	1.0
1956-67	17	1.4
1968-78	84	8.4
1979-89	151	15.1
1990-99	217	21.7
2000-10	652	59.3
Total	1131	17.1

Table 1. Number of recorded sporadic cutaneous leishmaniasis cases since 1945.

Clinically, SCL is characterized in more than 90 % of patients by a small single ulcerated or lupoid lesion of the face that often lasts longer than one year and up to three years (Bel Hadj et al., 1996; Ben Ismail & Ben Rachid, 1989; Chaffai et al, 1988; Masmoudi et al., 2007). On a parasitological level, amastigotes of *L. infantum* are smaller than those of *L. major*, usually less than 3µ , and promastigotes are difficult to maintain on NNN medium (Aoun et al., 2000, 2003).

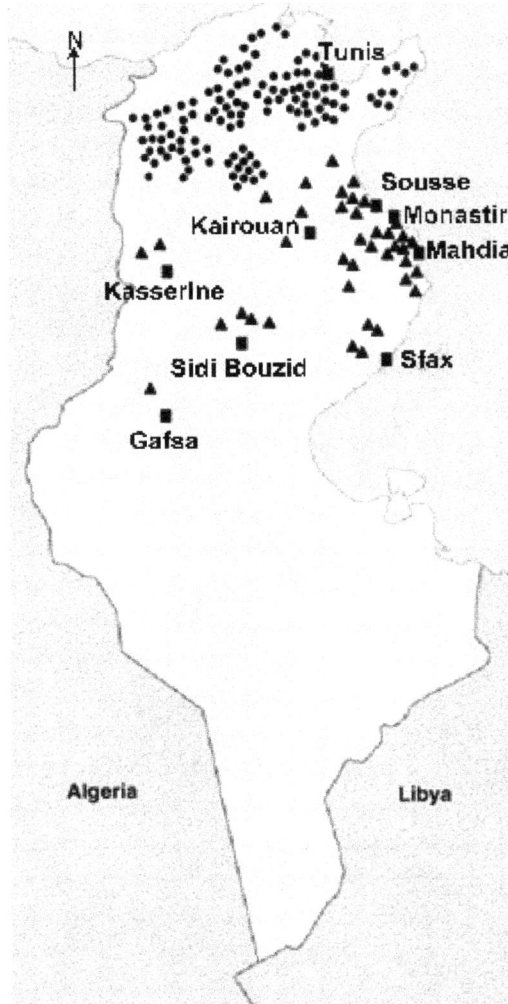

•: corresponds to the classical distribution of the cases; ▲: illustrates the emerging distribution of cases.

Fig. 3. Updated distribution of sporadic cutaneous leishmaniasis in Tunisia.

2.2 The chronic cutaneous leishmaniasis (CCL)

Formerly known as anthroponotic CL, CCL sporadically occurs in micro-foci located in the south-eastern presaharian and saharian areas of Tunisia. Its distribution is rural, sub-urban and urban; and cases are reported from houses, farms, and even from troglodytes of Tataouine (Tataouine governorate) and Matmata (Gabès governorate), with a median annual incidence of 10 cases /year (Figure 4; Ben Ismail & Ben Rachid, 1989; Ben Rachid et al., 1983, 1992; Chadli et al., 1968). CCL was first reported in 1957 and nearly nothing was known about the disease before this date. In 1979, an outbreak involving 47 individuals arose in Tataouine; and the epidemiological investigation, which included the isoenzymatic typing of strains isolated from the patients, led to the identification of the parasite as the MON 8 zymodeme of *L. tropica*, named *L. killicki*, a species previously described in Kenya, Namibia, Yemen and, more recently in Algeria and Libya (Harrat et al., 2009; Rioux et al., 1986; Sang et al., 1994).

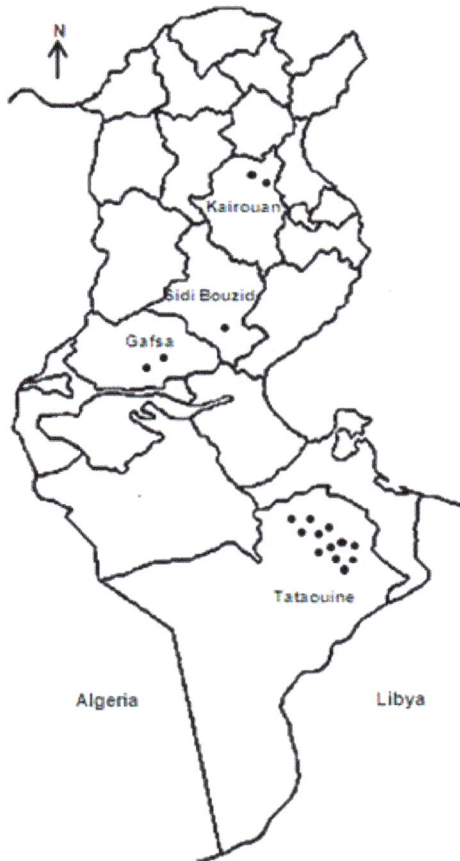

Fig. 4. Actual distribution of chronic cutaneous leishmaniasis.

Surprisingly, over the last decade, cases of CCL were reported in patients originating from areas where this form has never been previously reported, the first case being in a child from Meknassy in Sidi Bouzid governorate (Haouas et al., 2005). Later, additional cases were reported from Kairouan, Gafsa and Siliana governorates, very far from the classical foci of Tataouine (Aoun et al., 2008; Ben Abda et al., 2009; Bouratbine et al., 2005).

Hence the actual distribution and incidence of CCL need further investigations and obviously should be revised.

L. killicki is transmitted by *Phlebotomus sergenti*, but the reservoir is still debated. Median age of patients suffering of CCL is 21 years (Ben Abda et al., 2009; Ben Ismail & Ben Rachid, 1989). Clinically, CCL most often presents as single or very few lesions on the face or limbs, that are dry, extensive, and chronic, lasting for up to six years (Ben Abda et al., 2009; Ben Ismail & Ben Rachid., 1989; Chaffai et al., 1988; Masmoudi et al., 2007).

2.3 The zoonotic cutaneous leishmaniasis (ZCL)

ZCL is by far the most frequent and the most widely distributed form of CL in Tunisia where it constitutes a major public health problem. It is endemo-epidemic in extended areas of central and southern Tunisia (Figure 5). It is caused by *L. major* and transmitted by the zoo-anthropophilic *Phlebotomus papatasi* sandfly which is mainly encountered and caught in and around the rodent burrows, and less in and around human habitations (Ben Ismail et al., 1987b, 1987c; Ben Rachid et al., 1992; Ghrab et al., 2006; Helal et al., 1987). The reservoirs are rodents of the *Psammomys* and *Meriones* genera. The main one is *P. obesus*, a prolific diurnal rodent that is very abundant in arid and subsaharian areas. Its feeding requirements consist exclusively of chenopodiaceae (*Salicornia, Salsola, Atriplex*) that mainly grow in sandy, humid and salty soils unsuitable for agricultural purposes (Ben Ismail et al., 1987a; Ben Rachid et al., 1992; Fichet-Calvet et al., 2003). *Psammomys* infection rate may reach 100 %. The hygrophilic nocturnal rodents, *Meriones shawi* and *Meriones libycus* act as secondary reservoirs and are responsible of the spread of the disease because of their migratory habits. *Meriones* are granivorous and build their burrows in jujube trees (*Zizyphus*) surrounding cereal fields and often cause important agricultural damage (Ben Ismail & Ben Rachid, 1989; Ben Rachid et al., 1992). All *Leishmania* strains isolated so far from humans, rodents and phlebotomine vectors are of the zymodeme MON 25 (Aoun et al., 2008; Ben Abda et al., 2009; Ben Ismail et al., 1986; Haouas et al., 2007).

ZCL was first described in 1882 in and around Gafsa oases, and termed "clou de Gafsa" (Deperet & Bobinet, 1884). From this date and up to the beginning of the 20th century, many additional outbreaks were reported in the same area. Then, the disease continued to occur on a very sporadic mode, and nearly disappeared (Chadli et al., 1968; Vermeil, 1956).

In 1982, a large outbreak arose in Nasrallah delegation (Kairouan governorate), near to the recently completed Sidi-Saad dam (Ben Ammar et al., 1984). From there, the disease rapidly spread to cover large rural and sub-urban parts of the central and south-western neighbouring governorates, so that, by 1986, 10 governorates were involved (Figure 6). In season 1991-1992, ZCL extended further south-east to Medenine and Tataouine governorates. All along the outbreak, Sidi Bouzid, Gafsa and Kairouan governorates have remained the leading areas in terms of incidence (Anonymous). However, from the early 1990s and up to date, Tataouine, Tozeur, Médenine, Kébili, Gabès, Sfax and Kasserine have emerged as active and stable foci (Figure 5). In the last few years, some level of ZCL spread towards the north (Siliana, Béja, Le Kef, Tunis and Zaghouan governorates) was registered, which is somewhat surprising (Ben Abda et al., 2009).

The number of annual recorded cases rapidly grew from 182 cases in 1982 to > 18000 cases by 1987, > 65000 cases by 1999. Up to date, > 120000 cases were reported and the epidemic is still going on. It should be mentioned however, that the actual number of cases is supposed to be underestimated and would exceed 150000 cases (Chahed et al., 2002). The number of annual recorded cases greatly varied and ranged from 1129 cases in 1995 to > 15000 in 2004,

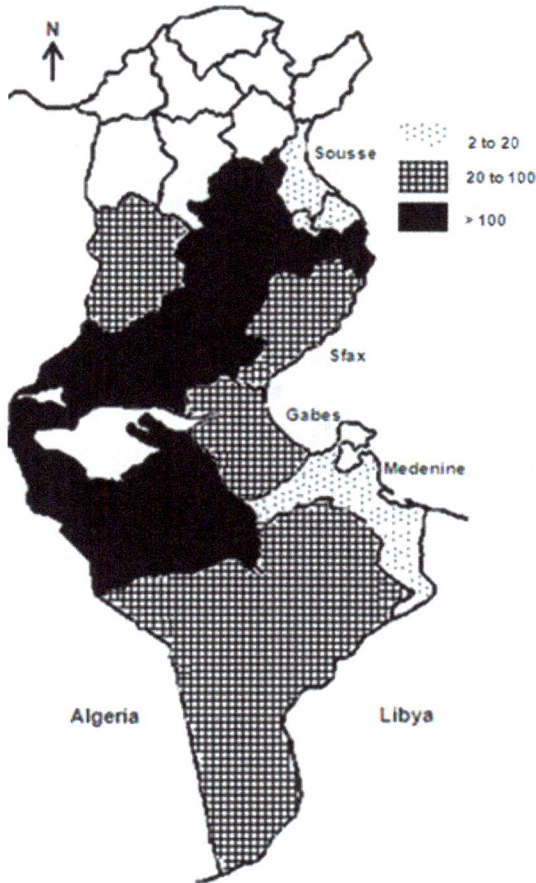

Fig. 5. Distribution of zoonotic cutaneous leishmaniasis according to incidence (expressed as $^0/_{00\,000}$).

with an average of 4700 cases/year (Figure 7). The annual incidence showed the same fluctuations. It ranged between 3 $^0/_{00\,000}$ in the less affected areas and > 500 in Kairouan, and > 1000 in Gafsa and Sidi Bouzid in 2004 (Anonymous). These fluctuations are at least in part related to the dynamics of rodents' populations. It was demonstrated that the distribution of *P. obesus* is of paramount importance in the epidemiology of the human disease (Ben Ismail et al., 1987a; Ben Ismail & Ben Rachid, 1989; Ben Salah et al., 2007; Fichet-Calvet et al., 2003). On the other hand, control programmes are undoubtedly very effective and beneficial in terms of incidence. Indeed, a rodent control project, consisting of ploughing lands with growing chenopods and reafforestation with acacia and other plants was launched in 1992 in Sidi Bouzid city and suburbs that resulted in a dramatic decrease in the incidence of the disease in the area; but the intensity of the epidemic grew again as soon as the control programme stopped (Figure 7). From the mid 2000s, similar control measures have been carried out again in Sidi Bouzid and then in Sidi El Heni delegation which is the main transmission focus in Sousse governorate, and led to an obvious decrease of incidence in both foci.

The ongoing outbreak that started in 1982 near the Sidi-Saad dam may be explained by the interruption, as a result of the construction of the dam, in the flooding that frequently occurred in the area and used to decimate a high proportion of rodents every year. In addition, the enrichment of the area's ground water helped the chenopodiaceae to grow abundantly, thereby increasing the food source of *Psammomys*. On the other hand, *Atriplex*, a plant grown in large quantities as a sheep fodder is much appreciated by *Psammomys*. Furthemore, humidity created by the dam is highly suitable for the sandflies.

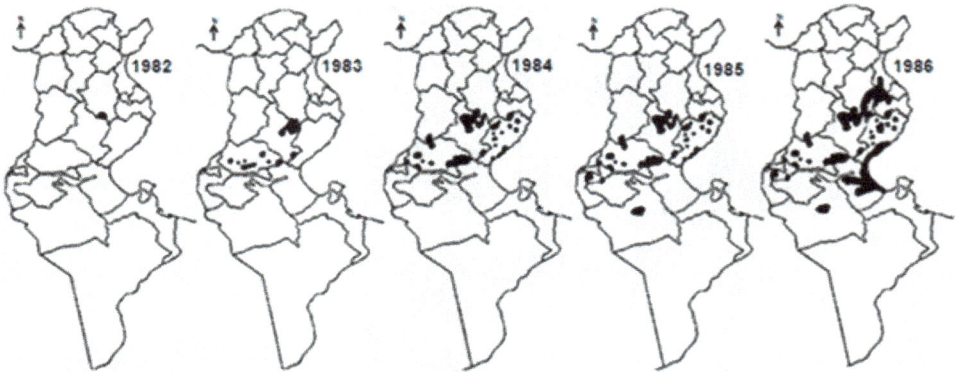

Fig. 6. Spread of zoonotic cutaneous leishmaniasis during the period 1982- 1986 (Ben Ismail R., unpublished).

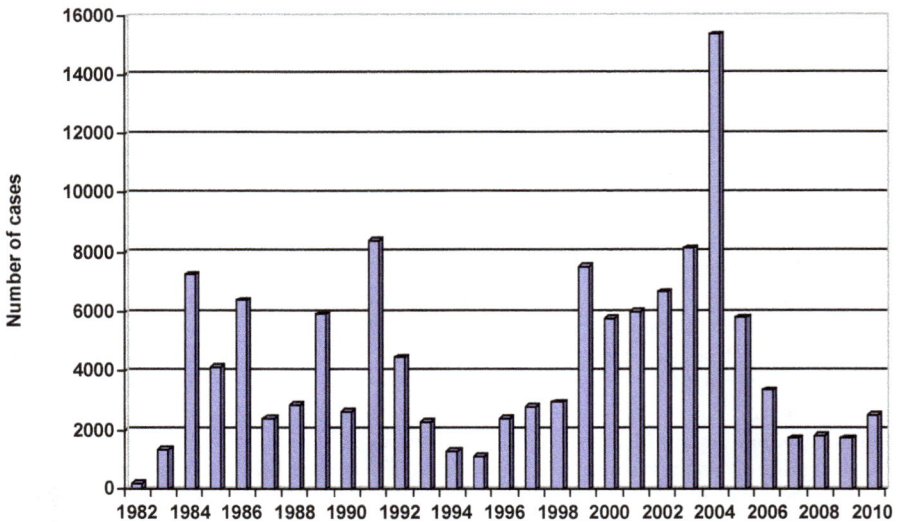

Fig. 7. Annual number of reported zoonotic cutaneous leishmaniasis cases at the national level from 1982 up to 2010.

One of the characteristics of ZCL is its marked seasonal occurence as most cases are observed between october and january (Ben Ismail & Ben Rachid 1989; Ben Rachid et al., 1992).
Clinically, ZCL most often presents as multiple, inflammatory ulcers on the face and the limbs that usually scar in less than 6-8 months, and affects all ages with a median of 24 years (Ben Abda et al., 2009; Ben Ismail & Ben Rachid, 1989; Chaffai et al., 1988; Masmoudi et al., 2007; Zakraoui et al., 1995).

2.4 Visceral leishmanasis (VL)

VL has been known to sporadically occur in Tunisia, since 1903 where the first case of mediterranean VL was described in a child living in the suburbs of Tunis. The disease is caused by *Leishmania infantum*, mostly zymodeme MON 1 and to a lesser extent zymodemes MON 24 and MON 80 (Aoun et al., 2001, 2008; Bel Hadj et al., 1996, 2000, 2002; Ben Ismail et al., 1986; Haouas et al., 2005; Kallel et al., 2008b). It is transmitted by *Phlebotomus perniciosus* sandfly, and the dog is the exclusive reservoir, with an infection prevalence rate ranging from 5% to 26 % (Ben Ismail et al., 1986; Ben Rachid et al., 1992; Bouratbine et al., 1998).
Since 1903, 2449 VL cases were reported in Tunisia (Table 2).

Period	Nb cases	Median/year
1903-1956	151	2.8
1957-1967	142	12.9
1968-1981	178	12.7
1982-1989	578	72.3
1990-2000	720	65.5
2001-2010	680	68.0
Total	2449	22.7

Table 2. Number of visceral leishmaniasis cases reported in Tunisia (1903-2010)

Up to 1981, incidence was low to moderate and nearly all cases were reported from Zaghouan, North-West (Le Kef, Béja, Jendouba, Siliana), Tunis and Sousse governorates, located in the humid, sub-humid and semi-arid zones (Anderson et al., 1934, 1938; Ben Ismail et al., 1986; Ben Rachid et al., 1983; Chadli et al., 1968; Khaldi et al., 1991; Nicolle, 1912; Vermeil, 1956). From the early 1980s, the incidence markedly increased and the disease progressed towards the south, mainly to Kairouan governorate and to a lesser extent to Sfax, Sidi Bouzid, Kasserine and Tozeur governorates, together with an increase in canine leishmaniasis (Ayadi et al., 1991; Bel Hadj et al., 1996; Ben Salah et al., 2000; Besbès et al., 1994; Bouratbine et al., 1998; Chargui et al., 2007; Pousse et al., 1995). Indeed, from the 1980s, the region of Kairouan emerged as a highly active VL focus, and by 1991-1992 it was recognized as the most active one, with 30 to 55 % of reported cases (Anonymous).
The distribution of VL is given in figure 8. Highest number of cases was reported in 1922 (n = 130), 1993 and 2006 (n = 122), and 2005 (n = 120). It is worth mentioning that VL has nearly disappeared between 1974 and 1980, as a result of the anti-malaria campaign which included extensive insecticide spraying (Ben Rachid et al., 1983). The disease sporadically occurs in rural and to a lesser extent in suburban areas and mainly affects children under five years, cases in immunocompetent adults being less than 5 % (Ben Ismail & Ben Rachid, 1989; Ben Rachid et al., 1983; Besbès et al., 1994; Bouratbine et al, 1998; Hammoud et al.,

2004; Pousse et al. 1995). In HIV Tunisian patients, VL is infrequent; it is best diagnosed by PCR (Kallel et al., 2007).

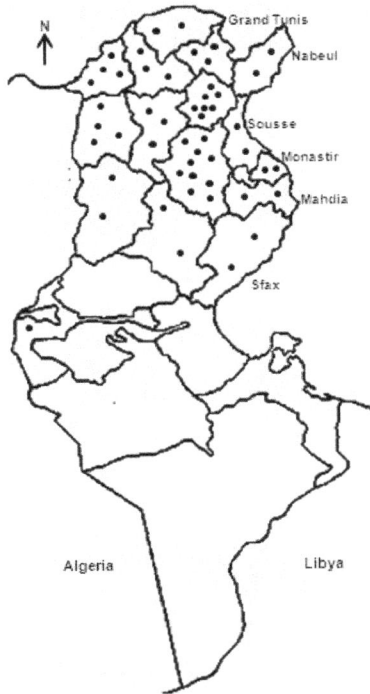

Fig. 8. Actual distribution of visceral leishmaniasis in Tunisia.

3. Materials and methods

The laboratory of parasitology of Sousse, the third major Tunisian city which is located in the central, coastal part of Tunisia, was first created in 1986. It can be considered as a central laboratory ensuring the diagnosis of parasitic diseases' cases including leishmaniasis, sent by generalists, dermatologists, pediatricians or hematologists either from the same hospital or other hospitals mainly from governorates of central Tunisia like Kairouan, Sidi Bouzid and Mahdia. Results are usually sent back to the referring doctors so the patients can be managed as appropriate. Since its creation, the laboratory has been involved in the diagnosis of all forms of leishmaniasis.

For purposes of this retrospective study, VL and CL patients' data, including age, sex, geographical origin and the likely place of contamination, clinical presentation and evolution without or after treatment were collected.

3.1 Diagnosis of cutaneous leishmaniasis

The diagnosis of CL is usually achieved by the demonstration of amastigotes in Giemsa-stained smears from the fluid obtained by scraping the edges of the cutaneous lesion with a sterile lancet. In addition, the size of the identified *Leishmania* is carefully evaluated, because small amastigotes (< 3μ) are evocative of *L. infantum* and *L. killicki* rather than *L. major* whose amastigotes are larger. Over the last decade, lesions evocative of CL but found negative in direct examination were further submitted to PCR technique, known to be more sensitive.

3.2 Diagnosis of visceral leishmaniasis
3.2.1 Parasitological diagnosis
Diagnosis of VL is usually based on the demonstration of amastigotes in Giemsa stained bone-marrow aspirates. However, in our laboratory, bone-marrow smears are mainly carried out and read in doubtful cases, because they usually are performed and interpreted by the haematologists and sometimes the pediatricians themselves and the results of the examination are later sent to us together with sera specimens.
For the purpose of parasitological diagnosis of VL, since 1996, we have been using the cytoconcentration of peripheral blood according to the technique of Petithory et al, 1997. Cytoconcentration is usually practiced first, and when positive the painful bone marrow aspiration is no more needed and the diagnosis of VL is established.

3.2.2 Serodiagnosis of leishmaniasis
All sera from suspected or confirmed VL cases are sent to our laboratory for serodiagnosis. Our reference technique is the fluorescent antibody test (FAT). It is carried out by using *Leishmania*-spot IF® slides (bioMerieux, France) on sera serially diluted starting from 1/100. Sera showing fluorescence at ≥ 1/200 dilution are considered positive.
In addition to FAT, we have been using, since 2003, the rK39 dipstick test (DST). The first one we used was from Inbios International, USA (kalazar detect®). Then, since 2007 and up to date, we have been using the Dia.Med IT Leish® (Dia Med, Switzerland), according to Saghrouni et al., 2009.

3.3 Culture of *Leishmania*
Our laboratory has mainly been involved in the culture of dermotropic *Leishmania*, even though isolates from VL bone-marrow aspirates were occasionally cultured.
Culture was mainly carried out for the purpose of typing strains by isoenzyme electrophoresis (IEE) technique. Media we have been using are the NNN (Nicolle Novy Mc Neal), the BHI (brain heart infusion agar) and the CRS (coagulated rabbit serum), the last being best for cutaneotropic *L. infantum* strains. *Leishmania* isolates were typed either in the IEE unit of the LEEP or in the laboratory of parasitology of the Faculty of Pharmacy, Monastir, where an IEE unit was set up in 2001.

3.4 Molecular biology
Up to 2008, our laboratory was not equipped for molecular biology techniques. In 2007, as part of a collaborative project on "molecular tools for accurate diagnosis and better assessment of leishmaniases", codirected by the LEEP and our own laboratory and financed by the IAEA, a molecular biology unit was set up in our department and has just started working. In the meanwhile we have been collaborating with the molecular biology unit of the LEEP, mainly for identifying *Leishmania* strains. The first study, conducted in 2005, aimed at identifying strains isolated from patients suspected for having SCL, by using K-DNA-PCR according to Smyth et al., 1992 and PCR-RFLP according to Guerbouj et al., 2001 (Ben Said et al., 2006).

Later, additional strains isolated from CL patients were typed by a novel Multiplex PCR (Saadi et al., in preparation) as part of the IAEA project that is still ongoing.

In addition, specimens from patients with lesions highly evocative of CL but found negative in parasitological examination were addressed for PCR to the laboratory of parasitology of the Faculty of Pharmacy, Monastir, where a molecular biology unit has just been set up. PCR was performed according to Chargui et al., 2005.

4. Results

4.1 Cutaneous leishmaniasis

Over the 25 year period study, 4329 patients were investigated for CL. Most of them were referred to our laboratory by the service of Dermatology of Farhat Hached hospital, Sousse. *Leishmania* parasites were demonstrated in 2087 cases (48.2%). In addition, out of 86 PCR performed on samples found negative in direct examination of dermal Giemsa stained smears, 17 were positive. So, the total number of CL cases diagnosed during the study period was 2104. Most of them were diagnosed during the last decade.

Out of the 2104 diagnosed cases 50 were confirmed or very likely SCL form. Fourteen came from areas known to be endemic for SCL (Le Kef, Jendouba, Siliana, Zaghouan and Bizerte governorates). The remaining 36 cases were from areas located in central Tunisian governorates where SCL has never been described: 13 were from Monastir, 12 from Sousse, 6 from Mahdia and 5 from Kairouan. Out of the 36 cases, 13 originated from areas known to be endemic for ZCL, in Kairouan, Mahdia and Sousse governorates. The age of patients ranged from to 5.5 to 63 years (median = 28.5 years). Twenty six were males and 24 were females (sex ratio M/F = 1.08).

In three patients, the isolate proved to be *L. killicki*. The first patient was a 5 year old child from Meknassi in Sidi Bouzid governorate where CCL was unknown. The second was a 30 year old woman from Ghomrassen, known to be endemic for CCL. The third patient was a 21 year old woman who came from Nasrallah, one of the most active ZCL foci in Kairouan governorate and from where no CCL cases were reported before.

All the remaining 2051 patients were suffering from ZCL. 1182 were females and 869 were males (sex ratio F/M = 1.36). Their age ranged from 1 month to 90 years (median = 28 years). The annual distribution of ZCL cases diagnosed over the 25 year period is shown in figure 9. The number of cases ranged from 5 in 1997 to 443 in 2004.

The place of contamination could be ascertained in 1873 out of the 2051 patients. In the 178 remaining cases, the geographical origin of contamination could not be determined with certainty because of multiple displacements of patients across two, three or more endemic areas. In addition, some patients were originating from Libya and Algeria and were not included in the analysis of the spatio-temporal distribution of ZCL cases.

The distribution of the 1873 ZCL cases according to the area where the contamination took place is given in table 3. Most of the patients came from Sidi Bouzid (610 = 32.6%), Mahdia (494 = 26.4%), Kairouan (369 = 19.7%), and Sousse (306 = 16.3%) governorates.

The distribution of cases according to delegations inside the four governorates mentioned above is shown in figure 10, and the annual distribution of diagnosed cases in figure 11. According to seasonal distribution 1745 (85.1 %) cases were diagnosed between October and February. All confirmed CL patients were treated with local or parenteral N-methylglucamine antimoniate (glucantime®) together with cryotherapy in those with few lesions. Most of treated patients responded well to antimonial treatment, and scarring of

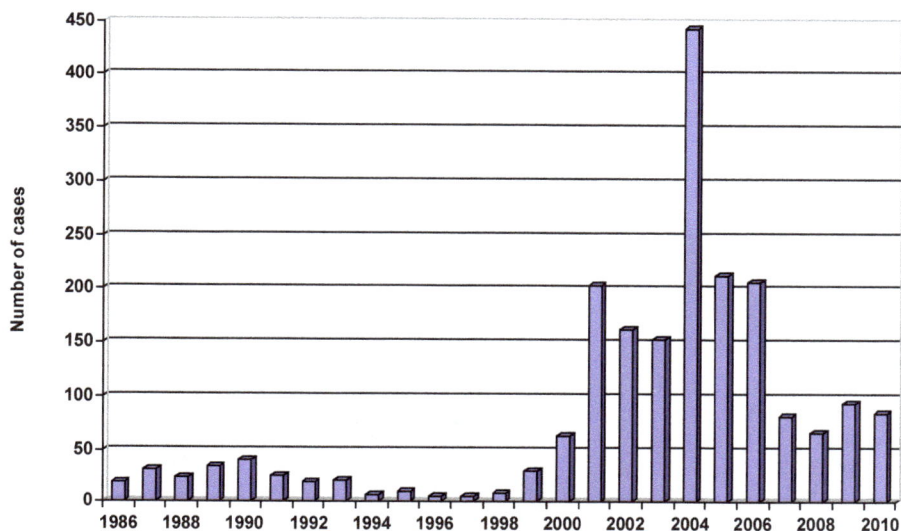

Fig. 9. Annual distribution of 2051 zoonotic cutaneous leishmaniasis cases (1986-2010).

Governorate	Delegation	Nb/delegation	Nb (% /governorate)
Sidi Bouzid	Ouled Haffouz	453	610 (32.6 %)
	Jelma	41	
	Sidi Bouzid city	33	
	Others	88	
Mahdia	Chorbène	321	494 (26.4 %)
	Souassi	54	
	Hbira	54	
	Ouled Chamekh	51	
	Others	14	
Kairouan	Nasrallah	127	369 (19.7 %)
	Bouhajla	56	
	Kairouan south	45	
	Hadjeb layoun	42	
	Others	99	
Sousse	Sidi El Heni	241	306 (16.3 %)
	Msaken	33	
	Others	32	
Others : Monastir, Gafsa, Kasserine, Sfax, Tataouine, Tozeur, Gabes, Kébili	-	-	94 (5%)
TOTAL	-	-	1873

Table 3. Distribution of 1873 zoonotic cutaneous leishmaniasis cases according to governorate and delegation.

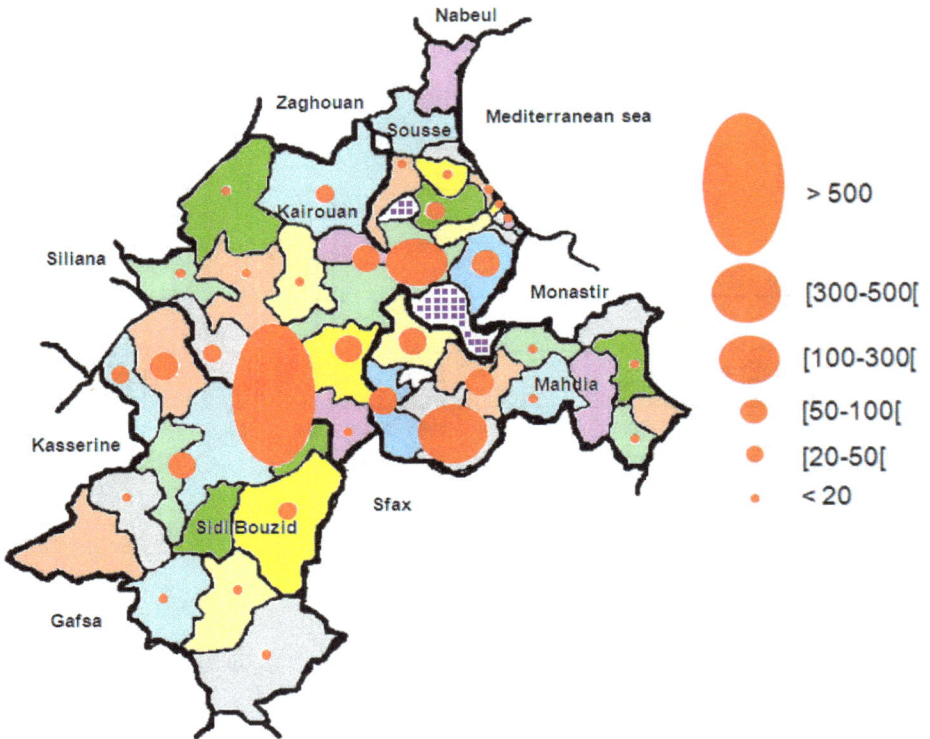

Fig. 10. Distribution of 1779 zoonotic cutaneous leishmaniasis cases diagnosed over the 25 year period originating from Sidi Bouzid, Mahdia, Kairouan and Sousse. The dots represent the number of cases. The limits of the governorates are shown in bold lines. The administrative district subdivisions are illustrated by different colours in each governorate.

lesions was obtained in a few weeks (one to three) after the treatment was initiated. However, in some patients, the outcome was unexpectedly atypical in that the lesions took much more delay to heal as demonstrated by the persistence of *Leishmania* in direct examination. In some adequately treated patients, the lesions persisted longer than one year and up to 4.5 years in one of them. In another patient, nearly 100 glucantime® injections were needed before the lesions resolved. In some additional cases, new lesions appeared while the patient was under specific treatment for previous ulcers. On the other hand, in many patients treated with *in situ* antimonial infiltrations, sporotrichoid nodules developed a few days or weeks later, next to the treated lesion.

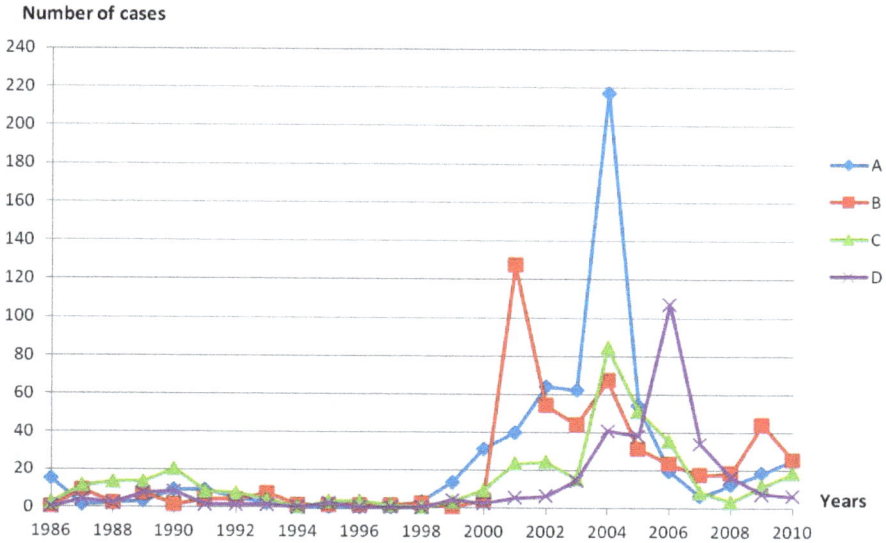

Fig. 11. Annual distribution of 1779 zoonotic cutaneous leishmaniasis cases in Sidi Bouzid (A), Mahdia (B), Kairouan (C) and Sousse (D) governorates (1986 to 2010).

4.2 Visceral leishmaniasis

Up to 2010, 2784 serum samples were addressed to our laboratory for suspected VL cases. Anti-*Leishmania* antibodies were demonstrated in 944 sera. FAT and rK39 DST were positive in 944 (99.2%) and 822 (87.1%) cases respectively. In all positive patients, VL was confirmed by the demonstration of amastigotes in bone marrow and/or cytocentrifuged blood and/or favourable outcome under antimonial treatment. In 8 confirmed VL cases, both serological tests were negative.

Thus, the total number of VL cases diagnosed over the 25 year period is 952.

Three hundred and eight blood samples were investigated by the cytoconcentration technique. Among them, 201 were from confirmed VL patients, and amastigotes were demonstrated in 88 (43.7%) of them. In six cases, bone marrow examination was also negative. Apart from the confirmed VL FAT negative cases, all the remaining negative sera were from patients suffering from diseases other than VL, mainly leukaemia and various haematological disorders. Nine hundred and thirty four of the VL patients were children, aged 2 months to 14 years (median: 26.8 months). Eighteen were adults aged 19 to 39 years (median: 25.9 years); one of them was a HIV+ woman. The number of annually diagnosed cases ranged from 14 cases in 2004 to 83 cases in 2005. The highest proportion of VL cases (60%) was from Kairouan governorate, known to include the most active foci of VL in Tunisia, followed by Sousse governorate and, to a lesser extent from other areas in central Tunisia (Mahdia, Monastir, Kasserine).

All confirmed VL patients were treated with glucantime®, usually a single 21 to 28 day course. The outcome was favourable in the majority of them. Death occurred in 18 (1.9%) patients. All were children. In 4 of them, no response to antimonials was observed despite an adequate treatment regimen. They were assumed to be resistant to antimonials even though the resistance could not be assessed by *in vitro* testing of the strain. In an additional child, initially treated by three successive courses of glucantime®, healing was ultimately obtained with ambisome® (liposomal amphotericin B).

4.3 Typing of *Leishmania* strains

Over the 25 year study period 103 *Leishmania* strains were typed by either IEE or PCR or both. More than 150 isolates were *in vitro* cultured. Fifteen of them were from bone-marrow aspirates in VL cases. All were typed by IEE and found to be *L. infantum*. Most cultured isolates were from CL patients. Eighty one of them could be maintained in culture media, cryopreserved and typed by IEE. The remaining isolates were either lost after repeated subculture or contaminated during sampling or subculturing. It should be mentioned that strains addressed to the laboratory of Monastir, were typed and identified at the zymodeme level, whereas those typed in the LEEP were only identified at the species level.

Sixty four isolates were typed by molecular techniques: 4 were typed by K-DNA-PCR and PCR-RFLP, and 60 by multiplex PCR.

Overall, 88 CL strains were typed by either IEE or PCR technique: 7 were *L. infantum*, 3 were *L. killicki* and 78 were *L. major*. All *L. major* strains that were typed at the zymodeme level were found to be *L. major* MON 25.

5. Discussion

One of the main characteristics of the four leishmaniasis forms occurring in Tunisia is their changing epidemiological pattern, which has continuously been described over the last 30 years. These changes mainly consisted of the spread of all forms of the disease from their initial endemic foci towards neighbouring or farther areas.

The VL which has long been confined to the northern parts of Tunisia showed a noticeable spread towards the central and southern parts of the country, where the disease has never been previously reported. The Kairouan governorate where VL was unknown till 1980, has progressively emerged as a highly endemic area and by the early 1990s, it became the most active focus in terms of incidence (Anonymous; Bel Hadj et al., 1996; Besbès et al., 1994; Bouratbine et al., 1998). These findings contrast with earlier periods where VL was mainly reported from Zaghouan, North-western and Tunis governorates and to a lesser extent from the central coastal region (Sousse) (Anderson et al., 1938; Ben Ismail et al., 1986; Ben Rachid et al., 1983; Chadli et al., 1968). In the same time, VL progressively spread further south to southern and central western governorates (Sfax, Sidi Bouzid, Kasserine, Tozeur) (Ayadi et al., 1991; Chargui et al., 2007). While spreading, the VL incidence markedly increased from a median of 12 to 68 annual recorded cases, 50 % of them being from Kairouan foci.

Similar trends were described in SCL which, up to 1980, was very rarely reported south to the Tunisian ridge ("dorsale"). From the early 1980s, and up to date, SCL has continuously been reported from central and southern parts of the country (Aoun et al., 2000, 2008; Ben Saïd et al., 2006; Kallel et al., 2005, 2008a).

ZCL was first reported on the end of the 19th century causing large outbreaks in Gafsa and neighbouring areas. Later, it has nearly disappeared for half a centrury; but reappeared again in 1982 causing a widespread epidemic that is still going on and constitutes a major public health problem in extended areas of the country, with up to date more than 150000 cases (Anonymous; Ben Abda et al., 2009; Ben Ismail & Ben Rachid, 1989).

CCL, known to be confined to limited areas in the presaharian region of Tataouine, has itself shown spread towards areas far from its original endemic foci, up to Kairouan governorate (Aoun et al., 2008; Haouas et al., 2005).

The described changes are supposed to mainly originate in the agricultural development and the ecological transformations that occurred in the concerned areas and led to a marked increase in irrigated surfaces that in turn helped the reservoirs (mainly rodents) and vectors to abundantly proliferate, and created biotopes very suitable for the *Leishmania* cycles to establish and amplify (Aoun et al., 2008; Ben Abda et al., 2009; Ben Salah et al., 2007). In addition, urbanization of previously rural areas made the populations' access to medical facilities easier, and consequently more and more leishmaniasis cases could be detected and diagnosed. The impact of climate change and variability on leishmaniasis (due to el Niño) was shown in Colombia and is associated to shifts in insect and animal distributions (Cardenas et al., 2008). This phenomenon was also shown to impact on the incidence of VL in Brazil and models were established to predict high risk years for VL (Franke et al., 2002). In Tunisia, the relationship between climate variability and leishmaniasis is not well studied. However, incidence rate of VL was shown to be positively correlated with mean yearly rainfall and continentality index; a rainy year is followed 2 years later by an increase in VL cases likely modulated by the intensity of transmission to dogs and by the influence on sandfly abundance (Ben-Ahmed et al., 2009). Distribution of sandflies classically associated to VL was also shown to be dependent on bioclimate (Zhioua et al., 2007), likewise for the distribution of *Phlebotomus papatasi*, the vector of ZCL (Chelbi et al., 2009).

Knowledge on the epidemiological patterns and trends in leishmaniasis has much increased over the last 3 decades mainly because of a better identification of the *Leishmania* species involved in the natural cycles of the parasite. This knowledge greatly benefited of the availability of techniques used in typing isolates obtained from humans or from reservoirs and sandflies. In this respect, IEE or molecular techniques allowed a more precise identification of the *Leishmania* at the species, zymodeme and genomic (schizodeme) level (Ben Hammouda et al., 2000; Ben Ismail et al., 1992; Ben Said et al., 2006; Guerbouj et al., 2007; Guizani et al., 1993, 1994a, 1994b; Guizani et al., 2002; Hanafi et al., 2001; Kallel et al., 2008b).

As far as zymodemes are concerned, it was shown that *L. major* was much more homogeneous than *L. infantum*. Indeed, all *L. major* strains obtained from humans, rodents and sandflies proved to be identical to the *L. major* MON 25 reference strain (Aoun et al., 2008 ; Ben Ismail et al., 1986; Haouas et al., 2007 ; Kallel et al., 2005). In contrast, at least three *L. infantum* zymodemes occur in Tunisia : i) the MON 1, mainly causing VL and to a lesser extent SCL ; ii) the MON 24, the most common agent of SCL, that also causes VL ; iii) the MON 80, which is very rarely isolated (Aoun et al., 1999, 2008; Bel Hadj et al., 2000, 2002; Gramiccia et al., 1991; Haouas et al., 2007). These findings show that a single zymodeme may cause quite different diseases; and raise the as yet poorly documented question of pathogenesis and virulence of strains in cause.   In addition, it was shown that the distribution of both MON 1 and MON 24 *L. infantum* zymodemes was different according to the geographical areas the patients originated from. Indeed, *L. infantum* MON 24 zymodeme was more frequently reported in VL cases from Kairouan governorate as compared to northern VL foci where MON 1 zymodeme is predominant.   This was attributed to the emergent character of Kairouan foci which may favour and select atypical or rare variants (Aoun et al., 2008; Ben Abda et al., 2009). Involvement of different sandfly species in transmission of different *L. infantum* parasites can not be excluded (Guerbouj et al. 2007). It is well established that different sandfly species belonging to the sub-genus *Larroussius* are involved in the transmission of *L. infantum*; in Tunisia clear association between sandfly species and bioclimate was demonstrated and presence of species of this subgenus in the different bioclimatic zones allowed explaining the extension of VL (Zhioua et al., 2007).

The reservoir of *L. killicki* is still debated. Some findings argue for its zoonotic origin as the disease is hypoendemic and frequently reported in rural populations. In addition, *L. killicki* in Kenya was isolated from hyracoides (Sang et al., 1994). However, CCL has also been reported from urban areas and from regions where *L. major* ZCL is highly prevalent and additional CCL cases were probably misdiagnosed. So, the CCL may be more frequent than previously thought. On the other hand, it was hypothesized that competition between *L. major* and *L. killicki* may lead to some degree of pressure exerted by the first species with a subsequent reduction in the incidence of the second one (Aoun et al., 2008). However, parasite identification still remains circumstantial; parasite isolation from cutaneous lesions is often contaminated by overgrowing microorganisms. In this situation, isolating and typing of much more additional strains is highly needed, in order to get further insight in the knowledge of the concerned *Leishmania* cycles.

Even though IEE has been demonstrated to be quite efficient in identifying isolates and still constitutes a reference tool, molecular techniques would be more relevant in assessing variability of strains, as even minor genomic variations may have important consequences on the epidemiological and the clinical levels. An additional advantage of the molecular techniques is their rapidity in that culture of isolates is no more needed. On the other hand, they are much adapted for both diagnostic (PCR, Multiplex PCR, Real time- PCR) and epidemiological (PCR-RFLP, Multiplex PCR, RAPD) purposes (Aoun et al., 2008; Bel Hadj et al., 2002; Ben Ismail et al., 1992; Ben Said et al., 2006; Chargui et al., 2005; Guerbouj et al., 2007; Guizani et al., 1994a, 1994b; Guizani et al., 2002; Hanafi et al., 2001; Saadi et al., in preparation). In addition, molecular techniques are specific and highly sensitive, allowing identification of parasite species hard to isolate or to maintain *in vitro* in culture or too scarce to be detected or cultured. It has been supposed that the dog is the reservoir of *L. infantum* MON 24 zymodeme and *P. perfiliewi* the phlebotomine vector. However, isolation of this zymodeme from either the dog or the sandfly has been unsuccessful, making the hypothesis questionable (Aoun et al., 2008). In this situation, molecular techniques would be much more suitable for this purpose. Using DNA tools, *P. langeroni* was found infected with *L. infantum* in an active transmission focus of SCL (Guerbouj et al., 2007). It may be concluded from all these findings that identification and typing of isolates are much needed in order to best assess the epidemiology and to investigate the diversity and changing patterns of leishmaniasis.

The incidence of leishmaniasis as reflected by the annually reported cases at the national level together with our own findings was shown to highly vary and fluctuate over the 25 year period study. These fluctuations were attributed first to the dynamics of the reservoirs' populations and sandflies, as a consequence of climatic variations, environmental and ecological changes occurring in the endemic areas (see section 2); and second, to the immunization, through the repeated outbreaks, of the infected human populations, that progressively makes previously infected people in the endemic area less receptive to the infection. This was best demonstrated in the ZCL form (Ben Salah et al., 2007).

In Tunisia, human activities, agricultural development and the subsequent ecological changes mainly benefited to rodents which dramatically proliferated in areas where their populations were previously too low for the *Leishmania* cycle to be completed. This can explain that ZCL is by far the predominant and the most widespread form of leishmaniasis in Tunisia, in terms of both incidence and geographical distribution. In addition, no sustained control programme for ZCL was carried out in most endemic areas, because of the difficulties that arose in the organization and the feasibility of such programmes. This made the ZCL epidemics still going on. It is worth mentioning however that control projects may be successful, as demonstrated by the results of those launched in 1992 in Sidi Bouzid area and again in the mid 2000s in Sidi Bouzid and Sidi El Heni, that led to an obvious decrease in the ZCL incidence over the mid 1990s in Sidi Bouzid and the last few years in both regions.

As compared to SCL, the spread of VL has been more important and obvious. This finding was related, among other factors, to the ecology of the phlebotomine vectors as it was shown that *P. perniciosus* (sub-genus *Larroussius*), the vector of MON 1 *L. infantum* zymodeme is more resistant to dry climate as compared to *P. perfiliewi*, the presumed vector of MON 24 zymodeme (Aoun et al., 2008 ; Ben Abda et al., 2009). Given the fact that presence and distribution of the different sandfly species generally associated to *L. infantum* transmission explained extension of VL (Zhioua et al., 2007) and that the extensions seem to concern in majority MON 24 parasites (Aoun et al., 2008; Ben Abda et al., 2009; Kallel et al., 2008a), explanations may well relate to parasite features not accounted for by the mere attribution to zymodemes and/or to differential distribution of reservoirs yet to identify.

Even though molecular techniques namely PCR and its variants have been increasingly used in the diagnosis of all forms of leishmaniasis, it is to be pointed out that conventional techniques should not be neglected. In VL, bone-marrow aspirate examination was shown to be sensitive enough, even though not optimal. Examination of cytoconcentrated peripheral blood was demonstrated to be positive in nearly 50 % of VL cases and was proposed to be carried out at first in order to avoid the painful bone-marrow puncture (Ben Said et al., 1998, Chemli et al., 2006). In serodiagnosis, FAT was found to be very efficient and suitable as its sensitivity exceeded 95 % and rK39 DST, even though less sensitive, very useful because it is highly specific, easy to perform and adapted to epidemiological investigations (Saghrouni et al., 2009). PCR is much more adapted to the diagnosis of the asymptomatic and subclinical forms of the disease because of its sensitivity and the scarcity of parasites in such situation. In CL, parasitological diagnosis by demonstrating amastigotes in dermal specimens is again very adequate, even though PCR was demonstrated to be more sensitive (Chargui et al., 2005). In contrast, serodiagnosis is much less useful in CL diagnosis as antibodies' amounts are often very low and results difficult to interpret.

One of the main objectives of this study was to assess whether the activity of our laboratory reflects the actual situation of the leishmaniases at the country level, and whether it could constitute an indicator of public health relevance. As far as VL is considered, most patients originating from Kairouan and Sousse governorates, where are located the most active foci, were investigated for serodiagnosis in our laboratory. So, we may conclude that our findings reflect the actual incidence of VL in the region. This is further confirmed by the comparison of our results to the statistics on the annually recorded cases of VL and edited by the primary health care direction of the Tunisian Ministry of Health (Anonymous). Obviously, our findings match these reports as highest number of registered cases at the national level was in 1992 (n = 130), 1993 (n = 122) and 2005 (n = 122); and highest number of cases diagnosed in our laboratory was as follows: 74 cases in 1992, 72 cases in 1993 and 83 cases in 2005. This is not surprising as nearly 50 % or more of VL cases originate from Kairouan governorate.

Concerning CL, we have to point out that first SCL cases from central Tunisia were diagnosed in our laboratory in patients with clinical presentation found to be evocative of this form, and amastigotes, very suggestive of *L. infantum* as compared to *L. major* because of their small size (Ben Saïd et al., 2006). As mentioned in section 2, additional cases were further reported and the spread of SCL towards central and southern Tunisia confirmed. Similarly, the first CCL case originating from outside the original foci of Tataouine area was again diagnosed in our laboratory (Haouas et al., 2005); and CCL spread was further confirmed by additional reports leading to the revised geographical distribution of the disease (Bouratbine et al., 2005; Aoun et al., 2008). In our laboratory, we used to diagnose ZCL since 1986. Up to the late 1990s, the number of diagnosed cases was too moderate as compared to that of ZCL reported cases in the endemic regions (Figures 7 & 9). This, for at least, the two following reasons: **i)** at the beginning of the outbreak, many patients suffering from ZCL were only clinically diagnosed, so that only a few of them were addressed to the laboratory for parasitological confirmation, **ii)** from the 1990s, a great number of families originating from ZCL endemic areas migrated and settled in Sousse city and suburbs, where they progressively constituted a large community. Most of them used to return back to their home of origin for summer holidays where, because continuously exposed to phlebotomine bites, many of them contract leishmaniasis which is later addressed to us for diagnosis. It is worth mentioning that a high proportion of this community originates from Sidi Khelif in Ouled Haffouz delegation, Sidi Bouzid; and and many of them were contaminated there and were later diagnosed in our laboratory. From 2000 and onwards, the number of ZCL patients who attended our laboratory for diagnosis dramatically increased. We consider that since this date the activity of our laboratory indirectly but adequately reflects the actual status of ZCL in central Tunisia, namely in Sidi Bouzid, Mahdia, Kairouan and Sousse governorates. This is best illustrated by our findings in 2004 where > 400 ZCL cases were diagnosed in our laboratory. In the same year, the highest incidence of ZCL (> 15000 cases) was registered at the national level, because of the three epidemic peaks that occurred in Sidi Bouzid (Sidi Bouzid city, Regueb, Menzel Bouzayène), Gafsa (Gafsa city, Sned, Mdhilla) and Kairouan (Nasrallah, Hajeb Layoun, Chrarda) governorates (Anonymous). The peak we registered in 2001 was due to an outbreak that arose in Chahda, a small locality in Chorbène delegation (Mahdia governorate). Indeed, more than 50 % of cases we diagnosed in 2001 were from this locality. A similar peak in Sidi El Heni delegation (Sousse governorate) was registered in 2006, with 107 cases. This peak was followed by a noticeable decrease as soon as control activities were carried out in the area. Similarly the decrease in ZCL incidence shown in our study over the last 5 years can be attributed to an important decrease in the transmission in Sidi Bouzid region where control activities were launched in the mid 2000s (Figure 9). This decrease was reflected on the national level over the same period (Figure 7). Last, our results confirm the seasonal occurrence of ZCL.

Our findings and results show that the activity of our laboratory reflects the situation of leishmaniasis at the regional level and at least in part at the national level, and may be an indicator of public health relevance. It may thus contribute to early alert of health authorities on changing epidemiological trends or emergence of leishmaniasis in the region. However, our activities may not reflect the actual situation and epidemiological changes occurring in farther endemic areas like Gafsa, Tozeur, Kébili, Médenine and Gabès known to include highly active foci because very few patients from these regions seek medical facilities in Sousse hospital. Work is in progress to identify and characterize the *Leishmania* parasites actually circulating in central Tunisia using molecular DNA techniques.

6. Acknowledgement

This work received financial support from IAEA (Project ref. TUN/6/012), and from the Ministry of Higher Education and Scientific Research (LR00SP04). We thank the staff of the LEEP, the laboratory of Parasitology of the Faculty of Pharmacy, Monastir and of the laboratory of Parasitology of Farhat Hached hospital, Sousse for their contribution.

7. References

Anderson, C. Chronique du kala-azar en Tunisie. *Arch. Inst.Pasteur Tunis* (1934), 23 : 455-464.

Anderson, C. Chronique du kala-azar.*Arch. Inst. Pasteur Tunis* (1938), 27 : 96-104.

Anonymous. Epidemiological Bulletins of the Direction of Primary Health care. Ministry of Health, Tunisia, 1980-2010.

Aoun, K., Bouratbine, A., Harrat, Z., Maherzi, A., Belkaid, M., Bousnina S. & Ben Ismail R. Confirmation of the presence of *Leishmania infantum* MON-80 in Tunisia. *Bul Soc Pathol Exot.* (1999), 92 : 29-30.

Aoun, K., Bouratbine, A., Harrat, Z., Guizani, I., Mokni, M., Bel Hadj Ali, S., Ben Osman, A., Belkaïd, M., Dellagi, K. & Ben Ismail, R. Epidemiologic and parasitologic data concerning sporadic cutaneous leishmaniasis in northern Tunisia. *Bull Soc Pathol Exot.* (2000), 93: 101-103.

Aoun, K., Bouratbine, A., Harrat, Z., Belkaïd, M. & Bel Hadj Ali S. Particular profile of the zymodemes of *Leishmania infantum* causing visceral in Tunisia. *Bull Soc Pathol Exot.* (2001), 94 : 375-377.

Aoun, K., Chahed, M.K., Mokni, M., Harrat, Z. & Bouratbine, A. Importance of amastigote forms morphology to differentiate *Leishmania infantum* and *Leishmania major* species. *Arch Inst Pasteur Tunis* (2003), 80 : 53-56.

Aoun. K., Amri. F., Chouihi. E., Haouas, N., Bedoui, K., Benikhelef, R. & Bouratbine, A. Epidemiology of *Leishmania (L) infantum, L. major* and *L. killicki* in Tunisia : results and analysis of the identification of 226 human and canine isolates. *Bull Soc Pathol Exot.* (2008), 101: 323-328.

Ayadi, A., Ben Ismail, R. & Ben Rachid, M.S. Spread of *Leishmania infantum* Kala-azar transmission area towards central and southern Tunisia. *Arch Ins Pasteur Tunis* (1991), 68 : 269-273.

Bel Hadj, S., Djaiet – Baraket, Z., Jemli, B., Ben Osman, A. & Chaker, E. Visceral and cutaneous leishmaniasis of the North. *Bull Soc Pathol exot,* (1996), 89: 269-273.

Bel Hadj, S., Pratlong, F., Mahjoub, H., Toumi, N.H., Azaiez, R., Dedet, J.P. & Chaker, E. Infantile visceral leishmaniasis from *Leishmania infantum* Mon-24 : a reality in Tunisia. *Bull Soc Pathol Exot.* (2000), 93: 12-13.

Bel Hadj, S., Pratlong, F., Toumi, N.H., Kallel, K., Mahjoub, H., Babba, H., Azaiez, R., Dedet, JP. & Chaker, E. Visceral leishmaniasis in Tunisia: result of the isoenzymatic characterization of 65 *Leishmania infantum* strains. *Trans R Soc Trop Med Hyg.* (2002), 96: 627-630.

Bel Hadj, S., Pratlong, F., Hammami, M., Kallel, K., Dedet, JP. & Chaker, E. Human cutaneous leishmaniasis due to *Leishmania infantum* in the Sidi Bourouis focus (Northern Tunisia): epidemiological study and isoenzymatic characterization of the parasites. *Acta Trop.* (2003), 85: 83-86.

Ben Abda, I., Aoun, K., Ben Alaya, N., Bousslimi, N., Mokni, M. & Bouratbine, A. Curent epidemiological, clinical and parasitological data concerning cutaneous leishmaniasis in Tunisia. *Revue Tunisiennne d'Infectiologie* (2009), 2: 31-36.

Ben-Ahmed, K., Aoun, K., Jeddi, F., Ghrab, J., El-Aroui, M.A. & Bouratbine, A. Visceral leishmaniasis in Tunisia: spatial distribution and association with climatic factors. *Am J Trop Med Hyg.* (2009), 81: 40-5.

Ben Ammar, R., Ben Ismail, R., Helal, H., Bacha-Hamba, D., Chaouch, A., Bouden, I. & Ben Rachid, M.S. A new focus of rural cutaneous leishmaniasis in Sidi Saad area (Tunisia). *Bull Soc Fr Parasitol.* (1984), 2: 9-12.

Ben Hammouda, A., Guizani, I., Jedidi, S., Dellagi, K. & Ben Ismail, R. *Leishmania infantum* species-specific kDNA probes: isolation an evaluation. *Arch Inst Pasteur Tunis.* (2000), 77: 37-43.

Ben Ismail, R., Gradoni, L., Gramiccia, M., Bettini, S., Ben Rachid, M.S. & Garraoui, A. Epidemic cutaneous leishmaniasis in Tunisia: biochemical characterization of parasites. *Trans R Soc Trop Med Hyg*, (1986), 80: 669-70.

Ben Ismail, R., Ben Rachid, M.S., Gradoni, L., Gramiccia, M., Helal, H. & Bach-Hamba, D. Zoonotic cutaneous leishmaniasis in Tunisia: study of the disease reservoir in the Douara area. *Ann Soc Belg Med Trop.* (1987a), 67: 335-343.

Ben Ismail, R., Gramiccia, M., Gradoni, L., Helal, H. & Ben Rachid, M.S. Isolation of *Leishmania major* from *Phlebotomus papatasi* in Tunisia. *Trans R Soc Trop Med Hyg.* (1987b), 81: 749.

Ben Ismail, R., Helal, H., Bach-Hamba, D. & Ben Rachid, M.S. Natural infestation of *Phlebotomus papatasi* in a focus of zoonotic cutaneous leismaniasis in Tunisia. *Bull Soc Pathol Exot.* (1987 c), 80: 613-614.

Ben Ismail, R. & Ben Rachid, M.S. Epidémiologie des leishmanioses en Tunisie, in : Maladies tropicales transmissibles. *AUPELF-UREF*, Paris, 1989, 73-80.

Ben Ismail, R., Smith, D.F., Ready, P.D., Ayadi, A., Gramiccia, M., Ben Osman, A. & Ben Rachid, M.S. Sporadic cutaneous leishmaniasis in north Tunisia: identification of the causative agent as *Leishmania infantum* by the use of a diagnostic deoxyribonucleic acid probe. *Trans R Soc Trop Med Hyg.* (1992), 86: 508-510.

Ben Rachid, M.S., Hamza, B., Tabbane, C., Gharbi, R., Jeridi, H. & Ben Saïd, M. Current status of leishmaniasis in Tunisia. *Ann Soc Belg Med Trop.* (1983), 63: 29-40.

Ben Rachid, M.S., Ben Ismail, R. & Ben Saïd, M. The ecology of visceral and cutaneous leishmaniasis in Tunisia. In: "Proceedings of the international worshop on leishmaniasis control strategies, 25-29 nov. 1991, Merida, Mexico, *IDRC and UPCH editors*, (1992, pp. 131-154.

Ben Saïd, M., Amri, F., Mili, A., Ardoin, F., Petithory, J.C. The cytoconcentration in the diagnosis of visceral leishmaniasis in immunocompetent children. *Bull Soc Fr Parasitol.* (1998), 16: 86-94.

Ben Saïd, M., Guerbouj, S., Saghrouni, F., Fathallah-Mili, A. & Guizani, I. Occurrence of *Leishmania infantum* cutaneous leishmaniasis in central Tunisia. *Trans R Soc Trop Med Hyg.* (2006), 100: 521-526.

Ben Salah, A., Ben Ismail, R., Amri, F., Chlif, S., Ben Rzig, F., Kharrat, H., Hadhri, H., Hassouna, M., & Dellagi, K. Investigation of the spread of human visceral leishmaniasis in central Tunisia. *Trans R Soc Trop Med Hyg.* (2000), 94: 382-386.

Ben Salah, A., Kamarianakis, Y., Chelif, S., Ben Alaya, N. & Prastacos, P. Zoonotic cutaneous leishmaniasis in central Tunisia : spatio temporal dynamics *Int J. Epidemiol.* (2007), 36: 991-1000.

Besbès, A., Pousse, H., Ben Saïd, M., Kharrat, H. & Ghenimi, L. Infantile visceral leishmaniasis in central Tunisia (report of 221 cases). *Med Mal Infect.* (1994), 24 : 628-634.

Bouratbine, A., Aoun, K., Chahed, M.K. & Ben Ismail, R. Epidemiological data on infantile visceral leishmaniasis in Tunisia. *Med Mal Infect.* (1998), 28 : 446-447.

Bouratbine, A., Aoun, K., Ghrab, J., Harrat, Z., Ezzedini, M.S. & Etlijani S. Spread of *Leishmania killicki* to Central and South-West Tunisia. *Parasite* (2005) 12: 59-63.

Cardenas, R., Sandoval, C.M., Rodríguez-Morales, A.J., Franco-Paredes, C. Impact of climate variability in the occurrence of leishmaniasis in northeastern Colombia. *Am J Trop Med Hyg.* (2006), 75: 273-7.

Chadli, A., Ben Rachid, M.S. & Fhaiel, A. Chroniques des leishmanioses en Tunisie. *Arch Inst Pasteur Tunis.* (1968), 45: 1-14.

Chaffai, M., Ben Rachid, M.S., Ben Ismail, R., Ben Osman, A. & Makni, N. Clinico-epidemiological forms of cutaneous leishmaniasis in Tunisia. *Ann Dermatol Vénéréol.* (1998), 115: 1255-1260.

Chahed, M.K., Hsairi, M., Bousnina, A., Achour, N., Bouratbine, A. & Hili, K. Assessment of the cutaneous leishmaniasis surveillance system in Tunisia. *Revue Tunisienne de la Santé Militaire.* (2002), 4: 40-47.

Chargui, N., Bastien, P., Kallel, K., Haouas, N., Akrout Messaadi, F, Masmoudi, A., Zili, J., Chaker, E., Othman, A.D., Azaiez, R., Crobu, L., Mezhoud, H. & Baba, H. Usefulness of PCR in the diagnosis of cutaneous leishmaniasis in Tunisia. *Trans R Soc Trop Med Hyg.* (2005), 99: 762-768.

Chargui, N., Haouas, N., Gorcii, M., Akrout Messaadi, F., Zribi, M. & Baba, H. Increase of canine leishmaniasis in a previously low-endemicity area in Tunisia. *Parasite.* (2007), 14: 247-251.

Chelbi I, Kaabi B, Béjaoui M, Derbali M, Zhioua E. Spatial correlation between *Phlebotomus papatasi* Scopoli (Diptera: Psychodidae) and incidence of zoonotic cutaneous leishmaniasis in Tunisia. *J Med Entomol.* (2009), 46: 400-2.

Chemli, J., Abroug, M., Fathallah, A., Abroug, S., Ben Said, M. & Harbi, A. Contribution of leucoconcentration in the diagnosis of kala-azar in Tunisia. *Med Mal Infect.* (2006), 36: 390-392.

Deperet, C. & Bobinet, E. Du bouton de Gafsa au camp de Sathonay. *Archs Med Pharm Milit.* (1884), 3: 296-302.

Fichet-Calvet, E., Jommaa, I., Ben Ismail, R. & Ashford, R.W. *Leishmania major* infection in the fat sand rat *Psammomys obesus* in Tunisia: interaction of host and parasite populations. *Ann Trop Med Parasitol.* (2003), 97: 593-603.

Franke CR, Ziller M, Staubach C, Latif M. Impact of the El Niño/Southern Oscillation on visceral leishmaniasis, Brazil. *Emerg Infect Dis.* (2002), 8: 914-7.

Ghrab, J., Rhim, A., Bach-Hamba, D., Chahed, M.K., Aoun, K., Nouira, S. & Bouratbine, A. Phlebotominae (Diptera: Psychodidae) of human leishmaniasis sites in Tunisia. *Parasite*. (2006), 13: 23-33.

Gramiccia, M., Ben Ismail, R., Gradoni, L., Ben Rachid, M.S. & Ben Said, M. A *Leishmania infantum* enzymatic variant, causative agent of cutaneous leishmaniasis in north Tunisia. *Trans R Soc Trop Med Hyg*. (1991), 85: 370-371.

Guerbouj, S., Victoir, K., Guizani, I., Seridi, N., Nuwayri-Salti, N., Belkaid, M., Ben Ismail, R., Le Ray, D. & Dujardin, JC. Gp63 gene polymorphism and population structure of *Leishmania donovani* complex: influence of the host selection pressure? *Parasitology*. (2001), 122: 25-35.

Guerbouj, S., Chemkhi, J., Kâabi, B., Rahali, A., Ben Ismail, R. & Guizani, I. Natural infection of the species *Phlebotomus Larroussius langeroni* (Diptera: Psychodidae) with *Leishmania infantum* in Tunisia. *Trans R Soc Trop Med Hyg*. (2007) 101: 372-377.

Guizani, I., Ben Hamouda, A., van Eys, G.J., Jedidi, S., Dellagi, K. & Ben Ismail, R. DNA probes development in Tunisia for the identification, the taxonomy and the eco-epidemiology of Old World *Leishmania* species. *Arch Inst Pasteur Tunis*. (1993), 70: 363-371.

Guizani, I., Ben Hamouda, A., Jedidi, S., Dellagi, K. & Ben Ismail, R. Molecular identification of *Leishmania*: development and application of DNA probes in Tunisia. *Arch Inst Pasteur Tunis*. (1994a), 71: 439-446.

Guizani, I., van Eys, G.J., Ben Ismail, R. & Dellagi, K. Use of recombinant DNA probes for species identification of Old World *Leishmania* isolates. *Am J Trop Med Hyg*. (1994b), 50: 632-640.

Guizani, I., Dellagi, K. & Ben Ismail, R. Random amplified polymorphic DNA technique for identification and differentiation of Old World *Leishmania* species. *Am J Trop Med Hyg*. (2002) 66: 152-156.

Haouas, N., Chargui, N., Chaker, E., Ben Said, M., Babba, H., Belhadj, S., Kallel, K., Pratlong, F., Dedet, JP., Mezhoud, H. & Azaiez, R. Anthroponotic cutaneous leishmaniasis in Tunisia: presence of *Leishmania killicki* outside its original focus of Tataouine. *Trans R Soc Trop Med Hyg*. (2005), 99: 499-501.

Haouas, N., Gorcii, M., Chargui, N., Aoun, K., Bouratbine, A., Messaadi Akrout F, Masmoudi, A., Zili, J., Ben Said, M., Pratlong, F., Dedet, JP., Mezhoud, H., Azaiez, R. & Babba, H. Leishmaniasis in central and southern Tunisia: current geographical distribution of zymodemes. *Parasite*. (2007), 14: 239-246.

Hammoud, M., Ben Hassine, L., Azzabi, S., Ben Abdelghani, K., Kooli, C., Kaouach, Z. & Khalfallah, N. Adult visceral leishmaniasis: about six cases. *Revue Tunisienne de la Santé Militaire*. (2004), 6: 54-57.

Hanafi, R., Barhoumi, M., Bel Hadj Ali, S., Guizani, I.. Molecular analysis of Old World *Leishmania* RAPD markers and development of a PCR assay selective for parasites of the *L. donovani* species complex. *Exp Parasitol*. (2001) 98: 90-99.

Harrat, Z., Boubidi, S.C., Pratlong, F., Benikhlef, R., Selt, B., Dedet, JP., Ravel, C. & Belkaid, M. Description of a dermatropic *Leishmania* close to *L. killicki* (Rioux, Lanotte & Pratlong 1986) in Algeria. *Trans R Soc Trop Med Hyg*. (2009), 103: 716-720.

Helal, H., Ben Ismail, R., Bach-Hamba, D., Sidhom, M., Bettini, S. & Ben Rachid, M.S. An epidemiological survey in the focus of zoonotic cutaneous leishmaniaisis

(*Leishmania major*) of Sidi Bouzid (Tunisia) in 1985. *Bull Soc Pathol Exot.* (1987), 80: 349-356.

Kallel, K., Pratlong, F., Belhadj, S., Cherif, F., Hammami, M., Dedet, JP. & Chaker, E. Cutaneous leishmaniasis in Tunisia: results of the iso-enzymatic characterization of 71 strains. *Ann Trop Med Parasitol.* (2005), 99: 11-19.

Kallel, K., Ammari, L., Kaouech, E., BelHadj, S., Anane, S., Kilani, B. & Chaker, E. Asymptomatic beading of *Leishmania infantum* among Tunisian HIV infected. *Pathol Biol.* (2007), 55: 521-524.

Kallel, K., Haouas, N., Pratlong, F., Kaouech, E., Bel Hadj, S., Anane, S., Dedet, JP., Babba, H. & Chaker, E. Cutaneous leishmaniasis caused by *Leishmania infantum* MON 24 in Tunisia : extension of the focus to the center of the country. *Bull Soc Pathol Exot.* (2008a), 101: 30-31.

Kallel, K., Pratlong, F., Belhadj, S., Cherif, F., Hammami, H. & Chaker, E. Isoenzyme variability of *Leishmania infantum* in Tunisia concerning 245 human strains. *Act Trop.* (2008b), 106: 132-136.

Khaldi, F., Achouri, E., Gharbi, A., Debabi, A. & Ben Naceur, B. Infantile visceral leishmaniasis. Data on hospitalized children cases from 1974 to 1988 in INSEE, Tunis. *Médecine Tropicale.* (1991), 51: 143-147.

Ladjimi, R. & Lakhoua, M. Premier cas de bouton d'orient dans la banlieue de Tunis. *Arch Inst Pasteur Tunis.* (1955), 32: 331-336.

Masmoudi, A., Ayadi, N., Boudaya, S., Mziou, T.J., Mseddi, M., Marrakchi, S. & Ayadi, A. Clinical polymorphism in cutaneous leishmaniasis of center of south Tunisia. *Bull Soc Pathol Exot.* (2007), 100: 36-40.

Nicolle C. Statistique des trente premières observations tunisiennes de kala-azar. *Arch Inst Pasteur Tunis.* (1912), 2: 65-67.

Nicolle, C. & Blanc, G. Extension de la région à bouton d'orient tunisienne. *Bull Soc Pathol Exot.* (1917), 10: 378-379.

Petithory, J.C., Ardoin, F., Ash, L.R., Vandemeulebroucke, E., Galeazzui, G., Dufour, M., Paugam, A. Microscopic diagnosis of blood parasites following a cytoconcentration technique. *Am J Trop Med Hyg.* (1997), 57 : 637-642.

Pousse, H., Besbès, A., Ben Said, M., Ghenimi, L. & Kharrat, H. Epidemiology of human visceral leishmaniasis in Tunisia. *J Trop Pediatr.* (1995), 41: 191-192.

Rioux, JA., Lanotte, G. & Pratlong, F. *Leishmania killicki* n.sp. (Kinetoplastida, Trypanosomatidae), in: *Leishmania, taxonomie et phylogenèse, applications éco-épidémiologiques.* IMEEE, Montpellier, 1986, 139-142.

Saghrouni, F., Gaied-Meksi, S., Fathallah, A., Amri, F., Ach, H., Guizani, I. & Ben Said, M. Immuno chromatographic rK39 strip test in the serodiagnosis of visceral leishmaniasis in Tunisia. *Trans R Soc Trop Med Hyg.* (2009), 103: 1273-1278.

Sang, D.K., Njeru, W.K. & Ashford, R.W. A zoonotic focus of cutaneous leishmaniasis due to *Leishmania tropica* at Utut, Rift Valley Province, Kenya. *Trans R Soc Trop Med Hyg.* (1994), 88: 35-37.

Smyth, A.J., Ghosh, A., Hassan, M.Q., Basu, D., De Bruijn, M.H.L., Adhya, S, Mallik, K.K. & Barker, D.C. Rapid and sensitive detection of *Leishmania* kinetoplast DNA from spleen and blood samples of kala-azar patients. *Parasitology.* (1992), 105: 183-192.

Vermeil, C. Chronique des leishmanioses en Tunisie. *Arch Inst Pasteur Tunis.* (1956), 33 : 195-201.

Zakraoui, H., Ben Salah, A., Ftaiti, A., Marrakchi, H., Zaatour, A., Zaafouri, B., Ahmadi, Z., Garraoui, A., Ben Osman, A. & Dellagi, K. Spontaneous course of lesions of *Leishmania major* cutaneous leishmaniasis in Tunisia. *Ann Dermatol Venereol.* (1995), 122: 405-407.

Zhioua, E., Kaabi, B. & Chelbi, I. Entomological investigations following the spread of visceral leishmaniasis in Tunisia. *J Vector Ecol.* (2007), 32: 371-374.

5

Toxoplasmosis: Advances and Vaccine Perspectives

Oscar Bruna-Romero[1], Dulcilene Mayrink de Oliveira[1]
and Valter Ferreira de Andrade-Neto[2,*]
*[1]Department of Microbiology, Instituto de Ciências Biológicas,
Universidade Federal de Minas Gerais – UFMG, Belo Horizonte-MG
[2]Department of Microbiology and Parasitology, Centro de Biociências,
Universidade Federal do Rio Grande do Norte – UFRN, Natal-RN
Brazil*

1. Introduction

Toxoplasma gondii was first identified more than 100 years ago in the tissues of birds and mammals. In 1908 Nicolle and Manceoux described it for the first time in the gundi (*Ctenodactylus gundi*), a North African rodent, in tachyzoite forms. At the same time, Splendore in Brazil, identified the parasite in rabbit tissues. Due to its bow-like shape (Greek: *Toxo* = Arc) the genus was named *Toxoplasma*. However, only in the 1970's was the complete life cycle known and the parasite recognized as a coccidian parasite (member of the phylum Apicomplexa). It is ubiquitous throughout the world and estimated to infect approximately half of the world's population. It is characterized by a polarized cell structure and two unique apical secretory organelles called micronemes and rhoptries.

Toxoplasma has a complex life cycle consisting of a sexual cycle in its feline definitive hosts and an asexual cycle in its intermediate hosts. The latter, including humans, can be infected by ingestion of oocysts shed in cat feces. Unlike most other Apicomplexan parasites, *Toxoplasma* can be transmitted between intermediate hosts by either vertical (via placenta) or horizontal (carnivorism) transmission.

Toxoplasma parasite is found in intermediate hosts in two interconvertable stages: bradyzoites and tachyzoites. Bradyzoites, a dormant form, are slow-growing, transmissible and encysted. Infections with bradyzoite-containing cysts occur upon ingestion of undercooked meat. The wall of these cysts is digested inside the host stomach and the released bradyzoites, which are resistant to gastric peptidases, subsequently invade the small intestine. There, they convert into tachyzoites, the rapidly growing, disease-causing form that can infect most nucleated cells, replicate inside a parasitophorous vacuole, egress, and then infect neighboring cells. These tachyzoites activate a potent host immune response that eliminates most of the parasites. Some tachyzoites, however, escape destruction and convert back into bradyzoites. In the absence of an adequate immune response, tachyzoites

---

* Corresponding Author

will grow unabated and cause tissue destruction, which can be severe and even fatal. However, the inflammatory immune response induced by tachyzoites can cause immune-mediated tissue destruction. Therefore, a subtle balance between inducing and evading the immune response is crucial for *Toxoplasma* to establish a chronic infection.

The success of *Toxoplasma* as a widespread pathogen is due to the ease in which it can be transmitted between intermediate hosts. Humans do not play a major role in transmission; consequently, pathogenesis in humans is the indirect result of adaptations to infection in other hosts and treatment of human infections is unlikely to lead to the spread of drug resistance.

Once inside a host, the parasite develops powerful tools to modulate its host cell and develop into a chronic infection that can evade the host's immune system as well as all known anti-toxoplasmatic drugs. The ability of the parasite to replicate within a host cell, evade immune responses and undergo bradyzoite development requires the parasite to effectively modulate its host.

Toxoplasmosis remains a major health concern in pregnancy, where it causes severe birth defects or miscarriage, and in immunocompromised hosts. Thus, new toxoplasmosis control strategies are needed. The development of effective human and veterinary vaccines against toxoplasmosis is a relevant goal for Public Health (Gazzinelli *et al.* 1996; Pifer and Yarovinsky 2011). Even if new therapeutic drugs, with less hypersensitivity and toxicity-related events, are developed, not only for acute *T. gondii* infection but also for the currently untreatable latent bradyzoite form of the parasite, a prophylactic vaccine against the disease would still be the best option from the financial, epidemiological, and social points of view. A vaccine would decrease the enormous costs of diagnosis/treatment, the premature loss of lives, the extensive rates of dissemination as well as the social impact of the disease. One major fact that suggests the possibility of vaccination against toxoplasmosis is that primary infection with the *T. gondii* parasite elicits protective immunity against re-infection in most individuals.

2. Mechanisms of protective immunity against toxoplasmosis

Immune responses during the early stages of *T. gondii* infection are characterized by activation of innate mechanisms mediated by macrophages and dendritic cells (DC) (Gazzinelli *et al.* 1996; Pifer and Yarovinsky 2011). These cells are activated in mice (not yet known how in humans) after parasite internalization, by engagement of endosomal toll-like receptor 11 (and probably others) with tachyzoite products, which drives subsequent production of interleukin-12 (IL-12) and tumor necrosis factor alpha (TNF-α). In turn, IL-12 activates natural killer (NK) cells (Denkers *et al.* 1993) to secrete gamma interferon (IFN-γ) (Gazzinelli *et al.* 1994), which then acts as stimulus for T-cell activation and, in synergy with TNF-α, mediates killing of tachyzoites by macrophages through enhanced production of free oxygen radicals and nitric oxide (NO).

Acquired immunity against *T. gondii* develops afterward, and is characterized by strong CD4+ and CD8+ T cell activity (Gazzinelli *et al.* 1992). The cytokine IFN-γ continues to be central in resistance to the parasite during the successive acute and chronic stages of infection, driving the differentiation of CD4+ T lymphocytes specific for parasite antigens to a helper T cell type (Th1) cytokine profile. More important, the newly generated CD8+ T cells become crucial to control parasite replication, not only by serving as additional sources of IFN-γ but also by developing cytotoxic activity against infected cells, eliminating parasite factories and thus preventing reactivation of infection (Denkers *et al.* 1993; Denkers and Gazzinelli 1998; Bhopale 2003). Whether B cells also play a role in protection against this parasite is not clear, but studies have generated indirect evidences that IgG antibodies may be important for protection (Kang *et al.* 2000). B cell-deficient mice have shown increased susceptibility to brain inflammatory pathology in chronic infections with the parasite, despite presenting similar levels of serum and tissue pro-inflammatory cytokines, such as IFN-γ. Furthermore, adoptive transfer of polyclonal anti- *T. gondii* IgG antibodies to these mice prevented both pathology and mortality.

3. Major toxoplasma vaccines and candidates studied to date

To reproduce what the immune system does naturally to protect hosts against *T. gondii* infection (and re-infection), researchers have attempted several strategies for vaccination. These include the use of whole parasites (attenuated in different ways), soluble parasite antigens, recombinant purified proteins (subunit vaccines) or recombinant live vectors that express heterologous antigen(s) within host organisms (figure 1). Currently, some of these tools are also being used in combination, as part of prime-boost immunization protocols. Below is a review of current's state of the art of most of these technologies.

3.1 Whole-parasite attenuated vaccines

Sporulated oocysts (sporozoite-containing cysts) from the environment or tissue cysts (bradyzoite-containing cysts) from infected animals are the two major sources of infection with *T. gondii* (figure 2). However, vaccine candidates that include sporozoites or sporozoite antigens have traditionally been less studied because of the ease of access to bradyzoites and tachyzoites, e.g. using animal brain cysts or acutely infected animal peritoneal lavage/cell cultures, respectively. As a result, the first *T. gondii* whole-parasite experimental vaccines were mainly based on attenuated tachyzoites/bradyzoites, in particular those generated by inactivation or irradiation. Inactive parasites were used for immunization of experimental animals from 1956 (Cutchins and Warren 1956) to 1972 (Krahenbuhl *et al.* 1972) with not much success. In contrast, gamma-irradiated *T. gondii* tachyzoites were successfully tested as experimental vaccines in 1975 (Seah and Hucal 1975), in part after taking the idea from the pioneering irradiated-sporozoite malaria vaccines, which were initially tested in the 1960s and 70s (Nussenzweig *et al.* 1967; Gwadz *et al.* 1979). In the 1975 report, all animals inoculated with highly irradiated *T. gondii* parasites survived, were free of tissue cysts and were solidly protected against a subsequent rechallenge. Later, a few reports (Dubey *et al.* 1996; Omata *et al.* 1996; Dubey *et al.* 1998) have also used irradiated sporozoites (under the form of sporulated oocysts) to vaccinate mice, cats and pigs against toxoplasmosis, but in contrast to tachyzoites, results were not very encouraging, though some protection was also observed.

Other attempts to induce protection against toxoplasmosis with whole-parasite vaccines included the use of live attenuated parasites (tachyzoites) such as the S-48, the cps1-1, the temperature-sensitive TS-4, the MIC1-3 knock-out or the non-replicative Δrps13 strains (McLeod *et al.* 1988; Hakim *et al.* 1991; Buxton 1993; Gigley *et al.* 2009; Lu *et al.* 2009; Hutson

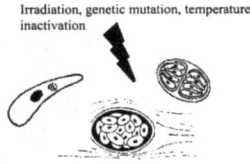

Irradiation, genetic mutation, temperature inactivation

Whole parasite vaccines

(+) Same key antigens.

(−) Reversion to pathogenic phenotype.

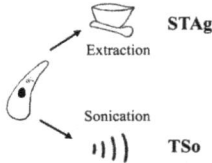

STAg

Extraction

Sonication

TSo

Immunogenic parasite extracts

(−) Partial protection; lack of standardization.

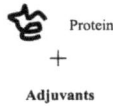

Protein

+

Adjuvants

Subunit vaccines

(−) Difficulties to induce high levels of T cells.

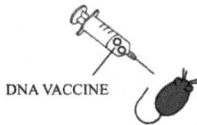

DNA VACCINE

Plasmid DNA vaccines

(+) Easy to obtain and efficient in small animals.

(−) Difficulties in transferring the success to larger animal models.

Recombinant bacterial vectors

(+) T cells and mucosal immunity induction.

(−) Protein modifications differ from parasite's. Virulence in immunocompromised hosts.

Recombinant viral vectors

(+) Mimic parasite antigen presentation inside host cells and efficiently stimulate T cell responses.

(−) Pre-existing immunity may preclude their use as vectors. Fear of reversion to virulence.

Fig. 1. Potential advantages (+) and concerns (-) of the major vaccination strategies used to immunize hosts against *T. gondii* infection. Abbreviations: STAg, Soluble Tachyzoite Antigen; TSo, Tachyzoites Sonicate.

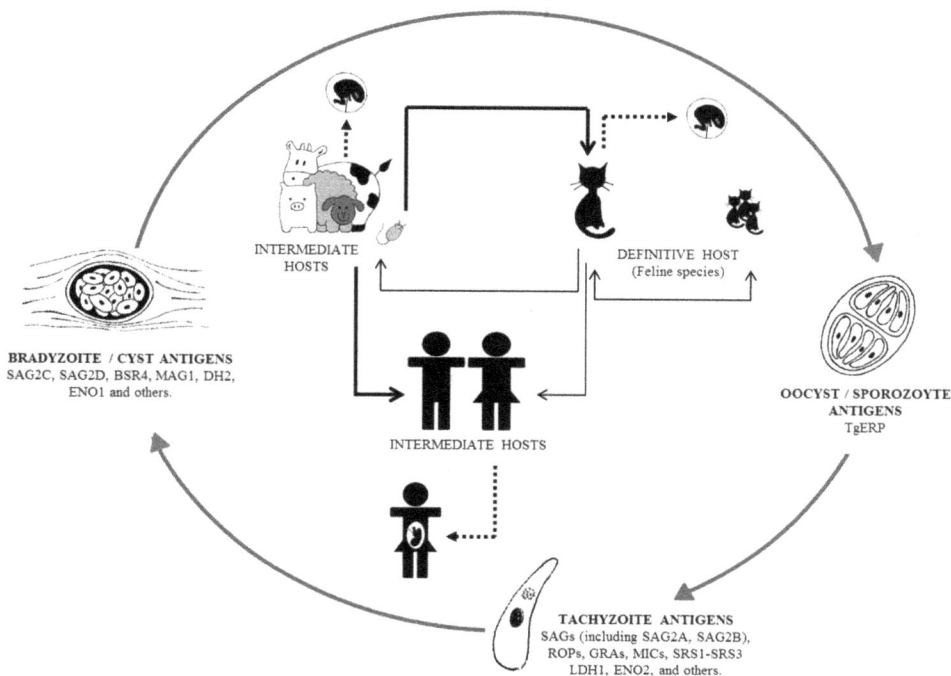

Fig. 2. Major *T. gondii* antigens identified to date in the different stages of the parasite´s life cycle and major routes of parasite transmission. Thin black arrow = horizontal transmission via oocysts; thick black arrow = horizontal transmission via tissue cysts; dotted arrows = vertical transmission via tachyzoites. Abbreviations: SAG, surface antigen; ROP, rhoptry protein; GRA, dense granules; MIC, microneme protein; SRS, SAG-related sequences; BSR, bradyzoite-specific recombinant; MAG, matrix antigen; LDH, lactate dehydrogenase; ENO, enolase; TgERP0, *T. gondii* embryogenesis-related protein.

et al. 2010; Mevelec *et al.* 2010). The only vaccine commercialized for veterinary purposes, Ovilis®Toxovax (Intervet/Schering-Plough Animal Health, UK), based on the incomplete parasite S-48 strain (not able to generate either tissue cysts or oocysts), began to be marketed in New Zealand and the United Kingdom in 1988 to control miscarriages provoked by *T. gondii* in sheep. Reduction in fetal loss and in formation of cysts in the meat used for consumption has been reported. This vaccine seems to reduce infection in sheep, which in free-range grazing are constantly exposed to oocyst contamination.

Interestingly, up to date, the most recent and technologically advanced recombinant vaccine formulations have reached, at best, the same levels of protective immunity induced by whole-parasite vaccines. Three main reasons may be responsible for that difference: (i) true protective antigens (or more plausibly antigen combinations) of the parasite have not yet been identified, (ii) while the whole organism and the recombinant vaccines contain the same antigenic sequences, the process by which the recombinant products are generated result in the loss of crucial features that are key for protein's immunogenicity (Crampton and Vanniasinkam 2007) or, finally, (iii) gamma-irradiated or otherwise attenuated parasites maintain metabolic functions, retain the capacity to invade mammalian cells, present antigens to the host's immune system and elicit cellular immunity and cytokine responses in a highly similar way to natural infection (Hiramoto *et al.* 2002), and exogenous recombinant antigens do not.

However, even though protection has been repeatedly demonstrated after immunization with whole-parasite vaccines, real concerns also exist regarding the use of this type of vaccines, in particular for uses other than veterinary immunization. The major fear is that attenuated parasites could revert to the pathogenic phenotype. For this reason, studies towards developing a human vaccine have focused on parasite extracts or recombinant technologies that use defined immunodominant antigens and delivery strategies.

3.2 Immunogenic parasite extracts

Identification and functional characterization of proteins of the tachyzoite stage of *T. gondii* has been the focus of extensive research, because antigens within this stage are presented to the immune system effectively during natural infection, forcing the parasite to enter (in less than two weeks) into the latent bradyzoite stage seeking for protection. This strategy results in physical parasite shielding by encystation and different, and much lower, antigen availability for the immune system.

The soluble tachyzoite antigen extract (STAg) was the first protein blend identified as source of protective products, before wide-scale proteomic analyses were available (Denkers *et al.* 1993; Yap *et al.* 1998). Protection with STAg is only partial, even when the very efficient CpG oligodeoxynucleotides are used as adjuvants (Yin *et al.* 2007). Similar partial protection was also induced by the *T. gondii* sonicate of tachyzoites (TSo), even when mixed with cholera toxin (CT, a mucosal adjuvant) for oral administration (Bourguin *et al.* 1991; Bourguin *et al.* 1993).

One of the reasons why immunogenic parasite extracts render non-protective immunity may be the diversification of immune responses amongst all the different antigens (immunodominant or not) present in those extracts. Additionally, the extraction process (in the case of STAg) may have eliminated some of the innate immunity activators, namely TLR agonists, present in the whole parasite. Current proteomic analyses (high-throughput 2-dimensional electrophoresis combined with mass spectrometry) have identified nine novel vaccine candidates within STAg (Ma *et al.* 2009) and we should see some of these promising antigens being tested *in vivo* as recombinant subunit or vectorised vaccines in the near future.

3.3 Individual antigens identified and used as subunit vaccines

Three major particularities characterize the difficulties found in the development of recombinant vaccines against toxoplasmosis; these are: (i) *T. gondii* is an unicellular protozoan parasite formed by thousands of different proteins, glycoproteins, lipoproteins, and other types of molecules that can become feasible candidate antigens for a vaccine, (ii) the parasite evolves into several different stages during its life cycle, with some of those stages (cysts) particularly protected against the action of the immune system and, in addition, the antigens of one stage may not be effective vaccines for subsequent stages, and (iii) numerous strains of the parasite coexist in nature, most of them with significant differences in antigenic sequences, pathogenicity and physiological behavior within the host. Thus, protection induced against one strain may not be either cross-reactive or sufficient to prevent infection by other strain(s).

Apprehension in using attenuated whole parasites for human (and in many countries also animal) vaccination has lead research´s efforts to the development of safer vaccines by means of the identification and subsequent experimental administration of individual antigens. In principle, for an efficient immunization against *T. gondii*, the best antigens to use in vaccines should be those that are excreted/secreted (ESA) from the parasite stages that invade the host, since those have been reported as the most relevant targets of immune responses during natural infection, which, in contrast to what is seen in other diseases, controls the parasite´s ability to spread and multiply.

The surface of the tachyzoite stage was the initial source of antigens tested as vaccines because of its accessibility. The abundant surface antigen 1 (SAG-1) was the initial and most widely studied tachyzoite antigen. Multiple other antigens (see figure 2) of the tachyzoite and bradyzoite stages of the parasite subsequently entered the vaccine development pipeline, and even sporozoite-specific antigens have recently begun to be identified in mice and humans (Hill *et al.* 2011). The use of all these antigens has been carefully reviewed by Jongert *et al.* (Jongert *et al.* 2009).

In brief, up-to-date a few bradyzoite antigens, such as the abundant BAG-1, BRAD-1, CST-1, SAG4A, SRS-9, BSR-4, or the bradyzoite/tachyzoite expressed protein MAG-1 and, innumerable tachyzoite antigens, including surface antigens (SAGs), dense granule (GRAs), rhoptries (ROPs) and microneme (MICs) antigens have been identified and used as vaccine candidates with relative success and mostly in small experimental animal models.

In humans, major T-cell antigens have yet to be identified (Boothroyd 2009) although recent tests using predicted CD8 epitopes derived from the most relevant mouse antigens could identify several reactive peptides presented by HLA-A02, A03 and B07 human major histocompatibility complex (MHC) molecules (Tan *et al.* 2010; Cong *et al.* 2011). Candidate proteins include 2 surface antigens (SAG1, and SUSA1, a surface marker specific to the slow-growing, bradyzoite form of *T. gondii*) and 7 secreted proteins (GRA2, GRA3, GRA6, GRA7, ROP2, ROP16, ROP18).

Recombinant proteins were the first and most obvious tools to induce immunity against *T. gondii* and antigens produced in bacteria or yeast cells were the first finely characterized molecules inoculated into experimental animals (Jongert *et al.* 2009). However, immunization with pure proteins did not show much success in terms of induction of protective immunity. Synthetic peptides encompassing antigenic epitopes were also tested as vaccine candidates (Duquesne *et al.* 1991), but with the same unfortunate fate. New combinations of antigens/adjuvants (specially the new generation of innate-stimulating adjuvants) aiming at inducing more adequate and stronger Th1/CTL responses are the paths to follow in order to improve the results obtained to date with these types of experimental vaccines.

3.4 Genetic vaccines: DNA molecules and live vectors

Proteins are excellent inducers of antibodies, but have some difficulties to induce high levels of T lymphocytes. Genetic vaccines, on the contrary, are highly efficient to induce antigen-specific T lymphocytes. This group of vaccines represents a number of novel technologies that involve direct delivery of genes encoding antigens of interest to host cells, which then serve as antigen factories and immune-related processing plants for the resulting products. The intracellular presence of these products facilitates further induction of antigen-specific cellular immune responses by means of the easier antigen presentation in association with MHC class I molecules, which efficiently primes CD8+ T lymphocyte responses. These novel vaccine technologies have therefore being used in clinical trials against a variety of pathogens for which this cellular immune profile renders protection (Barouch 2006). Immunization with DNA vaccines (almost exclusively bacterial plasmids because of the easy construction and multiplication, see Table 1) has traditionally been the first choice for experimental genetic vaccination against toxoplasmosis (Jongert *et al.* 2009). However, despite their successful application in many preclinical disease models, one of the most significant hurdles of DNA vaccine development has been transferring the success of inducing protective immunity in small animal models to larger animal models. The low potency of DNA vaccines in primates has so far precluded the development of most human health programs beyond Phase I clinical trials (Ulmer *et al.* 2006; Abdulhaqq and Weiner 2008). The reasons for the failure of DNA vaccines to induce potent immune responses in humans have not yet been elucidated. However, it is reasonable to assume that the low levels of overall antigen production, the inefficient cellular delivery of DNA plasmids and the insufficient stimulation of the innate immune system may be the major causes responsible for the lack of efficiency (Ulmer *et al.* 2006).

Vaccine candidate	Mouse strain	*T. gondii* chalange strain	Outcome of vaccination	References
pGRA4 + liposome, im	C57BL/6	ME49 tissue cysts, oral	Partial protection	Chen *et al.*, 2009
	BALB/c	RH tachyzoites, ip	No protection	Chen *et al.*, 2009
pSAG1 + pIL-18, im	BALB/c	RH tachyzoites, ip	Protection	Liu *et al.*, 2010
pSAG1, im	BALB/c	RH tachyzoites, ip	Partial protection	Liu *et al.*, 2010
pSAG1, im	BALB/c	RH tachyzoites, ip	No protection	Hoseinian Khosroshahi *et al.*, 2011
pROP2, im	BALB/c	RH tachyzoites, ip	No protection	Hoseinian Khosroshahi *et al.*, 2011
pSAG1 + pROP2, im	BALB/c	RH tachyzoites, ip	Partial protection	Hoseinian Khosroshahi *et al.*, 2011
pMIC3, im	BALB/c	RH tachyzoites, ip	Partial protection	Fang *et al.* 2009
pSCA/MIC3, im	BALB/c	RH tachyzoites, ip	Partial protection	Fang *et al.* 2009
pMIC3 + pGM-CSF, im	CBA/J	76K tissue cysts, oral	Protection	Ismael *et al.* 2003; Ismael *et al.*, 2009
pMIC3, sc	Kunming	RH tachyzoites, ip	Protection	Xiang *et al.* 2009
pT-ME (multi-epitope DNA), im	BALB/c	RH tachyzoites, ip	Protection	Liu *et al.*, 2009
	C57BL/6	RH tachyzoites, ip	Protection	Liu *et al.*, 2009
pEC2 (multi-epitope DNA), im	BALB/c	Prugniaud tissue cysts, oral	Partial protection	Rosenberg *et al.*, 2009
	BALB/c	Trousseau tissue cysts, oral	No protection	Rosenberg *et al.*, 2009
pEC3 (multi-epitope DNA), im	BALB/c	Prugniaud tissue cysts, oral	Partial protection	Rosenberg *et al.*, 2009
	BALB/c	Trousseau tissue cysts, oral	No protection	Rosenberg *et al.*, 2009
pSAG1-MIC4, in	BALB/c	RH tachyzoites, ip	Partial protection	Wang *et al.*, 2009
pSAG1-MIC4 + pCTA2/B, in	BALB/c	RH tachyzoites, ip	Protection	Wang *et al.*, 2009

Abbreviations: p, plasmid; im, intramuscular; ip, intraperitoneal; sc, subcutaneous; in, intranasal; pSCA, suicidal vector based on the SFV replicon; T-ME, $SAG1_{238-256}$, $SAG1_{281-320}$, $GRA1_{170-193}$, $GRA4_{331-345}$, $GRA4_{229-245}$, $GRA2_{171-185}$; EC2, MIC2-MIC3-SAG1; EC3, GRA3-GRA7-M2AP; CTA2/B, Cholera toxin A2 and B subunits.

Table 1. Major DNA vaccine candidates recently developed and tested against *T. gondii* infection

In order to increase the immunogenicity of DNA vaccines in large animal models, various methods have been tested including: (i) improvements in the design of the plasmid, e.g. by adding antigen-ubiquitination signals for improved immunoproteasome degradation and antigen presentation (Ishii *et al.* 2006), (ii) delivering multiple antigens at the same time (Beghetto *et al.* 2005; Mevelec *et al.* 2005; Jongert *et al.* 2007; Xue *et al.* 2008; Qu *et al.* 2009; Wang *et al.* 2009; Hoseinian Khosroshahi *et al.* 2011), (iii) using chemical adjuvants or immunomodulatory molecules formulated into microparticles or liposomes (van Drunen Littel-van den Hurk *et al.* 2004; Greenland and Letvin 2007), and (iv) using plasmid molecules as part of prime-boost immunization regimes (Doria-Rose and Haigwood 2003; Dunachie and Hill 2003; Dondji *et al.* 2005; Shang *et al.* 2009). However, at present, the low immunogenicity of DNA vaccines has forced researchers to find alternative immunization vectors, and recombinant bacterial or viral vectors, which carry and express DNA sequences into the host organisms more efficiently, have gradually substituted bacterial plasmids for experimental vaccination studies.

The use of bacteria as vehicles for genetic vaccination is an attractive and simple idea that derives from a number of intrinsic properties of the system. Live bacteria that contain recombinant plasmids encoding heterologous antigens of other pathogens have the potential of being oral delivery vectors for DNA vaccines in animal industry (Grillot-Courvalin *et al.* 1999; Grillot-Courvalin *et al.* 2002). In Table 2. we show two studies conducted by Qu *et al.* in which ICR mice were orally immunized with DNA vaccines encoding SAG1 and/or MIC3 antigens delivered by an attenuated *S. typhimurium* strain (Dam⁻ and PhoP⁻) at different doses, and challenged with 500 tachyzoites of *T. gondii* RH strain. Those studies show that oral administration of the attenuated bacteria could induce humoral and cellular immune responses, although they just elicited partial protection of animals (a maximum of 20% improvement in survival rate). Thus, new vectors and constructs have to be tested to consider this methodology as an applicable option.

Vaccine candidate	Mouse strain	*T. gondii* chalange strain	Outcome of vaccination	References
rPRV/SAG1, im	BALB/c	RH tachyzoites, ip	Partial protection	Liu *et al.*, 2008
pSAG1 (prime) + rPRV/SAG1 (boost), im	BALB/c	RH tachyzoites, ip	Protection	Shang *et al.*, 2009
BV-G/SAG1, im	BALB/c	RH tachyzoites, ip	Protection	Fang *et al.*, 2010
rFLU/SAG2 (prime), in + rAd/SAG2 (boost), sc	BALB/c	P-Br tissue cysts, oral	Protection	Machado *et al.*, 2010
S. typhimurium/pSAG1, oral	ICR	RH tachyzoites, ip	Partial protection	Qu *et al.*, 2008
S. typhimurium/pSAG1-MIC3, oral	ICR	RH tachyzoites, ip	Partial protection	Qu *et al.*, 2009

Abbreviations: p, plasmid; im, intramuscular; ip, intraperitoneal; sc, subcutaneous; in, intranasal; rPRV: recombinant pseudorabies virus; BV-G: recombinant baculovirus; rFLU: recombinant influenza A; rAd: recombinant adenovirus.

Table 2. Selected examples of live attenuated vectors expressing *Toxoplasma gondii* antigens currently in tests.

Viral vectors exhibit many advantages for the development of a vaccine against toxoplasmosis. In summary, viral vectors express foreign antigens directly inside host cells very efficiently; as a result they present antigen fragments in association with MHC molecules more proficiently and, subsequently, they better stimulate the required anti-toxoplasma T cell responses (Th1 and CTL) because they act as natural adjuvants and stimulate intracellular innate immunity receptors. In addition, they can be administrated through the natural route of infection, such as via nasal mucosa, and they are able to induce effective and long lasting immune responses.

Our group has tested adenoviruses and influenza viruses as feasible vaccine vectors against toxoplasmosis (Caetano et al. 2006; Machado et al. 2010; Mendes et al. 2011) and they have shown significant improvement in comparison with naked plasmid vaccines. For those studies we have focused on possible formulations and immunization protocols using T. gondii surface antigens (SAGs). These molecules are involved in host cell attachment and invasion, and their sequences are conserved among different strains of T. gondii, sharing a high degree of homology even between type I (pathogenic and lethal in mice) and type II/III strains (cystogenic). However, these favorable traits do not ensure that these antigens will end up displaying sufficient protective capacities, but the proofs-of-principle obtained with their use will surely be maintained for any other antigens that display better protective properties.

In Caetano et al. (Caetano et al. 2006), we generated three recombinant adenoviruses encoding genetically modified SAG1, SAG2 and SAG3, without the 3'-end GPI anchoring motifs to ensure secretion and subsequent induction of combined Th/CTL immune responses. BALB/c mice received rAd/SAG1, rAd/SAG2, rAd/SAG3, or a combination of the three viruses (rAdMIX) and were challenged with 100 live tachyzoites of the T. gondii RH strain or with 20 cysts of the P-Br strain. Adenovirus immunization elicited potent antibody responses against each protein and displayed a significant bias toward a Th1 profile. When comparing the three recombinant viruses, rAd/SAG2 was the most efficient in eliciting antigen-specific antibodies. A significant reduction in cysts loads in the brain was observed in animals challenged with the P-Br strain. Vaccination with a mixture of all viruses promoted the highest level of inhibition of cyst formation, about 80%. However, no protection was observed against tachyzoites of the highly virulent RH strain (Caetano et al. 2006).

In the study by Machado et al. (2010), we generated a recombinant Influenza A vector encoding SAG2 of T. gondii and explored an original heterologous prime-boost immunization protocol using influenza virus (rFLU/SAG2) and a recombinant adenovirus (rAd/SAG2). Influenza A viruses are promising but currently under-explored vectors, which display some advantageous features to be used as live recombinant vaccines, such as the ability to infect and activate antigen presenting cells as well as to present high immunogenicity at mucosal and systemic levels (Rocha et al. 2004; Machado et al. 2010). BALB/c mice primed with an intranasal rFLU/SAG2 dose and boosted with a subcutaneous rAd/SAG2 dose elicited both humoral and cellular immune responses specific for SAG2. Moreover, when immunized animals were challenged with the cystogenic P-Br strain of T. gondii, they displayed up to 85% of reduction in parasite burden. These results demonstrate the potential use of recombinant influenza and adenoviruses in vaccination protocols to protect against oral challenge with T. gondii (Machado et al. 2010), although there is room for improvement.

Literature shows that, for other diseases, there is a good reproducibility of results when transferring experimental results obtained by immunization with some viral vectors (in particular adenoviruses) from small experimental animals to larger animal models or humans. We expect this to be also true for the experimental vaccines generated against toxoplasmosis, so that we can see some encouraging results in the near future.

4. Conclusion

Recombinant subunit vaccines (proteins in adjuvants, DNA vaccines and recombinant live vectors) are the present trends for the development of a vaccine against Toxoplasmosis. A myriad of parasite antigens have been described and researchers are testing them in many animal models of the disease. It is our belief that, more than the description of new parasite antigens that could be used in a final vaccine formulation, one of the major issues for the next future is to develop and test highly antigenic formulations using currently known antigens. Developing this type of formulations requires a deep knowledge of the immune system's antigen processing and presentation pathways, proficiency in the use of molecular biology techniques to adapt the parasite antigen sequences to enter those pathways, and using the new generation of adjuvants and delivery vectors in a manner that can best stimulate the pretended anti-parasite Th1 cellular (and probably humoral) immune responses. The options and combinations are so broad, and yet untested, that several years of research will be needed before we can decide which combination will be more adequate [antigen(s) + adjuvant(s) + vector(s)] or what will be the most efficient immunization protocol (single dose, multiple dose, homologous or heterologous prime-boost, etc.).

Finally, we would like to call attention to the fact that a possible result of the immunization/protection tests may actually be the achievement of a cost-effective vaccine that may be suitable for large-scale production and use. Then, one key question will arise for the future, regarding the correct use of that vaccine. In principle, the vaccine should be applied to animals, because preventing oocyst shedding by cats and tissue cyst formation in meat-producing animals should have great impact on both environmental contamination and public health. But this intervention could pose a risk because of the loss of herd immunity against the parasite and the resurgence of a different profile of *Toxoplasma*-related pathologies because of the primo-infection of non-vaccinated adults traveling to other countries or regions instead of kids or young adults being infected at its home places. To solve this, a possibility would be the universal vaccination of all children against toxoplasmosis, although this might end up being not feasible in practice or even might not be considered as a priority. Researchers should include these topics amongst those to be discussed in the forthcoming years within the field of vaccine development against toxoplasmosis.

5. References

Abdulhaqq, S. A. and D. B. Weiner (2008). "DNA vaccines: developing new strategies to enhance immune responses." *Immunol Res* 42(1-3): 219-232.

Andre, F. E., R. Booy, et al. (2008). "Vaccination greatly reduces disease, disability, death and inequity worldwide." *Bull World Health Organ* 86(2): 140-146.

Barouch, D. H. (2006). "Rational design of gene-based vaccines." *J Pathol* 208(2): 283-289.

Beghetto, E., H. V. Nielsen, et al. (2005). "A combination of antigenic regions of Toxoplasma gondii microneme proteins induces protective immunity against oral infection with parasite cysts." *J Infect Dis* 191(4): 637-645.

Bhopale, G. M. (2003). "Development of a vaccine for toxoplasmosis: current status." *Microbes Infect* 5(5): 457-462.

Boothroyd, J. C. (2009). "Toxoplasma gondii: 25 years and 25 major advances for the field." *Int J Parasitol* 39(8): 935-946.

Bourguin, I., T. Chardes, et al. (1993). "Oral immunization with Toxoplasma gondii antigens in association with cholera toxin induces enhanced protective and cell-mediated immunity in C57BL/6 mice." *Infect Immun* 61(5): 2082-2088.

Bourguin, I., T. Chardes, et al. (1991). "Amplification of the secretory IgA response to Toxoplasma gondii using cholera toxin." *FEMS Microbiol Lett* 65(3): 265-271.

Buxton, D. (1993). "Toxoplasmosis: the first commercial vaccine." *Parasitol Today* 9(9): 335-337.

Caetano, B. C., O. Bruna-Romero, et al. (2006). "Vaccination with replication-deficient recombinant adenoviruses encoding the main surface antigens of toxoplasma gondii induces immune response and protection against infection in mice." *Hum Gene Ther* 17(4): 415-426.

Chen, R., S. H. Lu, et al. (2009). "Protective effect of DNA-mediated immunization with liposome-encapsulated GRA4 against infection of Toxoplasma gondii." *J Zhejiang Univ Sci B* 10(7): 512-521.

Cong, H., E. J. Mui, et al. (2011). "Towards an immunosense vaccine to prevent toxoplasmosis: protective Toxoplasma gondii epitopes restricted by HLA-A*0201." *Vaccine* 29(4): 754-762.

Crampton, A. and T. Vanniasinkam (2007). "Parasite vaccines: the new generation." *Infect Genet Evol* 7(5): 664-673.

Cutchins, E. C. and J. Warren (1956). "Immunity patterns in the guinea pig following Toxoplasma infection and vaccination with killed Toxoplasma." *Am J Trop Med Hyg* 5(2): 197-209.

Denkers, E. Y. and R. T. Gazzinelli (1998). "Regulation and function of T-cell-mediated immunity during Toxoplasma gondii infection." *Clin Microbiol Rev* 11(4): 569-588.

Denkers, E. Y., R. T. Gazzinelli, et al. (1993). "Bone marrow macrophages process exogenous Toxoplasma gondii polypeptides for recognition by parasite-specific cytolytic T lymphocytes." *J Immunol* 150(2): 517-526.

Denkers, E. Y., R. T. Gazzinelli, et al. (1993). "Emergence of NK1.1+ cells as effectors of IFN-gamma dependent immunity to Toxoplasma gondii in MHC class I-deficient mice." *J Exp Med* 178(5): 1465-1472.

Dondji, B., E. Perez-Jimenez, et al. (2005). "Heterologous prime-boost vaccination with the LACK antigen protects against murine visceral leishmaniasis." *Infect Immun* 73(8): 5286-5289.

Doria-Rose, N. A. and N. L. Haigwood (2003). "DNA vaccine strategies: candidates for immune modulation and immunization regimens." *Methods* 31(3): 207-216.

Dubey, J. P., M. C. Jenkins, et al. (1996). "Killing of Toxoplasma gondii oocysts by irradiation and protective immunity induced by vaccination with irradiated oocysts." *J Parasitol* 82(5): 724-727.

Dubey, J. P., J. K. Lunney, et al. (1998). "Immunity to toxoplasmosis in pigs fed irradiated Toxoplasma gondii oocysts." *J Parasitol* 84(4): 749-752.

Dunachie, S. J. and A. V. Hill (2003). "Prime-boost strategies for malaria vaccine development." *J Exp Biol* 206(Pt 21): 3771-3779.

Duquesne, V., C. Auriault, et al. (1991). "Identification of T cell epitopes within a 23-kD antigen (P24) of Toxoplasma gondii." *Clin Exp Immunol* 84(3): 527-534.

Fang, R., H. Feng, et al. (2010). "Construction and immunogenicity of pseudotype baculovirus expressing Toxoplasma gondii SAG1 protein in BALB/c mice model." *Vaccine* 28(7): 1803-1807.

Fang, R., H. Nie, et al. (2009). "Protective immune response in BALB/c mice induced by a suicidal DNA vaccine of the MIC3 gene of Toxoplasma gondii." *Vet Parasitol* 164(2-4): 134-140.

Gazzinelli, R., Y. Xu, et al. (1992). "Simultaneous depletion of CD4+ and CD8+ T lymphocytes is required to reactivate chronic infection with Toxoplasma gondii." *J Immunol* 149(1): 175-180.

Gazzinelli, R. T., D. Amichay, et al. (1996). "Role of macrophage-derived cytokines in the induction and regulation of cell-mediated immunity to Toxoplasma gondii." *Curr Top Microbiol Immunol* 219: 127-139.

Gazzinelli, R. T., M. Wysocka, et al. (1994). "Parasite-induced IL-12 stimulates early IFN-gamma synthesis and resistance during acute infection with Toxoplasma gondii." *J Immunol* 153(6): 2533-2543.

Gigley, J. P., B. A. Fox, et al. (2009). "Long-term immunity to lethal acute or chronic type II Toxoplasma gondii infection is effectively induced in genetically susceptible C57BL/6 mice by immunization with an attenuated type I vaccine strain." *Infect Immun* 77(12): 5380-5388.

Greenland, J. R. and N. L. Letvin (2007). "Chemical adjuvants for plasmid DNA vaccines." *Vaccine* 25(19): 3731-3741.

Grillot-Courvalin, C., S. Goussard, et al. (1999). "Bacteria as gene delivery vectors for mammalian cells." *Curr Opin Biotechnol* 10(5): 477-481.

Grillot-Courvalin, C., S. Goussard, et al. (2002). "Wild-type intracellular bacteria deliver DNA into mammalian cells." *Cell Microbiol* 4(3): 177-186.

Gwadz, R. W., A. H. Cochrane, et al. (1979). "Preliminary studies on vaccination of rhesus monkeys with irradiated sporozoites of Plasmodium knowlesi and characterization of surface antigens of these parasites." *Bull World Health Organ* 57 Suppl 1: 165-173.

Hakim, F. T., R. T. Gazzinelli, et al. (1991). "CD8+ T cells from mice vaccinated against Toxoplasma gondii are cytotoxic for parasite-infected or antigen-pulsed host cells." *J Immunol* 147(7): 2310-2316.

Hill, D., C. Coss, et al. (2011). "Identification of a sporozoite-specific antigen from Toxoplasma gondii." *J Parasitol* 97(2): 328-337.

Hiramoto, R. M., A. J. Galisteo, et al. (2002). "200 Gy sterilised Toxoplasma gondii tachyzoites maintain metabolic functions and mammalian cell invasion, eliciting cellular immunity and cytokine response similar to natural infection in mice." *Vaccine* 20(16): 2072-2081.

Hoseinian Khosroshahi, K., F. Ghaffarifar, et al. (2011). "Evaluation of the immune response induced by DNA vaccine cocktail expressing complete SAG1 and ROP2 genes against toxoplasmosis." *Vaccine* 29(4): 778-783.

Hutson, S. L., E. Mui, et al. (2010). "T. gondii RP promoters & knockdown reveal molecular pathways associated with proliferation and cell-cycle arrest." *PLoS One* 5(11): e14057.

Ishii, K., H. Hisaeda, et al. (2006). "The involvement of immunoproteasomes in induction of MHC class I-restricted immunity targeting Toxoplasma SAG1." *Microbes Infect* 8(4): 1045-1053.

Ismael, A. B., D. Hedhli, et al. (2009). "Further analysis of protection induced by the MIC3 DNA vaccine against T. gondii: CD4 and CD8 T cells are the major effectors of the MIC3 DNA vaccine-induced protection, both Lectin-like and EGF-like domains of MIC3 conferred protection." *Vaccine* 27(22): 2959-2966.

Ismael, A. B., D. Sekkai, et al. (2003). "The MIC3 gene of Toxoplasma gondii is a novel potent vaccine candidate against toxoplasmosis." *Infect Immun* 71(11): 6222-6228.

Jongert, E., S. de Craeye, et al. (2007). "GRA7 provides protective immunity in cocktail DNA vaccines against Toxoplasma gondii." *Parasite Immunol* 29(9): 445-453.

Jongert, E., C. W. Roberts, et al. (2009). "Vaccines against Toxoplasma gondii: challenges and opportunities." *Mem Inst Oswaldo Cruz* 104(2): 252-266.

Kang, H., J. S. Remington, et al. (2000). "Decreased resistance of B cell-deficient mice to infection with Toxoplasma gondii despite unimpaired expression of IFN-gamma, TNF-alpha, and inducible nitric oxide synthase." *J Immunol* 164(5): 2629-2634.

Krahenbuhl, J. L., J. Ruskin, et al. (1972). "The use of killed vaccines in immunization against an intracellular parasite: Toxoplasma gondii." *J Immunol* 108(2): 425-431.

Liu, Q., S. Gao, et al. (2008). "A recombinant pseudorabies virus expressing TgSAG1 protects against challenge with the virulent Toxoplasma gondii RH strain and pseudorabies in BALB/c mice." *Microbes Infect* 10(12-13): 1355-1362.

Liu, Q., L. Shang, et al. (2010). "The protective effect of a Toxoplasma gondii SAG1 plasmid DNA vaccine in mice is enhanced with IL-18." *Res Vet Sci* 89(1): 93-97.

Liu, S., L. Shi, et al. (2009). "Evaluation of protective effect of multi-epitope DNA vaccine encoding six antigen segments of Toxoplasma gondii in mice." *Parasitol Res* 105(1): 267-274.

Lu, F., S. Huang, et al. (2009). "The temperature-sensitive mutants of Toxoplasma gondii and ocular toxoplasmosis." *Vaccine* 27(4): 573-580.

Ma, G. Y., J. Z. Zhang, et al. (2009). "Toxoplasma gondii: proteomic analysis of antigenicity of soluble tachyzoite antigen." *Exp Parasitol* 122(1): 41-46.

Machado, A. V., B. C. Caetano, et al. (2010). "Prime and boost immunization with influenza and adenovirus encoding the Toxoplasma gondii surface antigen 2 (SAG2) induces strong protective immunity." *Vaccine* 28(18): 3247-3256.

McLeod, R., J. K. Frenkel, et al. (1988). "Subcutaneous and intestinal vaccination with tachyzoites of Toxoplasma gondii and acquisition of immunity to peroral and congenital toxoplasma challenge." *J Immunol* 140(5): 1632-1637.

Mendes, E. A., B. C. Caetano, et al. (2011). "MyD88-dependent protective immunity elicited by adenovirus 5 expressing the surface antigen 1 from Toxoplasma gondii is mediated by CD8(+) T lymphocytes." *Vaccine* 29(27): 4476-4484.

Mevelec, M. N., D. Bout, et al. (2005). "Evaluation of protective effect of DNA vaccination with genes encoding antigens GRA4 and SAG1 associated with GM-CSF plasmid, against acute, chronical and congenital toxoplasmosis in mice." *Vaccine* 23(36): 4489-4499.

Mevelec, M. N., C. Ducournau, et al. (2010). "Mic1-3 Knockout Toxoplasma gondii is a good candidate for a vaccine against T. gondii-induced abortion in sheep." *Vet Res* 41(4): 49.

Nussenzweig, R. S., J. Vanderberg, et al. (1967). "Protective immunity produced by the injection of x-irradiated sporozoites of plasmodium berghei." *Nature* 216(5111): 160-162.

Omata, Y., Y. Aihara, et al. (1996). "Toxoplasma gondii: experimental infection in cats vaccinated with 60Co-irradiated tachyzoites." *Vet Parasitol* 65(3-4): 173-183.

Pifer, R. and F. Yarovinsky (2011). "Innate responses to Toxoplasma gondii in mice and humans." *Trends Parasitol.*

Qu, D., S. Wang, et al. (2008). "Protective effect of a DNA vaccine delivered in attenuated Salmonella typhimurium against Toxoplasma gondii infection in mice." *Vaccine* 26(35): 4541-4548.

Qu, D., H. Yu, et al. (2009). "Induction of protective immunity by multiantigenic DNA vaccine delivered in attenuated Salmonella typhimurium against Toxoplasma gondii infection in mice." *Vet Parasitol* 166(3-4): 220-227.

Rocha, C. D., B. C. Caetano, et al. (2004). "Recombinant viruses as tools to induce protective cellular immunity against infectious diseases." *Int Microbiol* 7(2): 83-94.

Rosenberg, C., S. De Craeye, et al. (2009). "Induction of partial protection against infection with Toxoplasma gondii genotype II by DNA vaccination with recombinant chimeric tachyzoite antigens." *Vaccine* 27(18): 2489-2498.

Seah, S. K. and G. Hucal (1975). "The use of irradiated vaccine in immunization against experimental murine toxoplasmosis." *Can J Microbiol* 21(9): 1379-1385.

Shang, L., Q. Liu, et al. (2009). "Protection in mice immunized with a heterologous prime-boost regime using DNA and recombinant pseudorabies expressing TgSAG1 against Toxoplasma gondii challenge." *Vaccine* 27(21): 2741-2745.

Tan, T. G., E. Mui, et al. (2010). "Identification of T. gondii epitopes, adjuvants, and host genetic factors that influence protection of mice and humans." *Vaccine* 28(23): 3977-3989.

Ulmer, J. B., B. Wahren, et al. (2006). "Gene-based vaccines: recent technical and clinical advances." *Trends Mol Med* 12(5): 216-222.

van Drunen Littel-van den Hurk, S., S. L. Babiuk, et al. (2004). "Strategies for improved formulation and delivery of DNA vaccines to veterinary target species." *Immunol Rev* 199: 113-125.

Wang, H., S. He, et al. (2009). "Toxoplasma gondii: protective effect of an intranasal SAG1 and MIC4 DNA vaccine in mice." *Exp Parasitol* 122(3): 226-232.

Xiang, W., Z. Qiong, et al. (2009). "The location of invasion-related protein MIC3 of Toxoplasma gondii and protective effect of its DNA vaccine in mice." *Vet Parasitol* 166(1-2): 1-7.

Xue, M., S. He, et al. (2008). "Evaluation of the immune response elicited by multi-antigenic DNA vaccine expressing SAG1, ROP2 and GRA2 against Toxoplasma gondii." *Parasitol Int* 57(4): 424-429.

Yap, G. S., T. Scharton-Kersten, et al. (1998). "Partially protective vaccination permits the development of latency in a normally virulent strain of Toxoplasma gondii." *Infect Immun* 66(9): 4382-4388.

Yin, G. R., X. L. Meng, et al. (2007). "[Intranasal immunization with mucosal complex vaccine protects mice against Toxoplasma gondii]." *Zhongguo Ji Sheng Chong Xue Yu Ji Sheng Chong Bing Za Zhi* 25(4): 290-294.

6

Screening of the Prevalence of Antibodies to the Tick *Hyalomma lusitanicum* in a Province of Northern Spain

Consuelo Giménez Pardo and Lourdes Lledó García
Alcalá University
Spain

1. Introduction

In the recent decades it has been found the occurrence of a large number of hitherto unknown or undervalued pathogens, and they present a risk to health and human welfare. Almost all incidents caused by emerging pathogens have been attached to zoonotic agents, which expanded its host range and are capable of breaching the species barrier (Zeier et al., 2005). Besides the known diseases, new ones emerge or reemerge due to a variety of socioeconomic, health and environmental questions. This increase in communicable diseases has serious implications for public health and animal health (Chomel, 1998; Daszak et al., 2000, Cleaveland et al., 2001, Simpson, 2002; Daszak & Cunningham, 2003; Zeier et al., 2005; Cunningham, 2005; Blancou et al., 2005, Gibbs, 2005; Gortázar et al., 2007).

Emerging zoonoses are also a public health problem, the biggest threat to animal welfare, environmental quality and conservation of biodiversity (Daszak et al., 2000; Cunningham, 2005, Briones et al., 2002). The expected increase contact between humans and wildlife, caused by anthropogenic interference in the ecosystem, increase the emergence of pathogens originating in wildlife cycles, which can cross-infect man and animals (Bengis et al., 2004). Thus, wildlife is a constant source of "zoonotic pool" that plays a fundamental role in human exposure to infectious agents against novel animal (Morse, 1995).

In the recent past, the diseases of wild animals have been important only when they threatened livestock or human health (Daszak et al., 2000), but outbreaks in endangered species have led to them having more significant consideration. Currently, these diseases are booming, especially in the space where interaction occurs between wildlife and farm animals, including an increase in contact between them and the man (Simpson, 2002; Gortázar et al., 2007). Arthropod-borne diseases represent the most common zoonosis in relation to wildlife in the northern hemisphere, especially the Old World (Lindgren et al., 2000), so infectious agents are diverse and constantly growing, so their relationship would be endless (Bueno et al., 2009).

Wild animals and arthropod vectors play also important roles in the exposure of humans and domestic animals to animal-borne pathogens (Morse, 1995). Contact between humans and wild animals may occur when people venture into the latter's ecosystems, such contact in foreseen as a future generator of cross infestation, but the knowledge of ectoparasites, with special mention to ticks and their hosts' reservoirs that are located in many areas of world are unstudied. Ticks are vectors of disease have a wide range of pathogens (bacteria, rickettsia, viruses, protozoa and nematodes), affecting both domestic and wild animals, and humans with a zoonotic character. Ticks are considered as one of the most efficient arthropod vector role (Hillyard, 1996, Wall & Shearer, 1997).

In fact, it's known that ticks are vectors of transmission of a number of human viruses that causes Tick-borne meningoencephalitis, Colorado tick fever and Crimean-Congo hemorrhagic fever, among others, bacteria (*Rickettsia* spp, *Anaplasma phagocytophilum*, *Borrelia burgdorferi* and *Francisella turalensis*, among others) (Lopez-Vélez & Molina, 2005; Toledo et al., 2009) and protozoan pathogens including parasites (Lledó et al., 2010) and control of ticks and tick-borne diseases is a major component of animal health programes for the protection of livestock. Over the ixodid tick species which are often found on humans exposed to infested vegetation *Amblyomma* species, *Dermacentor* spp, *Haemaphysalis* spp, *Ixodes* spp and *Hyalomma* spp are found (Estrada- Peña et al., 1999).

In this sense, Genus *Hyalomma* is a phylogenetically young group of ixodid ticks. As proposed Kolonin (2009), domestication and the development of cattle-breeding stimulated the evolution and biological progress of this group. These transformations continue to this day, as is apparent from the great number of intraspecific forms. *Hyalomma* ticks (Figure 1) are medium to large sized, with prominent mouthparts. Most species are 3 hosts, but there are also 1 and 2 hosts. Some species of this genus can use 1, 2 or 3 hosts to develop according to the host they found. The life cycle can last between 3-4 months and more than a year, depending on species and climate. The nymphs and adults stay overwinter in cracks and crevices between the stones of walls and barns, or uncultivated grasslands. Adults are found throughout the year, although the parasite load is higher in spring and summer, parasitizing deer and wild boar. Larvae and nymphs parasitize rabbits and are more prevalent in spring. Though this genus is usually restricted to the Mediterranean region, one of the species, *Hyalomma lusitanicum,* Koch 1844 (*Ixodoidea: Ixodida*) has a widespread distribution in some regions of Southern Spain, from which is introduced by wild animals (Encinas-Grandes, 1986).

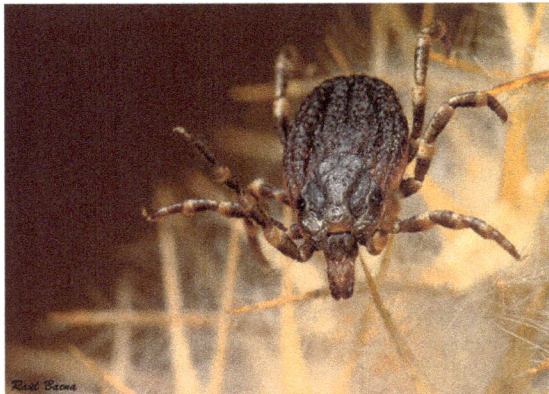

Fig. 1. Adult of Hyalomma lusitanicum

This ixodid tick is also located in the Burgos province (north western Spain) (Cordero del Campillo et al., 1994), in areas mainly rural, though recreational activities attracting non-residents have increased in recent years (Figure 2). This tick is not the most prevalent tick in this area.

In this studied area, in the northern sector, the winters are cold and humid and the summers are cold. Vegetation under Atlantic influences consists in oakwood and beechwood, with brushwood. In the southern sector is submediterranean and shows similar winter but hottest summers. Vegetation consists in gall-oak groes and holm-oak wood, being brush scarce (Roman et al., 1996; Dominguez, 2004). Mean summer temperatures in this area range between 16 and 20°C, while mean winter temperatures range between 2 and 5°C. Rainfall is usually high in winter at some 900-1100 mm/year. Altitude is ranging between 600-800 meters on the plateau. Climatic differences among different areas of Spain are responsible of both, the diversity of tick species and the circulation of tick-borne pathogens.

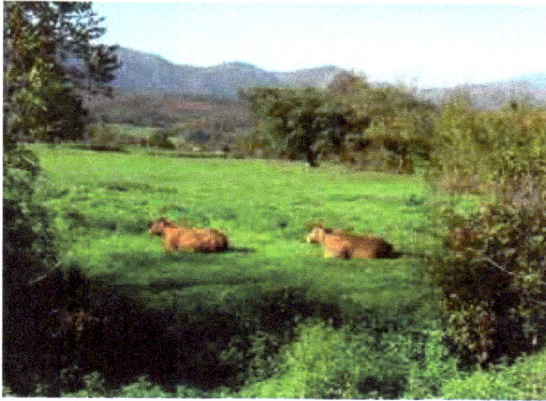

Fig. 2. Landscape of the studied area

While ticks have a clear geographical distribution in relation to climate, temperature, humidity and like attitude, climate change and global warming have influenced the geographical distribution of ticks. So, some groups as Experts from the International Scientific Working Group (ISW-TBE) on Central European encephalitis transmitted by ticks (Tick-Borne Encephalitis) warn of the first detection of these arthropods in areas above 1,500 m above sea level.

In Spain, it looks to be *Ixodes ricinus* the most abundant and widespread tick in the Basque Country (Northern Spain) (Barandika et al., 2006) and some authors (Toledo et al., 2009) have observed that one of the most abundant species in Central regions of Spain in terms of infection and tick abundance is *Hyalomma lusitanicum*. However, as happens with other ectoparasites and their host-reservoirs, are located in many areas of Spain that are unstudied or missstudied.

In this sense, the genus *Hyalomma* is one of the vectors for *Theileria annulata* that causes Mediterranean theileriosis, and produces considerable economic losses in cattle (Viseras & Garcia Fernandez., 1999) though in terms of public health, this tick is considered as not anthropophilic.

Tick bites are generally painless and many people may not even notice the bite and may never find the tick if it falls off. The majority of individuals with tick bites develop no symptoms, and many do not remember getting bitten. The direct damage caused by ticks depends on the number, species and location of the parasites. However, the most harmful effects on animal and public health are derived from indirect vector character (Hillyard, 1996, Wall & Shearer, 1997; Encinas et al., 1999, Sonenshine et al., 2002). Damage can be divided, according to the scope of the consequences, cutaneous and systemic. We can point to the inflammatory reaction in the fixation point, which causes itching, scratching, excoriations and self-harm. The reaction can spread awareness of the antigenic components of saliva, causing even anaphylactic shock. The bites often become infected with pyogenic agents such as *Staphylococcus aureus*, not ruling out the occurrence of myiasis (Wall & Shearer, 1997; Encinas et al., 1999, Wall, 2007).Systemic effects include tick paralysis is caused by a neurotoxin secreted by the females of some species, producing a neuromuscular blockade (Sonenshine et al., 2002). *Ixodes ricinus* and *Haemaphysalis punctata* are two species in our area involved in the process of paralysis (Hillyard, 1996, Wall & Shearer, 1997; Encinas et al., 1999). The mechanical transmission of pathogens from sepsis occurs in tick infestation in lambs or calves (Kettle, 1995), not neglecting the effects of blood loss. In this sense, a female has been eating packed up to 4 g of blood, so intense in parasites are common anemias (Encinas et al., 1999).

When ticks bite at time of the attachment they inoculate saliva and occasionally, a neurotoxin secreted at the time of attachment. Saliva in feeding ticks is rich in several biochemical components including various enzymes (Sauer et al., 1995; Giménez-Pardo & Martínez-Grueiro, 2008). Immunogenic and pathogenic proteins enter in the mammalian host during feeding via the tick salivary gland (Kaufman 1989). Their saliva secretions during bites are capable to produce toxicoses and allergic reactions, and in animals it's known that ticks are capable to induce a high humoral immune response (Perez-Sanchez et al., 1992). In human tick attachment are brief and sometimes, are immature forms which introduce a low quantity of antigens which are not enough to induce a good humoral response.

In this paper we i) study the preliminary humoral response in humans, employing antigens from male and female *Hyalomma lusitanicum* tick as a previous work to know if this tick could in a future be capable to bite humans in rural regions being implicated in the transmission of human pathogens and ii) observe differences between males and females in the response that could induce when they bite humans. For this, it was assayed a panel of human sera of different days post bitten by indirect enzyme-linked immunoabsorbent assay technique. This study was carried out in Burgos province (Spain) and results are compared with those obtained from general population and without history of tick bites.

2. Material and methods

2.1 Parasites

465 unfed adult ticks (males and females) were collected from vegetation in spring and each one was identified by binocular lens. Males (190) were separated from females (275) and processed individually. Specimens were immersed in 70% alcohol for ten minutes rinsed for 30 seconds in Milli-Q water and dried in a filter paper. Each ixodid tick was transferred in PBS-saline (10mM PBS pH 7.2, 146mM NaCl) in a Potter-Elvejem on an ice bath and homogenized. Extracts were removed in eppendorf tubes and centrifuged for 1min at 500 rpm to deposit cuticle fragments and tissue rests. Supernatants were collected and centrifuged in new eppendorf at 14000 rpm for 5 min, filtered through a 0.22µm filter (Millipore) and the resultant one were again filtered through a 0.22µm filter. This whole tick extract was collected and the protein concentration determined using the technique of Bradford (Bradford, 1976) and subsequently adjusted to 1mg/ml for females and 0.635 mg/ml for males using PBS-saline.

2.2 Human sera

The study was carried out on two population groups: sera from people who had been bitten by ticks and serum samples from the general population with no history of tick bites as control group. For the first group, 42 samples of human serum from 23 patients bitten by ticks were randomly collected from patients to the Burgos Health Centres (Figure 2), and the following information was recorded for each person: age, sex, occupation and area of residence. A serum sample was withdrawn from all bitten patients at the time of consultation and the patients were asked to return to provide another sample at 15-20 days later. All residents living in the study area are people related to livestock, or have pets in their care. They are people with an epidemiological history of tick bite, but without identification of the same. For the second group, serum from 97 people was obtained from the general population presented to healthcare centres for reasons unrelated to infectious diseases. All samples were aliquoted and conserved at -20°C until use. The survey was performed with the consent of the subjects included in the study, and in compliance with the ethical standards of Alcalá de Henares University´s Comitte on Human experimentation, as well as with the Helsinki Declaration of 1975 as revised in 2004.

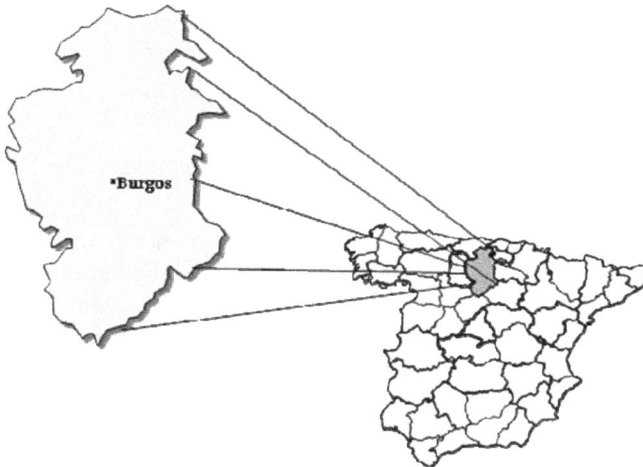

Fig. 3. Location in the Spain map the Burgos province

2.3 ELISA reactions

An indirect ELISA technique was used to detect anti-ticks Abs (IgG, IgM, IgE) in the samples. As antigens were used protein extracts from both males and females of *H. lusitanicum*. ELISA plates were coated with 1μg of antigen per well diluted in 0.1M carbonate/bicarbonate buffer, pH 9.6 and incubated at 4°C overnight. It was realized three washes in 0.05% PBS-Tween 20. After incubation with 0.05% PBS-Tween 20-1% casein for 1h at 37° and the subsequent washes, 100μl per well of human sera diluted at 1/50 for IgG, 1/20 for IgM and 1/10 for IgE in 0.05% PBS-Tween-20 and incubated for 1h at 37°C was added. After the subsequent washes, peroxidase-labeled anti-human immunoglobulin antibodies were also diluted in 0.05% PBS-Tween at 1/4000 for both anti-IgG (CalBiochem), anti-IgM (CalBiochem) and 1/500 for anti-IgE (CalBiochem), incubated for 1h at 37°C. ABTS (2-2´-Azino bis(3-Ethylbenzhia-zoline-6-sulfonic acid) and H_2O_2 were used as substrates. Reactions were stopped after with 3N sulphuric acid and results were read on a spectrophotometer at 405nm. On each ELISA plate were included negative controls sera obtained from people that never have been bitten by any tick. Experiences were done in triplicate (or more depending on the sera volume). The sample sera were considered positive when their optical density surpased a treshold calculated as the mean optical density of the negative control sera plus three times the standard deviation (mean OD+3δ). The same parameters were employed when it was referred to the general population.

3. Results

Twenty three of the patients presented at the Burgos Health Services for tick bites were asymptomatic at the time of sampling. Of these patients, 12 were males and 11 were females (Table 1).

	Age-groups (years)		
	0-10	**11-59**	**60-97**
Males (%)	2 (8.69)	4 (17.39)	6 (26.08)
Females (%)	2 (8.69)	8 (34.78)	1 (4.34)

Table 1. Characteristics of the patients attended for tick bites in this study

Nine patients were bled once, 13 patients were bled two times and 1 patient was bled in three occasions. All patients were bitten by unknown tick species and in 9 of them the serum samples were withdrawn more than 21 days after the tick bite (Table 2). There was no relation between the tick bite and the age, profession or place where the patient lived.

Of the patients studied, 4 had Abs (IgG) against both *H. lusitanicum* male and female antigens and two of them reacted only with male but not with female whole tick antigen as indicated in Table 2. Two sera showed Abs (IgG) against female but not male *H. lusitanicum* antigens.

Because ticks could have been removed from people in the first 48h post-attachment and even in the case of an effective transmission, the patients could have been bled before the synthesis of the anti-tick Abs have occurred, low values of IgM were found. Afterall, sera from three patients were considered positive against female antigens.

Serum from one patient was positive against male antigens of *Hyalomma lusitanicum*. Two patients showed IgM positive as only response and this fact indicate a possible acute case of *H. lusitanicum* bitten (see in Table 2).

Antibodies to IgE were analyzed in those sera that were positive against both male and female antigens, but we have not observed response to anti-IgE, neither male nor female *H. lusitanicum* antigens.

Relative to the general unexposed population, none of the sera studied were positive against female antigens of *H. lusitanicum* though when sera were assayed against male antigens, one serum was positive (see in Table 3).

Patient (n°)	Sera (n°)	Days (p.b)[1]	IgG (X±SE)		IgM (X±SE)	
			Female (Ag)	Males(Ag)	Females(Ag)	Males(Ag)
1	5		1.235±0.046	2.194±0.144	0.140±0.014	0.112±0.031
2	6		0.856±0.021	0.785±0.074	0.086±0.002	0.163±0.043
	7		0.975±0.077	1.098±0.207	0.079±0.022	0.165±0.022
3	8		1.270±0.094	1.224± 0.161	0.059±0.009	0.148±0.002
4	9		1.760±0.058	1.903±0.165	0.102±0.017	0.122±0.028
5	17a	17	1.044±0.015	0.928±0.133	0.106±0.009	0.144±0.038
	17b		0.816±0.040	0.499±0.062	0.100±0.026	0.057±0.027
6	23a		0.946±0.113	1.199±0.132	0.399±0.025	0.023±0.002
	23b	25	1.291±0.201	1.268±0.111	0.350±0.033	0.144±0.046
7	36a		0.724±0.067	0.445±0.095	0.060±0.001	0.050±0.007
	36b	11	1.442±0.124	1.229±0.024	0.046±0.010	0.134±0.019
	50	20	1.033±0.061	0.516±0.036	0.050±0.012	0.121±0.021
8	80		1.450±0.050	1.359±0.072	0.068±0.012	0.166±0.015
	79		1.443±0.190	1.250±0.138	0.107±0.004	0.187±0.005
9	81		1.161±0.093	0.674±0.066	0.023±0.004	0.150±0.016
	82		0.404±0.042	0	0.062±0.004	0.175±0.031
10	84		0.926±0.112	0.707±0.166	0.041±0.010	0.173±0.042
	83		1.241±0.011	0	0.040±0.004	0.171±0.039
11	189		1.256±0.187	1.040±0.140	0.100±0.011	0.166±0.041
	190	22	1.378±0.184	1.136±0.031	0.099±0.004	0.166±0.040
12	270		0.743±0.042	0.714±0.120	0.137±0.002	0.226±0.039
	271	33	0.872±0.009	0.626±0.176	0.146±0.016	0.238±0.025
13	272		1.289±0.161	1.164±0.038	0.068±0.004	0.060±0.007
	273	25	1.057±0.074	0.766±0.072	0.077±0.010	0.097±0.009
14	279		1.991±0.018	2.139±0.031	0.150±0.010	0.228±0.017
	280	30	2.152±0.029	1.767±0.029	0.119±0.009	0.290±0.032
15	258		1.730±0.047	1.876±0.205	0.091±0.009	0.256±0.032
	259	13	1.750±0.051	1.496±0.150	0.107±0.007	0.259±0.045
16	290		1.625±0.095	1.936±0.088	0.136±0.011	0.371±0.025
	291	27	1.628±0.070	1.864±0.101	0.114±0.007	0.316±0.020
17	293		1.283±0.033	0.931±0.078	0.029±0.0007	0.055±0.002
18	303		0.854±0.073	0.324±0.047	0.089±0.014	0.159±0.009
	304	18	0.883±0.074	0.517±0.046	0.055±0.007	0.156±0.018
19	308		1.531±0.070	1.104±0.070	0.030±0.012	0.134±0.006
	309	20	1.309±0.098	0.833±0.045	0.054±0.008	0.110±0.025
20	313		0.974±0.019	0.310±0.026	0.149±0.010	0.109±0.015
21	314		1.589±0.241	0.512±0.044	0.101±0.014	0.077±0.010
	315	24	1.891±0.055	0.493±0.007	0.120±0.010	0.116±0.026
22	388		0.624±0.054	0.309±0.037	0.100±0.005	0.111±0.009
	389	22	0.664±0.070	0.088±0.026	0.063±0.007	0.127±0.021
23	354		1.072±0.239	1.096±0.026	0.121±0.014	0.195±0.014
	355	25	1.711±0.054	0.251±0.077	0.237±0.028	0.214±0.009
Control sera (n=8)			0.996±0.149	0.782±0.098	0.086±0.013	0.149±0.021

Table 2. Reactivity of the human sera from the patients bitten by unspecific ticks, against the *Hyalomma lusitanicum* (male or female) whole antigens.

Sera (n°) (n=3)	IgG (X±SE)		Sera (n°) (n=3)	IgG (X±SE)	
	Females	Males		Females	Males
1	1.036±0.096	0.608±0.015	49	0.650±0.047	0.966±0.058
2	0.897±0.149	0.895±0.048	50	0.585±0.072	0.967±0.036
3	0.465±0.014	1.140±0.053	51	0.276±0.013	**1.75±0.025**
4	0.377±0.016	0.896±0.015	52	0.296±0.030	0.763±0.031
5	0.887±0.096	0.643±0.100	53	0.479±0.046	0.570±0.053
6	1.031±0.077	0.802±0.055	54	0.346±0.014	0.700±0.176
7	0.279±0.043	0.593±0.088	55	0.299±0.005	0.676±0.022
8	0.915±0.055	0.898±0.038	56	0.817±0.015	0.605±0.127
9	0.630±0.043	0.425±0.045	58	0.343±0.021	1.225±0.067
10	0.544±0.024	0.650±0.088	59	0.415±0.098	0.525±0.037
11	0.378±0.056	0.802±0.065	60	0.349±0.042	0.519±0.123
12	0.311±0.008	0.606±0.060	61	0.434±0.010	0.492±0.035
13	0.447±0.061	0.554±0.025	62	0.430±0.012	1.023±0.008
14	0.117±0.024	0.176±0.009	63	0.325±0.041	0.585±0.103
15	0.386±0.017	0.884±0.060	64	1.040±0.024	1.156±0.193
16	0.778±0.093	0.527±0.103	65	0.824±0.140	0.685±0.015
17	1.019±0.114	0.613±0.038	66	0.424±0.012	0.722±0.094
18	0.938±0.045	0.666±0.030	67	0.498±0.066	1.476±0.055
19	0.234±0.007	0.314±0.017	68	1.077±0.081	1.004±0.082
20	0.485±0.089	0.614±0.055	69	0.927±0.068	0.800±0.172
22	0.671±0.048	0.466±0.045	70	0.234±0.042	0.461±0.107
24	0.473±0.055	0.211±0.026	71	0.323±0.014	0.891±0.200
26	0.383±0.055	0.250±0.058	72	0.876±0.030	0.446±0.130
28	0.389±0.041	0.555±0.082	73	0.524±0.060	ND
29	0.475±0.009	0.167±0.032	74	0.897±0.100	1.182±0.304
30	0.676±0.051	0.306±0.067	76	0.786±0.016	0.516±0.045
31	0.437±0.005	0.810±0.025	77	0.888±0.074	0.922±0.036
32	0.892±0.038	0.206±0.060	79	0.345±0.027	0.856±0.035
33	0.943±0.017	0.148±0.053	80	0.904±0.017	1.408±0.144
34	1.003±0.109	0.957±0.164	81	0.670±0.017	0.826±0.076
35	0.160±0.057	0.499±0.046	82	0.340±0.062	0.866±0.085
36	0.382±0.016	0.943±0.076	83	0.398±0.042	0.985±0.074
37	0.989±0.045	1.093±0.077	84	0.786±0.016	0.578±0.032
38	0.728±0.025	1.400±0.080	85	0.425±0.010	ND
39	0.224±0.055	1.306±0.080	86	0.212±0.007	0.777±0.060
40	0.752±0.067	0.970±0.136	87	0.322±0.061	0.671±0.016
41	0.699±0.018	0.506±0.052	89	1.013±0.117	0.926±0.103
42	0.556±0.019	1.043±0.228	90	0.408±0.091	0.950±0.176
43	0.238±0.013	0.928±0.155	91	0.649±0.062	0.946±0.066
44	0.389±0.029	1.012±0.147	92	0.891±0.016	0.966±0.117
45	0.894±0.084	1.184±0.065	93	0.574±0.084	1.054±0.056
46	0.785±0.089	1.320±0.077	94	0.218±0.057	0.658±0.035
47	0.476±0.011	1.382±0.120	95	0.609±0.055	1.053±0.127
48	0.528±0.033	0.857±0.106	96	0.438±0.055	1.462±0.250
Control sera ♀ (n=16)	0.570±0.045		Control sera ♂ (n=18)		0.780±0.194

Table 3. Results of the general population antibodies (IgG) against *Hyalomma lusitanicum* male and female antigens

4. Conclusion

Burgos is a province of the inner north western region of the Iberian Peninsula. Its climate is continental with cold dry winters and mild summers. Animal husbandry is a very important economical source and livestock parasitism of ticks is common in the region. *Hyalomma* spp. ticks are distributed in Africa, the Mediterranean climatic zone of southern Europe, and in Asia.

It is known that ticks are important pets and livestock transmitting tick-borrne diseases. In this sense, though humans are not the preferred hosts of *Hyalomma* ticks and are infrequently bitten in comparison to livestock, sporadic infection of people is usually caused by *Hyalomma* ticks.

In fact, Crimea-Congo Haemorrhagic Fever transmitted by *Hyalomma* spp occurs sporadically throughout many areas of Africa, Asia and Europe, but can cause mortality (Estrada-Peña & Jongejan., 1999). Recently a new group of spotted fever has been isolated from *Hyalomma marginatum marginatum* ticks in Morocco (Beati et al., 1997). In Europe have been detected genotipically similar organisms in Portugal (Beati et al., 1995), Croatia (Punda-Polic et al., 2002), Corsica (Matsumoto et al., 2004), Germany (Rumer et al., 2011) and in Spain (Fernández-Soto et al., 2003).

Hyalomma lusitanicum is called perinneal specie which is present on cattle year around. These parasitize domestic and wild animals and birds, and are usually abundant in semi-arid zones. Its distribution reflects peaks in May-June and October that corresponds to the periods of maximum activity of adults (Habela et al., 1999), but in winter specimens (males and females) remain fixed on their host without feeding (Yousfi-Monod & Aeschliman., 1986). Adult *Hyalomma* actively run out from their resting sites when a host approaches. Cattle, rabbits, hares and deer which are the hosts of *Hyalomma lusitanicum* are well represented in the studied region.

The frequency with which different tick species bite humans varies significantly from one zone to another and much it depends on the likelihood of humans entering their biotope (human contact with ticks for professional and recreational activities) and the tick affinity for humans. Climatic changes could be probable implicated in the northern establishment of ticks, but perhaps would be more dependent on the introduction of adult females on wild and domestic ruminants due to the uncontrolled movement of livestock as have been proposed recently Rumer et al., (2011) in which the only documented *Hyalomma* spp. tick in Germany was found on a human in the southern part of the country (Lake Constance area) in May 2006, but they did not ruled out the tick transportation from Spain.

However it is not easy to detect that a person has been bitten by a tick, because people may confuse the bite ticks or other arthropods that might be no elicit antibody response.

Ticks can inoculate a variety of active molecules during feeding that can block pain, reduce inflammation and suppress or modulate innate and specific acquired immune defences (Brossard & Wikel., 2004). But the duration of the tick attachment may be insufficient to allow for adequate amount of saliva to elicit a detectable antibody response. Sometimes happens that is necessary several tick exposures before the antibody response will be strongly enough to be detected by ELISA. Ticks deposit saliva at the site of their attachment to a host in order to inhibit haemostasis, inflammation and innate and adaptive immune responses but ticks are able to modulate their host's local haemostatic reactions (Carvalho et al., 2010)

As happens with other ticks in which salivary gland proteins are immunogenic (Sanders et al., 1996), our results have shown that *H. lusitanicum* has proteins (antigens) that stimulate the production of immunoglobulins in humans as well as the finding of a significant high prevalence in bitten patients by ticks respect to the control group (see in Tables 1 and 2). It would be very interesting to conduct an epidemiological study, in those sera that have positive results, if at any time have had a history of febrile illness of unknown etiology with or without rash.

As occurs with other genus or species of ticks capable to induce high responses, *H. lusitanicum* could share antigens with other ticks. It is easy to found that antigens can cross react with the antigens of a closely related species. This fact has been observed in several studies that have realized cross-resistance studies between *Dermacentor andersoni* and *Dermacentor variabilis* (McTier et al., 1981), *Hyalomma anatolicum anatolicum* and *Boophilus microplus* (Parmar et al., 1996), *H. a. anatolicum, Hyalomma dromedari* and *Boophilus microplus* (Kumar & Kondal., 1999) as well as between a series of other tick species (Brown & Askenase., 1984; Jaansen van Vuuren et al., 1992). In fact, the homology among several tick species suggests that possibly common antigen(s) may be suitable for a vaccine against some different ticks.

By other hand, though ticks are well known blood suckers, blood sources between males and females seem to be different and gene expressions in fedding males and females are also different (Aljamali et al., 2009). In fact the male blood meals may be digested and nutrients can be used for spermatogenesis. The host blood meal is necessary for egg production in female ticks (Sanders et al., 1996). As occurs with partially fed female *Ixodes ricinus* (Linnaeus, 1758), female and male *Amblyomma variegatum* (Fabricius, 1794) and *Rhipicephalus appendiculatus* Neumann, 1901 in which have been observed that exist species- and sex-specific differences in the effects of tick salivary gland antigens on human lymphocyte proliferation, our results, as can be seen in Table III, have demonstrated that exist differences in the human antibodies response against male and female *H. lusitanicum* antigens. This fact makes that both could be considered as susceptible to bite humans.

Since for each tick-borne disease there may be one or several vectors (Lane, 1994), perhaps this ixodid could be implicated as a vector susceptible of parasitizing humans. In this sense, other studies would in a future provide us about the frequency and which life cycle stages of this tick can infest humans as well as its role in the transmission of human pathogens as happened with those studies in which *Dermacentor marginatus* was recently demonstrated to be the vector in the transmission of *Rickettsia slovaca*, that causes the TIBOLA/DEBONEL disease in humans (Rehacek, 1984; Lakos., 1997; Raoult et al., 1997; Ibarra et al., 2006).

Until date, each tick species has preferred environmental conditions and biotopes that determine the geographical distribution of the ticks and the risk areas fro tick borne diseases, but day to day more research studies are going on in order to elucidate a higher diversity of ixodid tick species infesting humans potentially transmisors of underdiagnosed diseases.

In this sense, we consider it would be very interesting to educate primary care physicians in these areas, to be able to identify ticks and how clinicians should deal with patients who have been bitten by ticks, because it would be very interesting to discover potential transmitters of both old and new diseases. It is necessary to develop studies in which ticks removed from the patients must be directly preserved in ethanol and identified because the knowledge about tick species that are susceptible of parasitizing humans is essential for assessing the risks for people who become infected, we can detect pathogens and design measures to prevent infection.

5. Acknowledgment

We want to give thanks to Helga Barrios Vidal and Gema Cervantes Uría for their grateful help in developing this study.

6. References

Aljamali ,M.N.; Ramakrishnan, V.G.; Weng, H.; Tucker, J.S.; Sauer, J.R & Essenberg R.C. (2009). Microarray analysis of gene expression changes in feeding female and male lone star ticks, *Amblyomma americanum* (L). *Archieves of Insect Biochemistry and Physiology*, Vol. 71, N° 4 (August), pp. 236-253, ISSN 0739-4462.

Barandika, J.F.; Berriatua, E.; Barral, M.; Juste, R.A.; Anda, P & García-Pérez, A.L. (2006). Risk factors associated with ixodid ticks species distributions in the Basque region in Spain. *Medical and Veterinary Entomology*, Vol. 20, N° 2 (June), pp 177-188, ISSN 0269-283X.

Beati, L.; Kelly, P.J.; Matthewman, L.A.; Mason, P.R. & Raoult, D. (1995). Prevalence of rickettsia-like organisms and spotted fever group rickettsiae inticks (*Acari: Ixodidae*) from Zimbabwe. *Journal of Medical Entomology*, Vol. 32, N° 6 (November), pp. 787-792, ISSN 0022-2585.

Beati, L.; Meskini, M.; Thiers, B. & Raoult, D. (1997). *Rickettsia aeschlimannii* sp. nov., a new spotted fever group rickettsia associated with *Hyalomma marginatum ticks*. *International Journal of Systematic Bacteriology*, Vol. 47, N° 2 (April), pp. 548-554, ISSN 0020-7713.

Bengis, R.G.; Leighton, F,A.; Fischer, J.R.; Artois, M.; Mörner, T.& Tate, C.M. (2004). The role of wildlife in emerging and re-emerging zoonoses. *Revue Scientifique Technique (International Office of Epizootics)*, Vol. 23, N° 2, pp. 497-511, ISSN 0253-1933.

Blancou, J.; Chomel, B.B.; Belotto, A. & Meslin, F.X. (2005). Emerging or re-emerging bacterial zoonoses: facts of emergence, surveillance and control. *Veterinary Research*, Vol. 36, pp. 507-522, ISSN 0928-4249.

Bradford, M. (1976). A rapid and sensitive method for the quantitation of microgram of protein-dye binding. *Analytical Biochemistry*, Vol. 72, N° 1-2 (May), pp. 248-254, ISSN 0003-2697.

Briones, V.; Téllez, S.; Ballesteros, C.; González, S.; Bordes, I.; Domínguez L *et al.* (2002). Enfermedades transmisibles de los mamíferos silvestres. *Quercus*, Vol. 198, pp. 22-27, ISSN 0212-0054.

Brossard, M. & Wikel, S. K. (2004). Tick immunobiology. *Parasitology*, Vol. 129, Suppl 1, pp. 161-176, ISSN 0031-1820.

Brown, S.J & Askenase, P.W. (1984). Analysis of host components mediating immune resistance to ticks, p.1040-1050. In: D. A Griffiths and C. E Browman (eds). *Acarology VI*, Vol 2. Ellis Horwood, Chichester, ISBN 9780130054890.

Bueno, R; Moreno, J.; Oltra, M.T. & Jiménez, R. (2009). Artrópodos con interés vectorial en la salud pública en España. *Revista Española de Salud Pública*, Vol. 83, N° 2, pp. 201-214, ISSN: 2173-9110 .

Carvalho, W. A.; Maruyama, S. R.; Franzin, A. M.; Abatepaulo, A. R.; Anderson, J.M.; Ferreira, B. R.; Ribeiro, J.M.; Moré, D.D.; Augusto Mendes Maia, A.; Valenzuela, J. G.; Garcia, G. R. & de Miranda Santos, I. K. (2010). *Rhipicephalus* (Boophilus) *microplus*: clotting time in tick-infested skin varies according to local inflammation and gene expression patterns in tick salivary glands. *Experimental Parasitology*, Vol. 124, N° 4 (April), pp. 428-435, ISSN 0014-4894.

Chomel, B. (1998). New emerging zoonoses: a challenge and an opportunity for the veterinary profession. *Comparative Immunology, Microbiology and Infectious Diseases*, Vol. 21, N° 1 (March), pp. 1-14, ISSN 0147-9571.

Cleaveland, S.; Laurenso, M. K. & Taylor, H. (2001). Diseases of human and their domestic mammals: pathogen characteristics, host range and the risk of emergence. *Philosophical Transactionc Royal Society Londondon. Series B, Biological Sciences.*, Vol. 356, N° 1411 (July), pp. 991-999, ISSN 0080-4622.

Cordero del Campillo, M.; Castañón Ordóñez, L. & Reguera Feo, A. (1994). *Índice-Catálogo de Zooparásitos Ibéricos*,   p. 650.   Universidad de León, Spain,   ISBN 9788477194033, León.

Cunningham, A.A. (2005). A walk on the wild side emerging wildlife diseases. *British Medical Journal*, Vol. 331, N° 7527 (November), pp. 1214-1215, ISSN 2007-9999.

Daszak, P.; Cunningham, A. A. & Hyatt, A. D. (2000). Emerging infectious diseases of wildlife threats to biodiversity and human   health. *Science*, Vol. 287, N° 5452 (January), pp. 443-449, ISSN 0036-8075.

Daszak, P. & Cunningham, A. A. (2003). Anthropogenic change, biodiversity loss, and a new agenda for emerging diseases. *Journal of Parasitology*, Vol. 89 Suppl (April), pp. 37-41, ISSN 0022-3395.

Domínguez, G. (2004). North Spain (Burgos) wild mammals ectoparasites. *Parasite*, Vol. 11, pp. 262-272, ISSN 1776-1042.

Encinas-Grandes, A. (1986). Ticks of the province of Salamanca (Central/NW/Spain). Prevalence and parasitization Intensity in dogs and domestic ungulates. *Annales de Parasitologie Humaine et Comparée*, Vol. 61, N°1 (January), pp. 95-107, ISSN 0003-4150.

Encinas, A.; Oleaga, A. & Pérez, R. (1999). Garrapatas duras. En: Cordero del Campillo *et al.*, editores. *Parasitología Veterinaria.*, McGraw-Hill Interamericana; pp. 420-429, ISBN 9788448602369, Madrid.

Estrada-Peña, A. & Jongejan, F. (1999). Ticks feeding on humans: a review of records on human biting *Ixodoidea* with special reference to pathogen transmission. *Experimental and Applied Acarology*, Vol. 23, N° 9 (September), pp. 685-715, ISSN 0168-8162.

Fernández-Soto, P.; Encinas-Grandes, A. & Pérez-Sánchez, R. (2003). *Rickettsia aeschlimannii* in Spain: molecular evidence in *Hyalomma marginatum* and five other tick species that feed on humans. *Emerging and Infectious Diseases*, Vol. 9, N° 7 (July), pp. 889-890, ISSN 1080-6040.

Gibbs, E. P.J. (2005). Emerging zoonotic epidemics in the interconnected global community. *Veterinary Records*, Vol. 26, N° 22 (November), pp. 673-679, ISSN 0042-4900.

Giménez-Pardo, C. & Martínez-Grueiro, M. M. (2008). Some hydrolase activities from the tick *Hyalomma lusitanicum* Koch, 1844 (*Ixodoidea: Ixodida*). *Parasite*, Vol. 15, N° 4 (December), pp. 589-593, ISSN 1776-1042.

Gortázar, C.; Ferroglio, E.; Höfle, U.; Frölich, K.; Vicente, J. (2007). Diseases shared between wildlife and livestock: a European perspective. *European Journal of Wildlife Research*, Vol. 53, N° 4 (April), pp. 241-256, ISSN 1612-4642.

Habela, M.; Rol, J. A.; Antón, J. M.; Pena, J.; Cordero, E.; van Ham, I. & Jorge, E. (1999). Epidemiology of mediterranean theileriosis in Extremadura region, Spain. *Parassitologia*, Vol. 41, Suppl 1 (September), pp. 47-51, ISSN 0048-2951.

Hillyard, P. D. (1996). Ticks of north-west Europe. Synopses of the British fauna. Ed. Barnes KRS & Crothers JH: The Linnean Society of London and the Estuarine and Coastal Sciences Association, ISBN 978-1851532575, London.

Ibarra, V.; Oteo, J. A.; Portillo, A, Santibáñez, S.; Blanco, J. R.; Metola, L.; Eiros, J. M.; . &, Sanz, M. (2006). *Rickettsia slovaca* infection: DEBONEL/TIBOLA. *Annals of the New York Academy of Science.* Vol. 1078 (October), pp. 206-214, ISSN 0077-8923.

Jansen van Vuuren, A.M.; Crause, J.C.; Vershoor, J.A.; Spickett, A.M. & Neitz, A.N. (1992). The identification of a shared immunogen present in the salivary glands and gut of ixodid and argasid ticks. *Experimental and Applied Acarology* Vol. 15, N° 3, pp. 205-210, ISSN 0168-8162.

Kaufman W. (1989). Tick-host interaction: A synthesis of current concepts *Parasitology Today* Vol. 5, N° 2, pp. 47-56. ISSN 0169-4758.

Kettle, D.S. (1995). Medical and veterinary entomology. 2th ed. Cambridge: CAB International, ISBN : 0-851-98968-3.

Kolonin, G.V. (2009). Fauna of Ixodid ticks of the world (*Acari, Ixodidae*). Moscow, ISSN 0132-8077.

Kumar, S. & Kondal, J.K. (1999): Lack of immunological cross-reactivity of 36 kDa secretory salivary glands antigen of *Hyalomma anatolicum anatolicum* with *Hyalomma dromedary* and *Boophilus microplus* ticks. *Zentralblatt für Veterinärmedizin. Reihe* B. Vol. 46, N° 6 (august), pp. 405-410, ISSN 0514-7166.

Lane, S. L. (1994). Competence of ticks as vectors of microbial agents with an emphasis on *Borrellia burgdorferi*, p. 45-67. In: Sonen Shine, DE, Mather, TN. (eds), *Ecological dynamics of tick-borne zoonoses*, Oxford University Press, ISBN 978-0195073133, New York.

Lakos, A. (1997). Tick-borne lymphadenopathy, a new rickettsial disease. *The Lancet*. Vol. 350, N° 4 (October), pp. 1006, ISSN 0140-6736.

Lindgren, E.; Talleklint, L.; Polfeldt, T. (2000). Impact of climate change on the northern latitude limit and population density of the disease transmitting European tick *Ixodes ricinus*. *Environmental Health Perspectives*, Vol. 108, N° 2 (February), pp. 119-123, ISSN 0091-6765.

Lledó, L.; Giménez-Pardo, C.; Domínguez-Peñafiel, G; Sousa, R.; Gegundez-Cámara, M.I.; Casado, N. & Criado-Fornelio, A. (2010). Molecular detection of Hemoprotozoa and *Rickettsiae* sp in arthropods from wild animals in the Burgos province, Spain. *Vector-Borne and Zoonotic Diseases*, Vol. 10, N° 8 (October), pp. 735-738, ISSN 1530-3667.

López-Vélez, R. & Molina, R. (2005). Cambio climático en España y riesgo de enfermedades infecciosas y parasitarias transmitidas por artrópodos y roedores. *Revista Española de Salud Pública*, Vol. 79, N° 2, pp. 177-190, ISSN 1135-5727.

Matsumoto, K.; Parola, P.; Brouqui, P. & Raoult,D. (2004). *Rickettsia aeschlimannii* in *Hyalomma* ticks from Corsica. *European Journal of Clinical Microbiology and Infectious Diseases*, Vol. 23, N° 9 (August), pp. 732-734, ISSN 0934-9723.

McTier, T.L.; George, T.E. & Benett, S.N. (1981). Resistance and cross-resistance of guinea pigs to *Dermacentor andersoni* Stiles, *D. variabilis* (Say), *Amblyomma americanum* (Linnaeus) and *Ixodes scapularis* (Say). *Journal of Parasitology*, Vol. 67, N° 6 (December), pp. 813-832, ISSN: 1937-2345.

Morse, S. S. (1995). Factors in the emergence of infectious diseases. *Emerging Infectious Diseases*, Vol. 1, No. 1 (January-March), pp. 7-15, ISSN 1080-6040.

Parmar, A.; Grewal A.S. & Dhillon P. (1996). Immunological cross-reactivity between salivary gland proteins of *Hyalomma anatolicum anatolicum* and *Boophilus microplus* ticks. *Veterinary Immunology and Immunopathology*, Vol.1, N° 3-4 (June), pp. 345-352, ISSN 0165-2427.

Pérez-Sánchez, R.; Oleaga-Pérez, A. & Encinas-Grandes, A. (1992). Analysis of the specificity of the salivary antigens of *Ornithodoros erraticus* for the purpose of serological detection of swine farms harbouring the parasite. *Parasite Immunology*, Vol. 14, N° 2 (March), pp. 201-216, ISSN 0141-9838.

Punda-Polic, V.; Petrovec, M.; Trilar, T.; Duh, D.; Bradaric, N.; Klismanic, Z. & Basic-Zupanc, T. (2002). Detection and identification of spotted fever group rickettsiae in ticks collected in southern Croatia. *Experimental and Applied Acarology*, Vol. 28, N° 1-4, pp. 169-176, ISSN 0168-8162.

Raoult, D.; Berbis, P.; Roux, V.; Xu, W. & Maurin, M. (1997). A new tick-transmitted disease due to *Rickettsia slovaca*. *The Lancet*, Vol. 350, N° 12 (July), pp. 112-113, ISSN 0140-6736.

Rehacek, J. (1984).   *Rickettsia slovaca*, the organism and its ecology. *Acta Scientiarum Naturalium Academiae Scientiarum Bohemoslovacae* ,Vol. 18, No 2 pp. 1-50, ISSN 0032-8758.

Rolníková, T.; Kazimírová, M.; Buc, M. (2003). Modulation of human lymphocyte proliferation by salivary gland extracts of ixodid ticks (*Acari: Ixodidae*): effect of feeding stage and sex. *Folia Parasitologica*, Vol. 50, N° 4, pp. 305-12, ISSN 0015-5683.

Román, J; Román, L.; Ansola, L.M;, Palma, C. & Ventosa, R. (1996). Atlas de las aves nidificantes en la provincia de Burgos. Ed. Aldecoa,   ISBN 978-84-7009-485-9, Burgos.

Rumer, L.; Graser, E.; Hillebrand, T.; Talaska, T.; Dautel, H.; Mediannikov, O.; Roy-Chowdhury, P.; Sheshukova, O.; Donoso Mantke, O. & Niedrig, M. (2011). *Rickettsia aeschlimannii* in *Hyalomma marginatum* ticks, Germany. *Emerging Infectious Diseases* , Vol. 17, N° 2 (February), pp. 325-325, ISSN 1080-6040.

Sanders, M,L.; Scott, A. L.; Glass, G.E. & Schwartz, B.S. (1996). Salivary gland changes and host antibody responses associated with feeding of male lone star ticks (*Acari:Ixodidae*). *Journal of Medical Entomology*, Vol. 33, N° 4 (July), pp. 628-34, ISSN: 0022-2585.

Sauer, J.R.; McSwain, J.L.; Bowman, A.S. &. Essenberg, R.C. (1995). Tick salivary gland physiology. *Annual Review of Entomology*, Vol. 40, (January), pp. 245-267, ISSN: 0066-4170.

Simpson, V. R. (2002). Wild animals as reservoirs of infectious diseases in the UK. *The Veterinary Journal*, Vol. 163, N° 2 (March), pp. 128-146, ISSN: 1090-0233.

Sonenshine, D.; Lane, R. S. & Nicholson, W. L. (2002). Ticks (Ixodida). In: Mullen G & Durden L, editors. *Medical and Veterinary Entomology*, Elsevier Science, pp. 517-557, ISBN 978-0125104517, Orlando.

Toledo, A.; Olmeda, S.; Escudero, R.; Jado,I.; Valcárcel, F.; Casado-Nistal,M.; Rodríguez-Vargas, M.; Gil, H. & Anda, P. (2009). Tick-borne zoonotic bacteria in ticks collected from central Spain. *American Journal of Tropical Medicine and Hygiene*, Vol. 81, N° 1 (July), pp. 67-74, ISSN 0002-9637.

Valenzuela, J. G.(2004). Exploring tick saliva: from biochemistryto"sialomes" and functional genomics. *Parasitology*. Vol. 129, Suppl, pp. S83-S94, ISSN 0031-1820.

Viseras, J. & García-Fernández, P. (1999). Studies on theileriosis in Southern Spain. *Parassitologia*, Vol. 41, Suppl 1 (September),   pp. 111-115,   ISSN 0048-2951.

Wall, R. &   Shearer, D. (1997). *Veterinary Entomology: Arthropods Ectoparasites of Veterinary importance*. 1th edition, Chapman & Hall, ISBN 978-0412615108, London.

Wall, R. (2007).   Ectoparasites: Future challenges in a changing world. *Veterinary Parasitology*, Vol. 148, N° 1 (August), pp. 62-74, ISSN 0304-4017.

Yousfi-Monod, R. & Aeschlimann, A. (1986). Studies on ticks (Acarina: Ixodidae), parasites of cattle in west Algeria. I. Systematic survey and seasonal activity. *Annales de parasitologie humaine et comparee*, Vol. 61, N° 3, pp. 341-358, ISSN 0003-4150.

Zeier, M.; Handermann, M.; Bahr, U.; Rensch, B.; Müller, S.; Kehm, R, et al. (2005). New ecological aspect of hantavirus infection: A change of paradigm and challenge of prevention. *Virus Genes*, Vol. 3, N° 2 (March), pp. 157-180, ISSN 0920-8569.

7

Current Advances in Computational Strategies for Drug Discovery in Leishmaniasis

Andrés F. Flórez[1,2], Stanley Watowich[3] and Carlos Muskus[2]
[1]German Cancer Research Center (DKFZ)/ Division Theoretical
Systems Biology, Heidelberg
[2]Universidad de Antioquia/Programa de Estudio y Control de
Enfermedades Tropicales – PECET, Medellín
[3]University of Texas Medical Branch/Department of Biochemistry and Molecular Biology
and the Sealy Center for Structural Biology and Molecular Biophysics, Galveston
[1]Germany
[2]Colombia
[3]USA

1. Introduction

Leishmaniasis is a complex disease caused by several species of the *Leishmania* genus ranging in severity from cutaneous and mucocutaneous lesions to the chronic visceral form that if untreated adequately can cause death. It has a worldwide distribution in 98 countries and 85 out of 98 are developing or poor countries. One of the main problems in leishmaniasis is the limited number of drug options along with the adverse effects they can cause including death (Ahasan., et al. 1996; Sundar & Chakravarty 2010; Oliveira., et al. 2011). In addition, there are reports of treatment failures due to increased parasite resistance to the first drug of choice, the antimonials (Faraut-Gambarelli., et al. 1997; Goyeneche-Patino., et al. 2008). Second-choice drugs, such as amphotericin B, pentamidine, paromomycin, and more recently, miltefosine, have also toxic effects that require hospital management (Maltezou 2008; Oliveira., et al. 2011). Miltefosine, the only oral administered drug for leishmaniasis, has not been tested in many *Leishmania* species. Recently, a central nervous system toxicity was reported for liposomal amphotericin B therapy used to treat cutaneous leishmaniasis (Glasser & Murray 2011).

In the search for new drug targets in *Leishmania*, a group of proteins have been proposed based mainly on their known function, the expression level, and localization, or because they are involved in important metabolic processes in the parasite. Topoisomerases (Das., et al. 2008), kinases (de Azevedo & Soares 2009), proteins localized or targeted to lysosomes (Carrero-Lerida., et al. 2009) are some potential *Leishmania* drug targets. However, none of these protein targets have been used to successfully develop new drugs that can substitute the existing therapies.

Currently, the massive genome sequencing of many medically important microorganisms together with protein structure and drug databases and the development of new computational tools, will allow molecular targets and new drugs to be searched in a more rigorous manner. Three *Leishmania* genomes, *L. major*, *L. infantum* and *L. braziliensis*

(Peacock., et al. 2007) have been sequenced and annotated and a fourth species, *L. mexicana* and some *L. major* strains are in the process of being sequenced (GeneDB, http://www.genedb.org; University of Washington Genome Sequencing Center, http://genome.wustl.edu/gsc/gschmpg.html). The availability of these genomes and the annotated proteins can be used in a rational manner to predict novel drug targets and provide a basis to develop new drugs.

The computational prediction of drugs, in addition to the evaluation of drugs already synthesized and used in other diseases, must be coupled with automated in vitro assessment methodologies of these compounds. In this sense and in the case of *Leishmania*, the use of GFP (Varela., et al. 2009) or luciferase transgenic parasites (Lang., et al. 2005) coupled with techniques such as flow cytometry or fluorometry can be used to rapidly evaluate potential anti-leishmanial drugs. The WHO program for training in tropical diseases research has created a network based on reporter gene technology to foster the process of drug search not only against leishmaniasis but also against other diseases with limited therapeutic options.

2. Selection of drug targets

An initial step in the drug discovery process involves the search and selection of the drug target. This target is frequently a protein that is essential for the organism survival or critical for regulating a particular signaling pathway. In the specific case of parasites, the protein target when inhibited should impair or delay parasite viability. The classical approach of finding a new essential protein that can act as a potential target is the experimental characterization by using gene knockout or knock-down strategies in the target organism. Besides essentiality, some targets are selected for being specific for the pathogen; for example, the ergosterol pathway is present in fungi and *Leishmania spp*, but humans only contain the required enzymes for the synthesis of cholesterol. This is the reason why this pathway has been exploited for searching drugs against mycotic pathogens and also *Leishmania*. However, the experimental approach employing interference RNA (RNAi) is not feasible given *Leishmania* species do not carry the machinery for RNAi (Peacock., et al. 2007), with the exception of *Leishmania braziliensis* where some RNAi-associated genes have been found. In addition, depending on the parasite stage the essentiality of a particular protein could change dramatically. With all these constraints, a rational alternative for choosing effective targets is a more systematic study of the biology of the parasite, with the aim of uncovering important mechanisms that are not evident by studying descriptively isolated proteins. A starting point for this "systems view" of the parasite biology in the case of *Leishmania*, was the sequencing of its genome in 2005 (Ivens., et al. 2005). Since then, more high-throughput data have been generated, not at the same rate as other organisms but with important applications for drug discovery in tropical diseases. This leads to an important issue of data analysis, where computational tools can have a role in reducing the ocean of possibilities of finding a drug for this disease, making more efficient and less costly the experimental setup. In the following sections, we will describe the current computational methods that can be applied to find new drug targets, with special application to the *Leishmania* parasite.

2.1 Selection of targets by homology searching

The simplest approach for finding a drug target is the homology search of essential proteins. There are several organisms with available essential data at genome-wide level (Forsyth., et al. 2002; Kamath., et al. 2003; Hu., et al. 2007). In model organisms such as yeast, the phenotypic effects of deletion of particular genes have been shown (Giaever., et al. 2002) and more recently the study of genetic interactions on a large scale (Costanzo., et al. 2010). This has been used to elucidate redundancy and possibly some synergistic effects among genes. Therefore, it is possible to find orthologs in the organism of interest that could be essential by comparing its sequences against the list of essential genes in model organisms. The Database of Essential Genes (http://tubic.tju.edu.cn/deg/) (Zhang & Lin 2009) provides information of essential genes in prokaryotes and eukaryotes, and it is also possible to do a BLAST search with the protein of interest. This resource is useful for an exploratory search of essentiality of a particular protein. Another important resource, for drug target data, is the DrugBank database (http://www.drugbank.ca/) (Knox., et al. 2011), which can be used to extract drug-target interactions along with additional pharmacological data. The same strategy can be employed in this case; with the advantage that the homology search will also return possible drug candidates that can be tested on the protein found to have homology to the target in DrugBank.

This methodology has been applied in *Pseudomonas aeruginosa* (Sakharkar., et al. 2004) with the aim of detecting new drug targets, given this bacterium is an important problem in nosocomial settings due to the rapid generation of resistance. In *Leishmania,* drug targets can be also identified by this approach. Tools like BLAST or PSI-BLAST can be employed, with PSI-BLAST being more sensitive for detecting distant relationships among proteins (Altschul., et al. 1997). However, some false positives still can occur due to alignments that are optimal according to the algorithm but not biologically meaningful. The E value helps to detect those alignments that are significant. As an example, running a PSI-BLAST search with the *Leishmania major* proteome against the DrugBank database, one can find among the potential *Leishmania* orthologs to known targets, the protein *LmjF36.2430,* which is similar to the sterol 14- alpha demethylase in fungi. Drugs such as miconazole are known inhibitors of this enzyme. Interestingly, the protein *LmjF19.0450* belongs to the group of protein kinases conserved in other *Leishmania* species; it is constitutively expressed and has significant similarity to other kinase targets in cancer. These are simple cases of how a homology search can generate a list of potential drug targets using existing genomic data. The main advantage of this methodology is that it offers a quick overview of potential targets and second use of drugs. In addition, the STITCH 2 database (http://stitch.embl.de/) (Kuhn., et al. 2010) compiles known and predicted drug-target relationships jointly with biological information about targets in a network-based view.

Despite its simplicity, the homology search strategy has some caveats. Proteins inside the cell perform specific functions depending on their interactions, and these interactions can vary between species. Even if sequences are highly related, pathway conservation is not necessarily present. In addition, temporal regulation is important, as not all the interactions are active at the same time, which can further complicate the analysis. These problems highlight the importance of detecting targets by incorporating more detailed information about the molecular interactions.

2.2 Selection of targets by topological analysis of protein networks

In order to better understand complex pathogens such as *Leishmania* and to improve the efficiency of the drug discovery process, it is crucial to gain deeper knowledge about how protein interactions are established and how these interactions are regulated. This is a central issue for a more accurate definition of essentiality and biological robustness. These interactions can be described as a *network*, a representation commonly used to describe complex systems. The protein interaction network (interactome) describes all possible molecular interactions among proteins. The interactome is composed of *nodes* that represent the molecular components, in this case proteins, and *edges,* that are the interactions between components (Fig. 1). Depending on the biological function of the node, other types of networks can also be constructed; for example, gene networks involving transcription factors as nodes that regulate other genes by binding (edges) and metabolic networks where the nodes are the enzymes connected by the production of some metabolites. The study of networks comes from a mathematical discipline called *graph theory,* and the analysis of the interaction patterns in the network is defined as *network topology.*(Barabasi & Oltvai 2004)

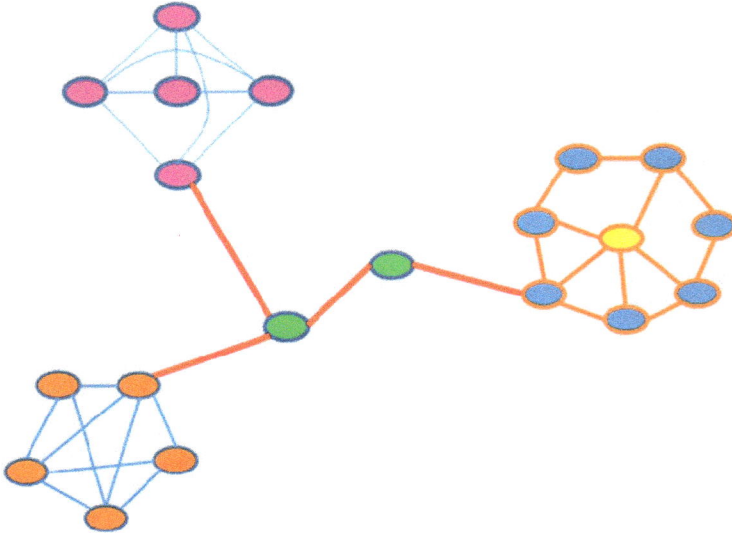

Fig. 1. Schematic representation of a protein network. Yellow circle corresponds to a hub protein, green circles correspond to bottleneck proteins connecting several sub-networks. Lines connecting circles represent the edges of the network.

To detect protein interactions in biological systems, large-scale methods have been developed that can map all possible pairwise interactions. Yeast two-hybrid is a popular technique of this kind, which was used to construct the first interactome (Uetz., et al. 2000). The technique involves the fusion of a protein with a transcription factor DNA-binding domain subunit. This protein is called the *bait.* The second protein is fused onto an activator domain subunit and it is called the *prey.* If the interaction between the bait and the prey is present, the two transcription factor subunits will come closer and the expression of the reporter gene is activated (Osman 2004). The most important limitation of this method is the presence of high number of false positives. However recent evidence has shown that a combination of experimental methods will reduce the number of false interactions (Dreze., et al. 2010).

The initial studies of the yeast interactome revealed that the network structure was not organized randomly, and in fact the organization pattern was similar to other experimentally-observed networks. This particular network structure was called *scale-free* and it was elucidated by analyzing the number of interactions (or degree distribution) of proteins in the yeast interactome, showing that some nodes were more highly connected than others, and those nodes were in relatively low frequency in the network. This scale-free structure followed a *power law* distribution for the node degree and it described the probability of a node having a certain degree. An interesting consequence of having a scale-free structure is that the network was robust against random deletion of nodes, but susceptible to the deletion of highly connected nodes or *hubs* (Jeong., et al. 2001). The hubs can be detected by measuring the connectivity or degree of the network. In addition, the scale-free network was also susceptible to deletion of other types of nodes that were not highly connected but control the flux of the network; these nodes were called *bottlenecks* (Yu., et al. 2007). A classical example of bottleneck nodes is the scaffold proteins (Good., et al. 2011); these proteins facilitate the communication between signalling pathways very efficiently, although sometimes they are not highly connected. Deleting a bottleneck node will disrupt cellular homeostasis by destroying communication between processes in the cell. This network biology approach becomes an important step in a systems level understanding of the biology of parasites like *Leishmania*, and it becomes very useful for detecting essential nodes that may constitute potential new drug targets.

2.2.1 Construction of the *Leishmania* protein interaction network

The analysis of the *Leishmania* protein network could lead to the discovery of new and effective drug targets. However, current protein interaction data in *Leishmania* have only focused on a few specific proteins, and at this time, no yeast two-hybrid data is available for this organism. Despite this limitation, the use of a computationally-predicted protein network from orthology-based methods is a good first step for the exploration of drug targets that may be more informative than a traditional homology search. The results described in the next section will focus on the current status of the predicted *Leishmania major* interactome and will give some directions for future experimental studies for network and target validation.

Even when protein domain sequences are conserved, multiple combinations of these domains enable an organism to rewire the interactome in different ways. This can overcome the problem of the context of the targets that influence essentiality and enable new hubs or protein targets to be detected. A common disadvantage is the bias towards detection of conserved interactions, which could be a caveat in the case of organism-specific interactions that may also be important for survival. These specific interactions will be only detected when more data becomes available, which will also allow existent predictions to be validated.

In our recent study (Florez., et al. 2010), the protein interaction network in *Leishmania major* was predicted using only the parasite protein sequences and several protein interaction databases, in particular iPfam (Finn., et al. 2005), PSIMAP (Park., et al. 2005) and PEIMAP. These databases included protein-protein interactions defined by analysis of structures of protein complexes and experimental data extracted from literature, including high-throughput experiments. From the structures, the analysis of interacting structural domains was mapped to the sequence, using the domain definition by Pfam (Finn., et al. 2006) and SCOP (Hubbard., et al. 1997). These two databases contained information of domains with a systematic classification for protein families. In this particular case the physical distance between adjacent domains within a complex was used as the criteria for the definition of interaction and it was stored in iPfam and PSIMAP databases. This strategy has been used in other organisms such as fungi and bacteria (He., et al. 2008; Kim., et al. 2008). The domain interaction analysis generated more diversity in the detection of possible interactions because modular exchange of protein domains allowed rewiring the network even if the isolated sequence of the domain was conserved. However, despite the high accuracy of this method, the prediction of protein interactions was limited as there was not an abundance of crystallized protein complexes. The PEIMAP database was also used, and it included sequences of protein interaction pairs detected by several methods, including co-immunoprecipitation (co-IP) and yeast two-hybrid.

To construct the *Leishmania major* network, protein sequences were extracted from the GeneDB database. This database included genomic and proteomic information of pathogens, including protozoan parasites. The protein sequences were aligned to the interacting domain pairs using PSI-BLAST against the SCOP 1.71 database with an E-value cutoff of 0.0001, as described previously (Kim., et al. 2008). The PSI-BLAST tool was used for the alignments because it had the advantage of detecting small conserved sequences, such as small domains that would be otherwise missed by using the standard BLASTP. The same strategy was applied for the alignments concerning the iPfam database. In this case, the domain assignment for the *Leishmania* proteins was carried out using the Pfam database (release 18.0) with the hmmpfam tool employed for the alignments. The final set of predicted interactions was carried out by homology search over the PEIMAP database using BLASTP, with a minimal cutoff of 40% sequence identity and 70% length coverage. The PEIMAP database included protein-protein interaction (PPI) information from six source databases: DIP (Xenarios., et al. 2000), BIND (Bader., et al. 2001), IntAct (Hermjakob., et al. 2004), MINT (Zanzoni., et al. 2002), HPRD(Peri., et al. 2004), and BioGrid (Stark., et al. 2006).

2.2.2 Filtering interactions by using a combined confidence score

As discussed earlier, the reliability of this analysis and its bias to certain types of protein interactions was dependent on the experimental method employed. Therefore, it was necessary to combine results from different databases to increase the coverage and the confidence of the predicted interactions. In the *Leishmania major* interactome, we used a simple scoring system to identify high confidence interactions. A previous study classified the experimental methods according to their reliability (Chua., et al. 2006), and we used this data in addition to the significance of the sequence alignments to calculate the confidence of the interactions. This scoring system was called the 'combined score' method, and it was applied for the confidence calculations in the STRING database (von Mering., et al. 2005). This database is useful for searching predicted protein interactions detected by other methods, although the definitions are beyond the scope of this chapter.

The score was calculated according to the formula (1):

$$score = 1 - \prod_{i \in E}(1 - R_i)^n \tag{1}$$

where *score* was the confidence value ranging from 0-1 with 1 equals to 100% accuracy, *E* was the set of methods under analysis (PEIMAP, PSIMAP, iPfam); R_i was the reliability of method *i*, and *n* was the number of interactions predicted by method *i*. The results of these calculations represented pairs of interactions with their respective confidence. With this information, it was possible to select those interactions that fulfilled a particular confidence threshold. In this case, a confidence score of 0.7 was chosen to select the core *Leishmania major* network. The threshold selection can vary depending on how strongly supported the interactions were required. For us, a 0.70 confidence value gave a smooth fit to the power law distribution and this was an important condition for reliable detection of hubs and bottlenecks.

2.2.3 Topological analysis of the network

Topological metrics such as clustering coefficient and mean shortest path help to describe global characteristics of the network. They measure the density of the connections within the network. Highly dense connected networks are characterized by modular components which also maintain the robustness of the network against failures. Biological networks tend to have a modular structure (Jeong., et al. 2001) and one additional way to test for reliability of the predicted network is by comparing the values of the clustering coefficient and mean shortest path to randomly generated networks with the same number of nodes and edges. These metrics should be statistically different between predicted and random networks. In the case of *Leishmania* network, 1,000 random networks were generated and the metrics calculated and compared to the original network.

The power law fitting for the definition of scale-free structure can be calculated using the plug-in Network Analyzer v.2.6.1(Assenov., et al. 2008) available in the platform Cytoscape (Shannon., et al. 2003). This platform includes a very advanced environment for network visualization and analysis. Network topology metrics, such as betweenness centrality, and connectivity were calculated using the Hubba server (http://hub.iis.sinica.edu.tw/ Hubbawebcite). (Lin., et al. 2008) A plug-in version of this tool in Cytoscape was recently made available. For the calculation of the metrics, the confidence scores of the interactions were used so the detection could be focused on the nodes most likely to be essential in the group of highly supported interactions. From this analysis, a potential list of targets was selected. However, it was possible that some proteins detected could also be conserved in terms of sequence and function among several organisms including humans. This becomes a problem if drugs targeting some of these proteins interfere with important biological process in humans, generating unwanted toxic effects. To avoid this, an additional filter was used for the list of predicted targets and it consisted of aligning the *Leishmania* proteins to the human proteins and excluding proteins that were conserved between these two species.

2.2.4 Prediction of protein function from network clusters

An important feature of network analysis was the prediction of protein function. The normal procedure for inferring function involved a homology search of the unknown protein versus a curated protein database such as UniProt (http://www.uniprot.org/). In some occasions, the detection of protein function was not feasible as significant similarity could not be found. When this approach failed, protein interaction network analysis helped to uncover potential functions. The prediction of protein function based on network analysis involved the assumption suggested by experimental data that interacting proteins tended to have related functions. This implied that it was possible to predict the function of neighboring nodes by clustering network modules and knowing the function of some of the nodes inside of the module. This analysis was carried out over the *Leishmania* network using the Markov Clustering (MCL) algorithm (Enright., et al. 2002) which has been demonstrated to be a robust and fast algorithm for detecting clusters or modules in protein networks (Brohee & van Helden 2006). The algorithm was implemented in the NeAT tool (Brohee., et al. 2008). For proteins of unknown function in the GeneDB database, we predicted their possible biological roles by evaluating the results of Gene Ontology terms for biological processes using the BinGO plug-in available in Cytoscape.

2.2.5 Selection of candidate drug targets from the network analysis

We constructed a protein-protein interaction (PPI) map, combining the results generated by PEIMAP, iPfam and PSIMAP (Fig. 2). The number of interactions detected for each database is described in (Table 1). By merging the data from the different approaches, bias to a specific class of interactions was avoided. The predicted network also contained isolated sub-networks which were difficult to analyze. These sub-networks appeared as a consequence of the inability to assign domains or from the lack of homology of those proteins to the known pairs of protein interactions. These sub-networks could be investigated by further experimental validation of the network. The total number of high confidence predicted interactions were 33,861 for 1,366 nodes

Number of Proteins	PEIMAP		PSIMAP		IPFAM	
8,335	Nodes	Edges	Nodes	Edges	Nodes	Edges
	718	14,839	3,184	158,984	2,336	50,398

Table 1. Number of nodes and predicted interactions for each database.

By using the topological metrics of connectivity and betweenness centrality we identified 384 potential targets. From these targets, those that had homology to human proteins were eliminated. This substantially reduced the number of potential targets, although higher specificity of drug effects was expected. As explained earlier, toxicity becomes a very important issue when designing or searching for a drug, since many clinical trials failed because of undesired and severe side effects. After this filter, the final number of targets was reduced to 142. Further filters can be applied to this list to select those targets that were most attractive for drug design (Table 2).

From the group of targets, 91 kinases were predicted as essential proteins in the network with no homology to the human kinome. Kinases are very important regulators of signaling in the cell, and in the case of *Leishmania*, kinases are crucial to enable the different metabolic changes needed to adapt to a human host. Perhaps by intensive pharmacological investigation, drugs that are very successful in treating cancer (e.g., Gleevec) could be used against *Leishmania* parasites. One particular example from the group of predicted kinases detected on the network is the protein LMPK (*LmjF36.6470*). This protein has been shown to be essential in *Leishmania mexicana* (Wiese 1998) and it has conserved orthologs in other species such as *L. amazonensis*, *L. major*, *L. tropica*, *L. aethiopica*, *L. donovani*, *L. infantum*, and *L. braziliensis* (Wiese & Gorcke 2001). Therefore, this kinase was an interesting candidate for experimental validation and possibly its upstream and down-stream interacting partners could also be inhibited by a combination of drugs. In addition, one of the challenges in this disease is to find a broad-spectrum drug that can have therapeutic effects on several *Leishmania* species that cause different forms of leishmaniasis. Further analysis of this target can help to elucidate drugs or combination of drugs that are active against amastigotes, the stage responsible for the disease in mammals. Three ABC transporters that were *Leishmania* specific -

LmjF34.0670, LmjF27.0470, LmjF32.2060 - were also predicted as essential. They confer resistance to antimonials and pentamidine by extruding the drug outside of the cell (Perez-Victoria., et al. 2002). Based upon our analysis, these proteins could be also interesting drug targets due to their role in the homeostasis of the intracellular parasite environment.

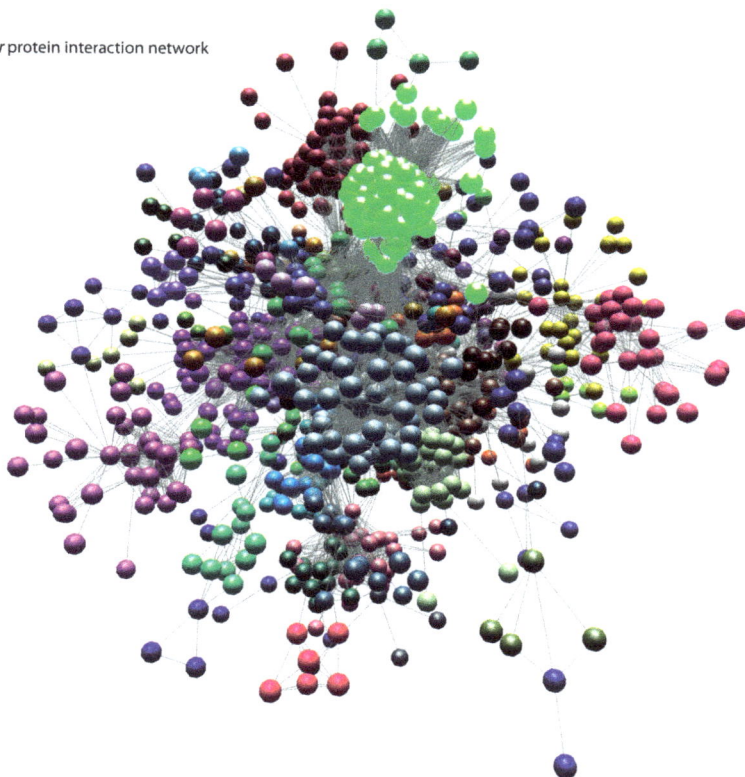

Leishmania major protein interaction network

Fig. 2. Visualization of the predicted *Leishmania major* interactome

GeneDB ID	Uniprot ID	Description
LmjF15.0770	Q4QFA8	Protein kinase.
LmjF07.0250	Q4QIR9	Protein kinase
LmjF11.0330	Q4QH47	PIF1 helicase-like protein
LmjF35.2450	Q4FWM4	Hypothetical protein conserved
LmjF25.1990	Q4Q9P0	Protein kinase
LmjF21.0853	Q4QCC1	Hypothetical protein conserved
LmjF27.1800	Q4FYE1	Protein kinase-like
LmjF35.1000	Q4FX16	Casein kinase I
LmjF26.0660	Q4Q9C8	Protein disulfide isomerase
LmjF25.2050	Q4Q9N4	Helicase-like protein

Table 2. Top 10 list of predicted targets from the *L. major* interactome.

It has been shown that modular organization is a prevalent feature in biology, and this modular organization of pathways can be used to infer protein function (Rives & Galitski 2003). We detected 63 clusters or modules in the network, and assigned potential biological processes to 263 proteins with no prior functional description. By examining the proportion of predicted targets by biological process, 64% of the proteins in the network were predicted to participate in the protein phosphorylation (GO:0006468). In addition, 8% of proteins were predicted to be involved in nucleosome assembly (GO:0006334), 4% in nucleic acid metabolic process (GO:0006139), 4% in electron transport (GO:0006118), 4% in transport processes (GO:0006810), and 2% in protein amino acid alkylation (GO:0006139). The remaining 14% of target proteins were distributed across processes with one protein per process. This result highlighted the importance of protein kinases as the main protein class to characterize and explore as drug targets in *Leishmania* parasites.

3. Selection of drug targets by metabolic flux balance analysis and *in silico* deletions

Proteins involved in metabolism constitute another important source of drug targets. The energetic balance in the cell is controlled by enzymes that regulate the transformation of substrates in a coordinated and efficient manner. These enzymes are needed specifically for producing energy or as building blocks for other molecules being essential for the viability of the organism. However, a different approach needs to be used for modeling metabolism because the interactions between enzymes depend upon the rate of turnover of molecules or *fluxes*, not specifically through physical interactions as described for the case of the interactome.

The reconstruction of metabolic networks is more established compared to interactome generation. Since glycolysis was elucidated in 1930, several metabolic pathways have been discovered in many organisms. Metabolic networks reconstructed from this source of data started with *E. coli* (Reed & Palsson 2003) and was followed later on by reconstructions in eukaryotic organisms such as *Saccharomyces cerevisiae* (Duarte., et al. 2004) and *Aspergillus niger* (David., et al. 2003). More recently, metabolic networks of *Plasmodium falciparum* (Plata., et al. 2010) and *Leishmania major* (Chavali., et al. 2008) were reconstructed with the aim of detecting drug targets, and some details about the network generation and analysis will be discussed.

In order to build a metabolic network it is necessary to list all the substances with their concentrations and the reactions between substances. In living systems these reactions are catalyzed by enzymes and the transport processes are carried out by transporters or channels. The reactions are influenced by the *stoichiometric coefficients* which denote the proportion of substrate and product molecules involved in a reaction. The reaction:

$$S1 + S1 \rightarrow 2P$$

describes the generation of product P from S1. Therefore, the stoichiometric coefficients for this particular reaction are -1,-1 and 2 respectively. For a metabolic network consisting of *m* substances and *r* reactions, the systems dynamics are described by *systems equations* (2) (or balance equations, since the balance of substrate production and degradation is considered):

$$\frac{dSi}{dt} = \sum_{j=1}^{r} n_{ij} v_j \qquad (2)$$

The term n_{ij} are the stoichiometric coefficients of metabolite i in reaction j. In this case, diffusion is not considered in the system. These equations can be applied to compartments, where the flux between compartments has to be considered as a different reaction. The stoichiometric coefficients n_{ij} can be combined into the so-called *stoichiometric matrix*, where each column belongs to a reaction and each row to a substance (Klipp et al., 2005).

According to this, a mathematical model for a metabolic network can be described as a system with a vector $S = (S1, S2, ..., Sn)$ of concentration values for the different species, a vector $v = (v1, v2, ..., vr)$ of reaction rates and the stoichiometric matrix N. With these definitions, the balance equation (3) can be rewritten as follows:

$$\frac{dS}{dt} = Nv \qquad (3)$$

3.1 Predicted drug targets in the *Leishmania major* metabolic network

The total number of genes included in the network was 560, with 1,112 reactions and 1,101 metabolites. The process for the reconstruction involved different data sources, in particular literature and biological databases. Reaction stoichiometry and subcellular localization were also extracted by examining the existing literature. Some reactions were assigned as non-gene-associated to account for spontaneously generated metabolites. The gene-associated reactions were further adjusted according to the specified constraints.

Flux balance analysis is a method that has been used extensively to analyze metabolic networks. The important advantage of this method is that does not require detailed knowledge of the enzyme kinetics. The principle of the method relies on investigation of the fluxes that have the greatest influence in the growth (or production of biomass) by preserving a set of constraints such as physicochemical, thermodynamic, topological and environmental. In the case of the *Leishmania* model, constraints included reaction reversibility rules, promastigote/amastigote protein expression data, various medium conditions and prevalence of transport reactions across cellular compartments were used. The model was simulated under *steady state* conditions, which means that the net change of any metabolite in the network during time should be zero.

Virtual knockouts were carried out over the network with the aim to detect potential drug targets. The knockout genes were classified as being lethal (essential for survival), growth reducing, or with no effect. From this analysis, only 12% of single knockouts were predicted as lethal and 10% as growth reducing. Approximately 83% of all lethal genes belonged to three metabolic processes: lipid, carbohydrate or amino-acid metabolism, highlighting how critical these are to general function.

From the group of lethal genes, the authors selected those that were exclusive or without human orthologs as potential candidates (a strategy that was also employed for the interactome analysis). The gene *LmjF05.0350*, which encodes for trypanothione reductase, was lethal *in silico*. This enzyme participates in the reduction of oxidative agents by using trypanothione and this molecule is only present in kinetoplastids. This enzyme has been studied extensively as drug target, confirming the predictions of the mathematical model (Eberle., et al. 2011). *LmjF31.2940* and *LmjF21.0845*, encoding for squalene synthase and hypoxanthine-guanine phosphoribosyltransferase respectively, were also predicted as lethal in the network. The squalene synthase inhibitors affect the sterol biosynthesis pathway, taking advantage of the trypanosomatid requirement for specific endogenous sterols (e.g.

ergosterol). Interestingly, proteins belonging to this process in *Leishmania* were also detected by homology and interactome analysis showing consistency between methods.

Double knockouts were also simulated to identify lethal combination of genes. Out of 152,520 double deletions, 19,341 were lethal. From this group, 19,285 double deletions were trivial lethal, which means that at least one of the genes involved was lethal in a single deletion. There were 56 non-trivial lethal double deletions that could be interesting to test experimentally. The main participation of these double knockouts was in the lipid and carbohydrate metabolism with 57.6% of the genes in these groups. One explanation for the large number of double deletions that were not essential is the high degree of redundancy in the network. These results show the utility of a different methodology that uses mathematical modeling for the detection of essential genes in metabolism.

4. Discovery of new drugs using virtual screening

Once the protein target is identified, the next step is finding an effective and non-toxic inhibitor that can be administrated in human patients. However, the process for identifying compounds, as in the case for drug targets, requires expensive equipment for testing millions of chemicals with a final result of few *hits* that can advance in further drug development stages. This process is unpractical and time consuming. A computational strategy has been used to improve the drug search by using computational chemistry to select those compounds that are likely to work in the experimental setting, this computational technique is called *virtual screening*. The aim of this technique is to identify novel small molecules that could bind the target of interest. This is carried out by *docking* compound libraries over the protein structure of the target, using optimization algorithms that search for the best conformation of the target and the ligand, which by definition has the lowest conformational energy (McInnes 2007). The libraries are usually compounds available from chemical vendors or predicted in some cases.

The procedure for virtual screening involves the selection of the target as a first step. The target can be chosen by the results from RNAi screenings or from computational approaches as the ones previously described. The target must have a 3D structure with an acceptable resolution, which is critical for the accuracy of the predictions. The structures determined by experimental methods can be easily accessed through the Protein Data Bank (PDB; http://www.pdb.org/). This database contains protein structures from different organisms determined by X-ray crystallography or NMR methods. In addition, predicted structures by homology-modeling methods can be found in the ModBase database (http://modbase.compbio.ucsf.edu/) (Pieper., et al. 2009). In contrast, the resources for compounds or *ligands* are restricted due to patent protection. However an interesting resource that contains millions of ligands ready to use for virtual screening experiments is the ZINC database (http://zinc.docking.org/) (Irwin & Shoichet 2005). This database includes commercial ligands and it is also free for academic use. This combination of resources of protein structures and ligand databases facilitates enormously the development of virtual screening projects which can be very productive for finding new drugs, especially for neglected diseases such as leishmaniasis.

The tools employed for virtual screening are also very diverse. One very popular tool is AutoDock (Goodsell., et al. 1996), which was developed by the Scripps Institute and used in several virtual screening projects, demonstrating good performance and accuracy. However, a recent study (Chang., et al. 2010) compared the accuracy and reproducibility of AutoDock against a recently developed tool, also freely available, called AutoDock Vina (Trott & Olson 2010). The experiments consisted of screening ligands with known activity against the HIV protease and *decoys* or non-binders. Autodock Vina performed very well in terms of speed, being ~10 times faster, and more accurate in ranking larger molecules compared to AutoDock. We are currently using AutoDock Vina in a virtual screening project called "Drug Search for Leishmaniasis" in association with IBM-World Community Grid (http://www.worldcommunitygrid.org/research/dsfl/overview.do) to speed up the process of finding new active compounds.

As an example of the application of this strategy in *Leishmania*, a recent study demonstrated the utility of virtual screening to identify potential MAPK inhibitors. The target, MAPK was first modeled by using *homology modeling* techniques. Essentially, the technique predicts the 3D structure of a particular protein by finding sequence homology to a model protein with experimentally determined structure. This model was refined by molecular dynamics. Structural features, such as ATP binding pocket, phosphorylation lip, and common docking site were identified. Virtual screening was carried out using this target with several compounds from the class of ATP inhibitors. Interestingly, the docking analysis suggested that the indirubin class of molecules could act as putative inhibitors of *Leishmania* MAPK. By testing this result experimentally, the authors found reasonably good correlation between *in vitro* activity and calculated binding energy for indirubin class of inhibitors obtained in the virtual screening study. These molecules make strong hydrogen bonding interactions with Lys43, Arg57, Asp155, Glu94, and Ile96 amino acid residues of the *Leishmania* MAPK model. These residues belong to the catalytic domain and inhibition of the catalytic domain leads to impaired kinase activity (Awale., et al. 2010). This is a clear example of the synergy between computational and experimental methods to accelerate drug discovery.

5. Selection of new drugs using machine learning techniques

The *Leishmania* proteome is estimated to contain ~8,150 proteins based on the annotated genome of the sequenced species (Peacock., et al. 2007). However, fewer than 150 proteins have 3D structures in the PDB. This limits the use of docking-based strategies to search for anti-Leishmania compounds. An alternative strategy to associate active compounds with *Leishmania* targets is by using machine learning techniques. This approach is intended to find patterns on protein targets such as domains, post-translational modifications etc, that can be linked to a specific class of compounds. This system will "learn" these patterns and when challenged by proteins from the organism of interest it will predict the potential association for a particular compound. Two studies have applied this strategy to a particular set of protein targets (Bulashevska., et al. 2009; Thangudu., et al. 2010), employing the different techniques such as support vector machines (SVM) and Bayesian classifiers (BC). As a perspective, these methods could also be applied for drug search in *Leishmania;* however, the definition of protein patterns would be critical for establishing robust drug-target relationships.

6. Experimental approaches for drug testing in Leishmania

Several *in vitro* assays to test *Leishmania* susceptibility to new potential inhibitors have been developed for the two stages of *Leishmania*, namely promastigotes and amastigotes. These two stages are morphologically and biochemically different and these differences are likely responsible for their differing susceptibility to proven anti-leishmanial compounds. Assays developed with intracellular amastigotes have the advantage of being more "disease appropriate" since this is the stage responsible for mammalian disease. In addition, an intracellular *in vitro* model resembles the natural event when the parasite is in the mammalian host. Axenic amastigotes are also employed, although a more efficient alternative is the use of intracellular fluorescent or bioluminescent amastigotes.

The effectiveness of compounds to kill the parasites has been evaluated using different methodological approaches. Several years ago, direct parasite counting was the most used method (Gaspar., et al. 1992; Chan-Bacab., et al. 2003; Khan., et al. 2003). However, this method lacked accuracy and precision, likely due to human errors. This made necessary to develop new automated methods based on colorimetric, radioactive, fluorescent and luminometer detection (Fumarola., et al. 2004). Colorimetric methods like MTT [3-(4,5-dimethylthiazol-2-yl)2,5-diphenyltetrazolium bromide] have been used frequently. Recently, these methods are being replaced by transgenic parasites with reporter genes that do not interfere with cellular mitochondria. Parasites genetically engineered to express green fluorescent protein (GFP) or luciferase, have been developed and are currently used in automatized protocols involving flow cytometer or luminometer.

On the other hand, it is important to measure cytotoxicity to evaluate the possibility that a compound might produce side effects in humans. Mammalian or mouse cell lines are usually employed in these assays. The most used cells are U-937 human histiocytes, TPH-1 human peripheral blood monocytes, and hamster peritoneal macrophages (Robledo., et al. 1999; Weniger., et al. 2001; Varela., et al. 2009; Taylor., et al. 2010). To increase the selectivity of promising drugs, liposomal formulations of the compounds may be evaluated in order to reduce the toxicity as was observed for amphotericin B (Mehta., et al. 1985; Lopez-Berestein 1987).

The leishmanicidal activity of compounds that show high anti-leishmanial activity and low toxicity for mammalian cells *in vitro*, is next evaluated *in vivo*. This is normally performed in mouse or the golden hamster (*Mesocricetus auratus*) models depending on the *Leishmania* subgenus (Travi., et al. 2002). Monkey models can also used but these studies are limited to only a few laboratories worldwide (Grimaldi., et al. 2010).

7. Conclusion

Through the current chapter, the more relevant techniques for finding drugs and targets employing computational approaches were described. Special considerations should be made when using the homology searching approach for finding drug targets as the context of protein interactions is important for the definition of essentiality. Protein interaction network analysis together with metabolic flux balance analysis are becoming useful alternatives to understand protein function and to systematically select drug targets. The selection of new inhibitory compounds can be done by using virtual screening. Predicted structures can also be used in virtual screening when experimentally derived structures are absent. Finally, machine learning techniques are a promising option to search for anti-leishmanial drugs, especially when experimental or predicted structures are not available, as may occur with many *Leishmania* proteins. It is important to state that any computational analysis is considered exploratory, and experimental validation is necessary to guide final decisions about potential compounds that can advance to the next stage of drug discovery. However, by using computational tools the search space for drugs and targets is reduced, allowing more focused experiments that could reduce the cost and time of drug development.

8. Acknowledgment

This book chapter was supported by Colciencias, through the projects with the following contracts and codes: Contract 538 with code 111549326124 and contract 197 with code 111551929015.

9. References

Ahasan, H. A., M. A. Chowdhury, M. A. Azhar, A. K. Rafiqueuddin & K. A. Azad (1996). "Deaths in visceral leishmaniasis (Kala-azar) during treatment." *Med J Malaysia* 51(1): 29-32.

Altschul, S. F., T. L. Madden, A. A. Schaffer, J. Zhang, Z. Zhang, W. Miller & D. J. Lipman (1997). "Gapped BLAST and PSI-BLAST: a new generation of protein database search programs." *Nucleic Acids Res* 25(17): 3389-3402.

Assenov, Y., F. Ramirez, S. E. Schelhorn, T. Lengauer & M. Albrecht (2008). "Computing topological parameters of biological networks." *Bioinformatics* 24(2): 282-284.

Awale, M., V. Kumar, P. Saravanan & C. G. Mohan (2010). "Homology modeling and atomic level binding study of Leishmania MAPK with inhibitors." *J Mol Model* 16(3): 475-488.

Bader, G. D., I. Donaldson, C. Wolting, B. F. Ouellette, T. Pawson & C. W. Hogue (2001). "BIND--The Biomolecular Interaction Network Database." *Nucleic Acids Res* 29(1): 242-245.

Barabasi, A. L. & Z. N. Oltvai (2004). "Network biology: understanding the cell's functional organization." *Nat Rev Genet* 5(2): 101-113.

Brohee, S., K. Faust, G. Lima-Mendez, G. Vanderstocken & J. van Helden (2008). "Network Analysis Tools: from biological networks to clusters and pathways." *Nat Protoc* 3(10): 1616-1629.

Brohee, S. & J. van Helden (2006). "Evaluation of clustering algorithms for protein-protein interaction networks." *BMC Bioinformatics* 7: 488.

Bulashevska, A., M. Stein, D. Jackson & R. Eils (2009). "Prediction of small molecule binding property of protein domains with Bayesian classifiers based on Markov chains." *Comput Biol Chem* 33(6): 457-460.

Carrero-Lerida, J., G. Perez-Moreno, V. M. Castillo-Acosta, L. M. Ruiz-Perez & D. Gonzalez-Pacanowska (2009). "Intracellular location of the early steps of the isoprenoid biosynthetic pathway in the trypanosomatids Leishmania major and Trypanosoma brucei." *Int J Parasitol* 39(3): 307-314.

Costanzo, M., A. Baryshnikova, J. Bellay, Y. Kim, E. D. Spear, C. S. Sevier, H. Ding, J. L. Koh, K. Toufighi, S. Mostafavi, J. Prinz, R. P. St Onge, B. VanderSluis, T. Makhnevych, F. J. Vizeacoumar, S. Alizadeh, S. Bahr, R. L. Brost, Y. Chen, M. Cokol, R. Deshpande, Z. Li, Z. Y. Lin, W. Liang, M. Marback, J. Paw, B. J. San Luis, E. Shuteriqi, A. H. Tong, N. van Dyk, I. M. Wallace, J. A. Whitney, M. T. Weirauch, G. Zhong, H. Zhu, W. A. Houry, M. Brudno, S. Ragibizadeh, B. Papp, C. Pal, F. P. Roth, G. Giaever, C. Nislow, O. G. Troyanskaya, H. Bussey, G. D. Bader, A. C. Gingras, Q. D. Morris, P. M. Kim, C. A. Kaiser, C. L. Myers, B. J. Andrews & C. Boone (2010). "The genetic landscape of a cell." *Science* 327(5964): 425-431.

Chan-Bacab, M. J., E. Balanza, E. Deharo, V. Munoz, R. D. Garcia & L. M. Pena-Rodriguez (2003). "Variation of leishmanicidal activity in four populations of Urechites andrieuxii." *J Ethnopharmacol* 86(2-3): 243-247.

Chang, M. W., C. Ayeni, S. Breuer & B. E. Torbett (2010). "Virtual screening for HIV protease inhibitors: a comparison of AutoDock 4 and Vina." *PLoS One* 5(8): e11955.

Chavali, A. K., J. D. Whittemore, J. A. Eddy, K. T. Williams & J. A. Papin (2008). "Systems analysis of metabolism in the pathogenic trypanosomatid Leishmania major." *Mol Syst Biol* 4: 177.

Chua, H. N., W. K. Sung & L. Wong (2006). "Exploiting indirect neighbours and topological weight to predict protein function from protein-protein interactions." *Bioinformatics* 22(13): 1623-1630.

Das, B. B., A. Ganguly & H. K. Majumder (2008). "DNA topoisomerases of Leishmania: the potential targets for anti-leishmanial therapy." *Adv Exp Med Biol* 625: 103-115.

David, H., M. Akesson & J. Nielsen (2003). "Reconstruction of the central carbon metabolism of Aspergillus niger." *Eur J Biochem* 270(21): 4243-4253.

de Azevedo, W. F., Jr. & M. B. Soares (2009). "Selection of targets for drug development against protozoan parasites." *Curr Drug Targets* 10(3): 193-201.

Dreze, M., D. Monachello, C. Lurin, M. E. Cusick, D. E. Hill, M. Vidal & P. Braun (2010). "High-quality binary interactome mapping." *Methods Enzymol* 470: 281-315.

Duarte, N. C., M. J. Herrgard & B. O. Palsson (2004). "Reconstruction and validation of Saccharomyces cerevisiae iND750, a fully compartmentalized genome-scale metabolic model." *Genome Res* 14(7): 1298-1309.

Eberle, C., B. S. Lauber, D. Fankhauser, M. Kaiser, R. Brun, R. L. Krauth-Siegel & F. Diederich (2011). "Improved inhibitors of trypanothione reductase by combination of motifs: synthesis, inhibitory potency, binding mode, and antiprotozoal activities." *ChemMedChem* 6(2): 292-301.

Enright, A. J., S. Van Dongen & C. A. Ouzounis (2002). "An efficient algorithm for large-scale detection of protein families." *Nucleic Acids Res* 30(7): 1575-1584.

Faraut-Gambarelli, F., R. Piarroux, M. Deniau, B. Giusiano, P. Marty, G. Michel, B. Faugere & H. Dumon (1997). "In vitro and in vivo resistance of Leishmania infantum to meglumine antimoniate: a study of 37 strains collected from patients with visceral leishmaniasis." *Antimicrob Agents Chemother* 41(4): 827-830.

Finn, R. D., M. Marshall & A. Bateman (2005). "iPfam: visualization of protein-protein interactions in PDB at domain and amino acid resolutions." *Bioinformatics* 21(3): 410-412.

Finn, R. D., J. Mistry, B. Schuster-Bockler, S. Griffiths-Jones, V. Hollich, T. Lassmann, S. Moxon, M. Marshall, A. Khanna, R. Durbin, S. R. Eddy, E. L. Sonnhammer & A. Bateman (2006). "Pfam: clans, web tools and services." *Nucleic Acids Res* 34(Database issue): D247-251.

Florez, A. F., D. Park, J. Bhak, B. C. Kim, A. Kuchinsky, J. H. Morris, J. Espinosa & C. Muskus (2010). "Protein network prediction and topological analysis in Leishmania major as a tool for drug target selection." *BMC Bioinformatics* 11: 484.

Forsyth, R. A., R. J. Haselbeck, K. L. Ohlsen, R. T. Yamamoto, H. Xu, J. D. Trawick, D. Wall, L. Wang, V. Brown-Driver, J. M. Froelich, K. G. C, P. King, M. McCarthy, C. Malone, B. Misiner, D. Robbins, Z. Tan, Z. Y. Zhu Zy, G. Carr, D. A. Mosca, C. Zamudio, J. G. Foulkes & J. W. Zyskind (2002). "A genome-wide strategy for the identification of essential genes in Staphylococcus aureus." *Mol Microbiol* 43(6): 1387-1400.

Fumarola, L., R. Spinelli & O. Brandonisio (2004). "In vitro assays for evaluation of drug activity against Leishmania spp." *Res Microbiol* 155(4): 224-230.

Gaspar, R., F. R. Opperdoes, V. Preat & M. Roland (1992). "Drug targeting with polyalkylcyanoacrylate nanoparticles: in vitro activity of primaquine-loaded nanoparticles against intracellular Leishmania donovani." *Ann Trop Med Parasitol* 86(1): 41-49.

Giaever, G., A. M. Chu, L. Ni, C. Connelly, L. Riles, S. Veronneau, S. Dow, A. Lucau-Danila, K. Anderson, B. Andre, A. P. Arkin, A. Astromoff, M. El-Bakkoury, R. Bangham, R. Benito, S. Brachat, S. Campanaro, M. Curtiss, K. Davis, A. Deutschbauer, K. D. Entian, P. Flaherty, F. Foury, D. J. Garfinkel, M. Gerstein, D. Gotte, U. Guldener, J. H. Hegemann, S. Hempel, Z. Herman, D. F. Jaramillo, D. E. Kelly, S. L. Kelly, P. Kotter, D. LaBonte, D. C. Lamb, N. Lan, H. Liang, H. Liao, L. Liu, C. Luo, M. Lussier, R. Mao, P. Menard, S. L. Ooi, J. L. Revuelta, C. J. Roberts, M. Rose, P. Ross-Macdonald, B. Scherens, G. Schimmack, B. Shafer, D. D. Shoemaker, S. Sookhai-Mahadeo, R. K. Storms, J. N. Strathern, G. Valle, M. Voet, G. Volckaert, C. Y. Wang, T. R. Ward, J. Wilhelmy, E. A. Winzeler, Y. Yang, G. Yen, E. Youngman, K. Yu, H. Bussey, J. D. Boeke, M. Snyder, P. Philippsen, R. W. Davis & M. Johnston (2002). "Functional profiling of the Saccharomyces cerevisiae genome." *Nature* 418(6896): 387-391.

Glasser, J. S. & C. K. Murray (2011). "Central nervous system toxicity associated with liposomal amphotericin B therapy for cutaneous leishmaniasis." *Am J Trop Med Hyg* 84(4): 566-568.

Good, M. C., J. G. Zalatan & W. A. Lim (2011). "Scaffold proteins: hubs for controlling the flow of cellular information." *Science* 332(6030): 680-686.

Goodsell, D. S., G. M. Morris & A. J. Olson (1996). "Automated docking of flexible ligands: applications of AutoDock." *J Mol Recognit* 9(1): 1-5.

Goyeneche-Patino, D. A., L. Valderrama, J. Walker & N. G. Saravia (2008). "Antimony resistance and trypanothione in experimentally selected and clinical strains of Leishmania panamensis." *Antimicrob Agents Chemother* 52(12): 4503-4506.

Grimaldi, G., Jr., R. Porrozzi, K. Friedrich, A. Teva, R. S. Marchevsky, F. Vieira, N. Miekeley & F. J. Paumgartten (2010). "Comparative efficacies of two antimony regimens to treat Leishmania braziliensis-induced cutaneous Leishmaniasis in rhesus macaques (Macaca mulatta)." *Antimicrob Agents Chemother* 54(1): 502-505.

He, F., Y. Zhang, H. Chen, Z. Zhang & Y. L. Peng (2008). "The prediction of protein-protein interaction networks in rice blast fungus." *BMC Genomics* 9: 519.

Hermjakob, H., L. Montecchi-Palazzi, C. Lewington, S. Mudali, S. Kerrien, S. Orchard, M. Vingron, B. Roechert, P. Roepstorff, A. Valencia, H. Margalit, J. Armstrong, A. Bairoch, G. Cesareni, D. Sherman & R. Apweiler (2004). "IntAct: an open source molecular interaction database." *Nucleic Acids Res* 32(Database issue): D452-455.

Hu, W., S. Sillaots, S. Lemieux, J. Davison, S. Kauffman, A. Breton, A. Linteau, C. Xin, J. Bowman, J. Becker, B. Jiang & T. Roemer (2007). "Essential gene identification and drug target prioritization in Aspergillus fumigatus." *PLoS Pathog* 3(3): e24.

Hubbard, T. J., A. G. Murzin, S. E. Brenner & C. Chothia (1997). "SCOP: a structural classification of proteins database." *Nucleic Acids Res* 25(1): 236-239.

Irwin, J. J. & B. K. Shoichet (2005). "ZINC--a free database of commercially available compounds for virtual screening." *J Chem Inf Model* 45(1): 177-182.

Ivens, A. C., C. S. Peacock, E. A. Worthey, L. Murphy, G. Aggarwal, M. Berriman, E. Sisk, M. A. Rajandream, E. Adlem, R. Aert, A. Anupama, Z. Apostolou, P. Attipoe, N. Bason, C. Bauser, A. Beck, S. M. Beverley, G. Bianchettin, K. Borzym, G. Bothe, C. V. Bruschi, M. Collins, E. Cadag, L. Ciarloni, C. Clayton, R. M. Coulson, A. Cronin, A. K. Cruz, R. M. Davies, J. De Gaudenzi, D. E. Dobson, A. Duesterhoeft, G. Fazelina, N. Fosker, A. C. Frasch, A. Fraser, M. Fuchs, C. Gabel, A. Goble, A. Goffeau, D. Harris, C. Hertz-Fowler, H. Hilbert, D. Horn, Y. Huang, S. Klages, A. Knights, M. Kube, N. Larke, L. Litvin, A.

Lord, T. Louie, M. Marra, D. Masuy, K. Matthews, S. Michaeli, J. C. Mottram, S. Muller-Auer, H. Munden, S. Nelson, H. Norbertczak, K. Oliver, S. O'Neil, M. Pentony, T. M. Pohl, C. Price, B. Purnelle, M. A. Quail, E. Rabbinowitsch, R. Reinhardt, M. Rieger, J. Rinta, J. Robben, L. Robertson, J. C. Ruiz, S. Rutter, D. Saunders, M. Schafer, J. Schein, D. C. Schwartz, K. Seeger, A. Seyler, S. Sharp, H. Shin, D. Sivam, R. Squares, S. Squares, V. Tosato, C. Vogt, G. Volckaert, R. Wambutt, T. Warren, H. Wedler, J. Woodward, S. Zhou, W. Zimmermann, D. F. Smith, J. M. Blackwell, K. D. Stuart, B. Barrell & P. J. Myler (2005). "The genome of the kinetoplastid parasite, Leishmania major." *Science* 309(5733): 436-442.

Jeong, H., S. P. Mason, A. L. Barabasi & Z. N. Oltvai (2001). "Lethality and centrality in protein networks." *Nature* 411(6833): 41-42.

Kamath, R. S., A. G. Fraser, Y. Dong, G. Poulin, R. Durbin, M. Gotta, A. Kanapin, N. Le Bot, S. Moreno, M. Sohrmann, D. P. Welchman, P. Zipperlen & J. Ahringer (2003). "Systematic functional analysis of the Caenorhabditis elegans genome using RNAi." *Nature* 421(6920): 231-237.

Khan, K. M., M. Rasheed, U. Zia, S. Hayat, F. Kaukab, M. I. Choudhary, R. Atta ur & S. Perveen (2003). "Synthesis and in vitro leishmanicidal activity of some hydrazides and their analogues." *Bioorg Med Chem* 11(7): 1381-1387.

Kim, J. G., D. Park, B. C. Kim, S. W. Cho, Y. T. Kim, Y. J. Park, H. J. Cho, H. Park, K. B. Kim, K. O. Yoon, S. J. Park, B. M. Lee & J. Bhak (2008). "Predicting the interactome of Xanthomonas oryzae pathovar oryzae for target selection and DB service." *BMC Bioinformatics* 9: 41.

Klipp, E., Herwig, R., Kowald, A.,Wierling, C. & Lehrach, H (2005). *Systems Biology in Practice: Concepts, Implementation and Application.* Wiley-VCH Verlag GmbH & Co. KGaA, ISBN: 9783527310784, Weinheim, Germany.

Knox, C., V. Law, T. Jewison, P. Liu, S. Ly, A. Frolkis, A. Pon, K. Banco, C. Mak, V. Neveu, Y. Djoumbou, R. Eisner, A. C. Guo & D. S. Wishart (2011). "DrugBank 3.0: a comprehensive resource for 'omics' research on drugs." *Nucleic Acids Res* 39(Database issue): D1035-1041.

Kuhn, M., D. Szklarczyk, A. Franceschini, M. Campillos, C. von Mering, L. J. Jensen, A. Beyer & P. Bork (2010). "STITCH 2: an interaction network database for small molecules and proteins." *Nucleic Acids Res* 38(Database issue): D552-556.

Lang, T., S. Goyard, M. Lebastard & G. Milon (2005). "Bioluminescent Leishmania expressing luciferase for rapid and high throughput screening of drugs acting on amastigote-harbouring macrophages and for quantitative real-time monitoring of parasitism features in living mice." *Cell Microbiol* 7(3): 383-392.

Lin, C. Y., C. H. Chin, H. H. Wu, S. H. Chen, C. W. Ho & M. T. Ko (2008). "Hubba: hub objects analyzer--a framework of interactome hubs identification for network biology." *Nucleic Acids Res* 36(Web Server issue): W438-443.

Lopez-Berestein, G. (1987). "Liposomes as carriers of antimicrobial agents." *Antimicrob Agents Chemother* 31(5): 675-678.

Maltezou, H. C. (2008). "Visceral leishmaniasis: advances in treatment." *Recent Pat Antiinfect Drug Discov* 3(3): 192-198.

McInnes, C. (2007). "Virtual screening strategies in drug discovery." *Curr Opin Chem Biol* 11(5): 494-502.

Mehta, R. T., G. Lopez-Berestein, R. L. Hopfer, K. Mehta, R. A. White & R. L. Juliano (1985). "Prophylaxis of murine candidiasis via application of liposome-encapsulated amphotericin B and a muramyl dipeptide analog, alone and in combination." *Antimicrob Agents Chemother* 28(4): 511-513.

Oliveira, L. F., A. O. Schubach, M. M. Martins, S. L. Passos, R. V. Oliveira, M. C. Marzochi & C. A. Andrade (2011). "Systematic review of the adverse effects of cutaneous leishmaniasis treatment in the New World." *Acta Trop* 118(2): 87-96.

Osman, A. (2004). "Yeast two-hybrid assay for studying protein-protein interactions." *Methods Mol Biol* 270: 403-422.

Park, D., S. Lee, D. Bolser, M. Schroeder, M. Lappe, D. Oh & J. Bhak (2005). "Comparative interactomics analysis of protein family interaction networks using PSIMAP (protein structural interactome map)." *Bioinformatics* 21(15): 3234-3240.

Peacock, C. S., K. Seeger, D. Harris, L. Murphy, J. C. Ruiz, M. A. Quail, N. Peters, E. Adlem, A. Tivey, M. Aslett, A. Kerhornou, A. Ivens, A. Fraser, M. A. Rajandream, T. Carver, H. Norbertczak, T. Chillingworth, Z. Hance, K. Jagels, S. Moule, D. Ormond, S. Rutter, R. Squares, S. Whitehead, E. Rabbinowitsch, C. Arrowsmith, B. White, S. Thurston, F. Bringaud, S. L. Baldauf, A. Faulconbridge, D. Jeffares, D. P. Depledge, S. O. Oyola, J. D. Hilley, L. O. Brito, L. R. Tosi, B. Barrell, A. K. Cruz, J. C. Mottram, D. F. Smith & M. Berriman (2007). "Comparative genomic analysis of three Leishmania species that cause diverse human disease." *Nat Genet* 39(7): 839-847.

Perez-Victoria, J. M., A. Di Pietro, D. Barron, A. G. Ravelo, S. Castanys & F. Gamarro (2002). "Multidrug resistance phenotype mediated by the P-glycoprotein-like transporter in Leishmania: a search for reversal agents." *Curr Drug Targets* 3(4): 311-333.

Peri, S., J. D. Navarro, T. Z. Kristiansen, R. Amanchy, V. Surendranath, B. Muthusamy, T. K. Gandhi, K. N. Chandrika, N. Deshpande, S. Suresh, B. P. Rashmi, K. Shanker, N. Padma, V. Niranjan, H. C. Harsha, N. Talreja, B. M. Vrushabendra, M. A. Ramya, A. J. Yatish, M. Joy, H. N. Shivashankar, M. P. Kavitha, M. Menezes, D. R. Choudhury, N. Ghosh, R. Saravana, S. Chandran, S. Mohan, C. K. Jonnalagadda, C. K. Prasad, C. Kumar-Sinha, K. S. Deshpande & A. Pandey (2004). "Human protein reference database as a discovery resource for proteomics." *Nucleic Acids Res* 32(Database issue): D497-501.

Pieper, U., N. Eswar, B. M. Webb, D. Eramian, L. Kelly, D. T. Barkan, H. Carter, P. Mankoo, R. Karchin, M. A. Marti-Renom, F. P. Davis & A. Sali (2009). "MODBASE, a database of annotated comparative protein structure models and associated resources." *Nucleic Acids Res* 37(Database issue): D347-354.

Plata, G., T. L. Hsiao, K. L. Olszewski, M. Llinas & D. Vitkup (2010). "Reconstruction and flux-balance analysis of the Plasmodium falciparum metabolic network." *Mol Syst Biol* 6: 408.

Reed, J. L. & B. O. Palsson (2003). "Thirteen years of building constraint-based in silico models of Escherichia coli." *J Bacteriol* 185(9): 2692-2699.

Rives, A. W. & T. Galitski (2003). "Modular organization of cellular networks." *Proc Natl Acad Sci U S A* 100(3): 1128-1133.

Robledo, S. M., A. Z. Valencia & N. G. Saravia (1999). "Sensitivity to Glucantime of Leishmania viannia isolated from patients prior to treatment." *J Parasitol* 85(2): 360-366.

Sakharkar, K. R., M. K. Sakharkar & V. T. Chow (2004). "A novel genomics approach for the identification of drug targets in pathogens, with special reference to Pseudomonas aeruginosa." *In Silico Biol* 4(3): 355-360.

Shannon, P., A. Markiel, O. Ozier, N. S. Baliga, J. T. Wang, D. Ramage, N. Amin, B. Schwikowski & T. Ideker (2003). "Cytoscape: a software environment for integrated models of biomolecular interaction networks." *Genome Res* 13(11): 2498-2504.

Stark, C., B. J. Breitkreutz, T. Reguly, L. Boucher, A. Breitkreutz & M. Tyers (2006). "BioGRID: a general repository for interaction datasets." *Nucleic Acids Res* 34(Database issue): D535-539.

Sundar, S. & J. Chakravarty (2010). "Antimony toxicity." *Int J Environ Res Public Health* 7(12): 4267-4277.

Taylor, V. M., D. L. Munoz, D. L. Cedeno, I. D. Velez, M. A. Jones & S. M. Robledo (2010). "Leishmania tarentolae: utility as an in vitro model for screening of antileishmanial agents." *Exp Parasitol* 126(4): 471-475.

Thangudu, R. R., M. Tyagi, B. A. Shoemaker, S. H. Bryant, A. R. Panchenko & T. Madej (2010). "Knowledge-based annotation of small molecule binding sites in proteins." *BMC Bioinformatics* 11: 365.

Travi, B. L., Y. Osorio, P. C. Melby, B. Chandrasekar, L. Arteaga & N. G. Saravia (2002). "Gender is a major determinant of the clinical evolution and immune response in hamsters infected with Leishmania spp." *Infect Immun* 70(5): 2288-2296.

Trott, O. & A. J. Olson (2010). "AutoDock Vina: improving the speed and accuracy of docking with a new scoring function, efficient optimization, and multithreading." *J Comput Chem* 31(2): 455-461.

Uetz, P., L. Giot, G. Cagney, T. A. Mansfield, R. S. Judson, J. R. Knight, D. Lockshon, V. Narayan, M. Srinivasan, P. Pochart, A. Qureshi-Emili, Y. Li, B. Godwin, D. Conover, T. Kalbfleisch, G. Vijayadamodar, M. Yang, M. Johnston, S. Fields & J. M. Rothberg (2000). "A comprehensive analysis of protein-protein interactions in Saccharomyces cerevisiae." *Nature* 403(6770): 623-627.

Varela, M. R., D. L. Munoz, S. M. Robledo, B. K. Kolli, S. Dutta, K. P. Chang & C. Muskus (2009). "Leishmania (Viannia) panamensis: an in vitro assay using the expression of GFP for screening of antileishmanial drug." *Exp Parasitol* 122(2): 134-139.

von Mering, C., L. J. Jensen, B. Snel, S. D. Hooper, M. Krupp, M. Foglierini, N. Jouffre, M. A. Huynen & P. Bork (2005). "STRING: known and predicted protein-protein associations, integrated and transferred across organisms." *Nucleic Acids Res* 33(Database issue): D433-437.

Weniger, B., S. Robledo, G. J. Arango, E. Deharo, R. Aragon, V. Munoz, J. Callapa, A. Lobstein & R. Anton (2001). "Antiprotozoal activities of Colombian plants." *J Ethnopharmacol* 78(2-3): 193-200.

Wiese, M. (1998). "A mitogen-activated protein (MAP) kinase homologue of Leishmania mexicana is essential for parasite survival in the infected host." *EMBO J* 17(9): 2619-2628.

Wiese, M. & I. Gorcke (2001). "Homologues of LMPK, a mitogen-activated protein kinase from Leishmania mexicana, in different Leishmania species." *Med Microbiol Immunol* 190(1-2): 19-22.

Xenarios, I., D. W. Rice, L. Salwinski, M. K. Baron, E. M. Marcotte & D. Eisenberg (2000). "DIP: the database of interacting proteins." *Nucleic Acids Res* 28(1): 289-291.

Yu, H., P. M. Kim, E. Sprecher, V. Trifonov & M. Gerstein (2007). "The importance of bottlenecks in protein networks: correlation with gene essentiality and expression dynamics." *PLoS Comput Biol* 3(4): e59.

Zanzoni, A., L. Montecchi-Palazzi, M. Quondam, G. Ausiello, M. Helmer-Citterich & G. Cesareni (2002). "MINT: a Molecular INTeraction database." *FEBS Lett* 513(1): 135-140.

Zhang, R. & Y. Lin (2009). "DEG 5.0, a database of essential genes in both prokaryotes and eukaryotes." *Nucleic Acids Res* 37(Database issue): D455-458.

8

Advances in Serological Diagnosis of Chagas' Disease by Using Recombinant Proteins

Iván S. Marcipar[1] and Claudia M. Lagier[2]
[1]*Laboratorio de Tecnología Inmunológica (LTI), Fac. Bioquímica y Cs. Biológicas,*
Universidad Nacional del Litoral
[2]*Instituto de Química Rosario (IQUIR-CONICET), División Química Analítica,*
Fac. Cs. Bioquímicas y Farmacéuticas, Universidad Nacional de Rosario
Argentina

1. Introduction

Chagas' disease is an infection caused by the parasite *Trypanosoma cruzi*, mainly occurring in American countries where the parasite vector bug, *Triatoma infestans*, is widespread. One hundred million individuals are currently under threaten of infection, as well as 16 million people are considered affected by the illness in Latin America alone.(Editorial, 2009) Considering indicators such as the disability-adjusted life years, DALY, and from a social point of view, Chagas' disease accounts for the third most important tropical illness of the World, following malaria and schistosomiasis.(Bitran *et al.*, 2009) Moreover, Chagas disease epidemiology nowadays impacts in non-endemic regions due to globalization, being the infection disseminated all over the world (Gascon *et al.* 2009). Certainly, the non-vectorial disease transmission (mother to child, transfusional and by organ transplantation) is the way the illness spreads in Europe, North America, Japan, and Australia, because many infected people have migrated from endemic regions to distant cities. (Bowling & Walter, 2009; Lescure *et al.*, 2009; Yadon & Schmunis, 2009)

The parasite distribution and living habits of rural Latin-American people have determined that the main transmission route is the vectorial one (via *Triatoma infestans*), leading to up 80% of human infection.(WHO, 2003) The main contagion way in urban areas arise from blood-transfusion, being responsible for 5-20% of the reported cases, while vertical transmission (mother-to-child) accounts for 2-10% of the infections.(Carlier & Torrico, 2003)

The infection transmission by oral route because of consumption of contaminated food and drinks is lower than that reported for the previously-mentioned routes.(Dias *et al.*, 2011) However, it has to be taken into account that the success of the non-oral infection prevention has increased the importance of the oral route of transmission.(Dias *et al.*, 2011; Nóbrega *et al.*, 2009) It is noteworthy that the acute outcome of the oral infection is particularly severe.(Bastos et al 2010).

From the clinical point of view, the illness presents variable unspecific symptoms, depending on its stage: the acute one, shortly after primary infection, and the chronic stage, which may last many years if the individual is not treated. Human infection typically appears with an incubation period of 4-10 days, which is generally asymptomatic. Afterwards, the infection may advance to the short acute phase, followed by the long-lasting chronic stage, which may occur in a syntomatic or asymptomatic way.

The acute stage of the infection usually lasts 2-4 months. When symptoms appear, these are often light and atypical. The infection proceeds generally unnoticed, and this prevents its diagnosis. Most of the patients recover within 3-5 months. However, global mortality during this phase reaches 5-10%,(WHO, 2002) and may be higher in children.(Pinto et al., 2004) Deaths can be caused by complications related to myocarditis and/or meningoencephalitis,(Pittella, 2009) which has been proved by the presence of the amastigote form of parasites in cardiac, skeletal, glial and soft tissue cells.(da Silveira et al., 2007)

The undetermined, chronic phase generally begins 8-10 weeks after the acute infection, and may last several years or even the whole life of the individual. The illness overtakes asymptomatically, and generally, infected individuals keep their full working capacity without being aware of the infection. However, during this stage, patients display positive serology for specific IgG antibodies and low parasitemia.(Coura, 2007) Over 50% of the infected individuals show themselves healthy and do not develop serious outcomes. In the other cases, the infection is often detected once its sequels appear, after 10-20 years of the first parasite entry. The illness features that mainly develop are cardiac, digestive and/or neurological damages. Chagas' pathologic alterations can be summarized as chronic myocarditis, 27%, esophageal or colonic expansion, 5%, and abnormalities of central nervous system, ca. 3%.(Teixeira et al., 2006) The most severe impact of the illness occurs during chronic phase, and after many years that the infection has been established, leading to high mortality rate among people who have develop cardiac pathology.(Rassi, Jr. et al., 2007)

Undoubtedly, the most effective alternative to prevent Chagas' disease spreading is to control vectorial and transfusional ways of transmissions. Nevertheless, once the individual has been infected by T. cruzi, he/she may be treated. Two main aspects are covered by therapy, aiming to eliminate the parasite with trypanocidal medication, and/or medicating to relief symptoms of the several clinical outlines of the illness. Nowadays, two chemicals are used as trypanocidal agents namely, nifurtimox (Lampit®, Bayer; 5-nitrofuran 3-methyl-4-(5'-nitrofurfurylideneamine) tetrahydro-4H-1,4-tiazine-1,1-dioxide) and benznidazole (Rochagan® and Radanil®, Roche; N-benzyl-2-nitroimidazole acetamide). When infection is treated during the acute stage, it has been reported that parasitemia disappeared in 60% of the cases and serology turned into negative. Nevertheless, the outcome after therapy is finished shows variable effectiveness percentages, depending mainly on the age of the individual and the geographical region.(Perez-Molina et al., 2009)

Currently, studies trying to expand the indicators on treatment effectiveness are in progress and will be accomplished by 2012.(Marin-Neto et al., 2008) Though these studies have not yet finished, there is a consensus on treating Chagas' disease, taking into account the clear-cut results when using trypanocidal medication with children, during the indeterminate phase of the infection.(Lescure et al., 2010;Perez-Molina et al., 2009;Sosa-Estani & Segura, 2006) It therefore follows that it is highly advisable to count with reliable methods to early diagnose the disease, since this may accelerate the patient treatment, helping to reduce the serious consequences that the long term infection may cause.

1.1 *T. cruzi* infection diagnostic during the different stages of the illness

The infection diagnosis is not a simple task because the features of the illness development as well as the immunological response of the host must be taken into account when performing the laboratory diagnosis. Different diagnostic methods are used, depending on the illness stage and the particular clinical entity of the patient.

The alternative ways to get acute Chagas' infection are mainly vectorial and vertical transmission, and the reactivation of the chronic disease in immunosuppressed individuals. Therefore, diagnosis at this stage limits to: *i)* the uncommon cases of symptomatic patients, *ii)* newborns delivered from chagasic mothers, and *iii)* immunosuppressed patients that have been previously diagnosed as infected.

In the above mentioned cases, parasites are usually, easily found in blood, therefore being their direct microscopic observation the chosen method for a safe diagnosis.(WHO, 2002;Rosenblatt, 2009) In contrast, indirect serological techniques present low sensitivity in recently infected individuals because humoral immune response is delayed.(Zuniga *et al.*, 2000) Moreover, even specific IgM immunoglobulin has a window period that requires up to several weeks to be produced at detectable concentrations. Other pitfalls such as the lack of IgM anti-*T. cruzi* commercial kits prevents from choosing serology as the infection diagnostic method. This methodology is only used when the parasite is not found in fresh blood smears, by Struot and/or microhematocrit methods.(Luquetti & Schmunis, 2010)

During the chronic phase, the *T. cruzi* infection diagnosis is required, *i)* as pregnancy or occupational routine control analysis -in countries where according legislation is in force-, *ii)* when in presence of a Chagas' compatible cardiopathy, *iii)* during transfusion and transplantation screening, and *iv)* to achieve a reliable illness prognosis of patients who were already diagnosed. One particular case among the latter ones is monitoring the antiparasitic treatment effectiveness.

Conversely to what happens in the acute phase, during the chronic infection, a significant humoral response is found in immunocompetent individuals, along with low parasite concentration in blood. Under these circumstances, indirect techniques are highly sensitive, while the direct ones fail. Hence, Chagas' disease serologic diagnoses intend to verify the occurrence of several specific antibodies against *T. cruzi*. However, conventional serology presents different sensitivity and selectivity, depending on the immunological technique used to perform the determination, and mainly in the nature of the antigen used to capture the specific antibodies.(Belluzo *et al.*, 2011)

In this Chapter, we will describe the most recent contributions of our and other groups to improve the analytical tools available to properly and safely diagnose Chagas' disease using recombinant proteins, in each one of the clinical entities mentioned above.

2. Conventional diagnosis of *T. cruzi* infection

Direct parasite detection in whole blood is the simplest, regular procedure used to diagnose acute infection whereas, indirect serological tests are the chosen ones to diagnose the undetermined, chronic state.(Rosenblatt, 2009;WHO, 2002)

2.1 Parasitological and serological diagnosis of acute entities

The direct microscopic observation of parasites from patients peripheral blood is the elected methodology to confirm acute infection. The Strout concentration method is the routinely performed parasitologic analysis in adults since more than 50 years,(Strout, 1962) and it has been reported about 95% sensitivity.(Freilij & Storino, 1994)

The other commonly used concentration method is the pediatric, more recent version, named the direct micromethod or microhematocrit, which requires a lower blood volume than Strout method, and is mainly used to diagnose congenital Chagas' disease and acute infection in children.(Freilij et al., 1983;Freilij & Altcheh, 1995) However, newborn babies usually present low parasitemia, therefore making difficult to perform a proper conventional parasitologic analysis. It is then recommended to perform serologic tests to diagnose the congenital infection. The evaluation of specific anti-T. cruzi IgA and IgM is not recommended due to the high rate of false-negative results in neonates.(Moya et al., 2005) Considering that maternal specific anti-T. cruzi IgG antibodies are commonly present in newborn circulating blood, even up to the ninth month, it is not advisable to perform serologic IgG determinations as routine, in newborns younger than 9 months old. In this line, if the micromethod is negative or if it has not been performed during the first months of life of the newborn, then congenital infection should be serologically diagnosed using peripheral blood not before the child is 9 months old, once maternal antibodies have disappeared.(Gomes et al., 2009) Following, when specific IgG presence is negative after the ninth month of life, then vertical transmission is ruled out. Alternatively, during the first months of life of babies, it is possible to forego results using other non-standard, more expensive techniques such as the polymerase chain reaction, PCR.(Diez et al., 2008) This technology is particularly preferred when the health center counts with the supplies to carry out the methodology.

Indirect parasitological methods are also used, mainly when the parasite is not easily found in samples. These methods are the hemoculture and xenodiagnosis, and consist of enriching the parasites present in the patient's blood sample, through allowing their replication.(Chiari et al., 1989) Both of these latter techniques are also used when diagnosing chronic infection. These methods demand long periods of time to arise to the results (weeks or months), together with other drawbacks. For example, xenodiagnostic method has the disadvantage of producing rather variable sensitivity results, 20-50%, alongside the requirement of a suitable building infrastructure and trained personnel to deal with insect breeding. Thus, this method is not commonly performed in basic health centers.(Luquetti & Schmunis, 2010)

When searching for reappearance of acute infection in immunosuppressed individuals under risk, negative serological results are not always associated with absence of the infection. This is a consequence of the immunological status of the patient that shows difficulties to produce detectable amounts of specific IgG. As mentioned previously, in the particular, difficult cases, expensive PCR techniques are the recommended diagnostic method.

2.2 Serological diagnosis of chronic entities

The widely used serological assays to diagnose T. cruzi infection in present clinical practice are indirect haemagglutination (IHA), indirect immunofluorescence (IIF), and enzyme-linked immunosorbent assay (ELISA).(WHO, 2002;Yadon & Schmunis, 2009) The analyst's choice of the particular technique depends on sanitary-authority recommendations, market impositions, and the lab-technician preference. This latter one is generally related to the methodology simplicity, and the personal confidence he/she has in a particular technique after having performed it for a long while.

IHA is an inexpensive technique, which is easy to be performed and interpreted, and it has been used for more than 50 years, therefore being appropriately settled among lab technicians. Similarly, IIF was developed in the sixties and presents equivalent features to IHA though, more skillful technicians are required to perform the analysis and produce accurate readings, as well as it needs a fluorescence microscope. IIF is a very sensitive, specific and cheap alternative for those who have the equipment and the trained personnel. However, regular health centers do not count with both of them.

ELISA is a more recent technique which was firstly described during 1975 to diagnose Chagas' disease,(Voller *et al.*, 1975) and its usage was settled just at the ends of the eighties. This technique has the advantage of being widely extended as a diagnostic tool of many infections. Therefore, most of regular laboratories have the required equipment and trained personnel to appropriately perform the analysis. Contrarily to IHA and IIF, ELISA may be performed with automatic equipment at large health institutions. Moreover, even though ELISA is more expensive than the other two techniques, its notable performance in terms of sensitivity and specificity, has made of this the preferred methodology to diagnose *T. cruzi* infection.(Saez-Alquezar *et al.*, 1997)

Recently, one very fast technique with a different format has been developed namely, lateral chromatography.(Ponce *et al.*, 2005;Barfield *et al.*, 2011) This methodology uses small volume samples such as one serum drop, and allows acquiring results in 15 min, therefore being useful to perform the test in the field, without the need of refrigerator to preserve the reagents. Several multicenter studies have demonstrated that a commercial lateral chromatography kit show more than 92% sensitivity, whereas specificity is ca. 96%.(Ponce *et al.*, 2005;Brutus *et al.*, 2008;Roddy *et al.*, 2008;Sosa-Estani *et al.*, 2008)

The fundamental problems of *T. cruzi* infection serological diagnostic methods are the lack of reproducibility that sometimes occur, deficient immunological reaction specificity, what produces false-positive results, and the occasional insufficient sensitivity translated into false-negative outcomes.

Chagasic infection serology tests may produce cross-reactions with antibodies produced during the course of other illnesses. In this line, unspecific reactivity has been described for infections caused by *T. cruzi* phylogenetically related microorganisms, such as *T. rangeli* and *Leishmania sp.*(Soto *et al.*, 1996;Araujo, 1986;Saez-Alquezar *et al.*, 2000) Moreover, other false-positive results due to cross-reactions have been described when testing samples from patients with autoimmune diseases,(Reiche *et al.*, 1996) or from individuals suffering from other acute infections or pregnant women who display an important, polyclonal unspecific response.(Konishi, 1993)

The clinical practice often finds an important number of inconsistent results regarding reproducibility and confidence when diagnosing chagasic infection. The lack of reproducibility and confident results has also been reported in a multicenter study.(Saez-Alquezar *et al.*, 1997) In this work, it was proved the deficiency of reagents standardization, what produced incongruent results when testing the same serum panel. Along the same direction, since the early nineties, several works accounted for the huge losses caused by disposal of whole blood reservoirs typified as undetermined for *T. cruzi* infection.(Carvalho *et al.*, 1993;Salles *et al.*, 1996;Saez-Alquezar *et al.*, 2000) Taking into account tests discrepancies, one of WHO recommendations states that *T. cruzi* infection must be diagnosed when the sample produces positive results by two different serological methods, whereas the undetermined condition is established for samples rendering dissimilar outcomes.

Traditionally, whole parasites, or extracts from laboratory strains of *T. cruzi* epimastigotes cultures, have been the source of antigens used for the serological infection diagnosis. However, this yields to complex protein mixtures of unknown composition, which display severe difficulties to be standardized, and additionally lead to false-positive results.

The diagnostic problems arising from serology deficient specificity, as well as the deprived reagents standardization, can be resolved through the use of defined antigens, such as the proteins obtained by molecular biology technology procedures.(Saez-Alquezar *et al.*, 2000;Umezawa *et al.*, 2003;Umezawa *et al.*, 2004;Aguirre *et al.*, 2006)

The following sections will be focused in this issue and the most important contributions that several research groups have recently made.

3. Use and prospects of recombinant DNA technology

Since the emergence of recombinant DNA technology, many protein molecules have been designed and prepared to eventually be assessed for serological diagnosis. The proteins obtained through this technology may be used as antigens to capture antibodies, to evaluate exclusively defined molecules, avoiding potential interferences from other components that usually occur when the antigens have been obtained by purifying native source proteins. (da Silveira *et al.*, 2001) It follows that the usage of recombinant proteins as antigens to detect or quantify specific antibodies markers of a disease permits enhancing the specificity of the immunological reaction involved, therefore leading to more accurate diagnosis.(Aguirre *et al.*, 2006;Camussone *et al.*, 2009)

In this methodology the proteins are usually prepared by heterologous expression, mainly in *Escherichia coli* cells.(da Silveira *et al.*, 2001) Sequences of *T. cruzi*-protein codifying-DNA are inserted in a bacterial plasmid, which is transformed in competent bacteria. The proteins encoded by the plasmid are expressed in the bacterial culture, and are afterward purified into a highly pure product. The advantage of the proteins thus obtained is that they are an entirely characterized antigen, which may be evaluated individually for antibody determination in different clinical conditions. The prepared antigens can therefore be characterized considering the clinical information they provide, and may then be used to prepare specific diagnostic reagents. These proteins count with one desired feature of diagnostic reagents, as it is that their production and evaluation can be highly standardized. From another point of view, recombinant antigens do not require manipulation of the infective agent as do the antigens obtained by purification procedures from rough cultures. This has been a significant progress when considering the characteristics of viral infective agents, for which reagents production has substantially switched to that derived from recombinant DNA technology. Not less important is the major saving financial benefit of these reagents. Indeed, once bacteria are transformed into competent, protein producing strain, they can be used to prepare substantial amounts of antigen with low cost of production.

Using this technology, many gene expression clones have been create, a fact that has made available the obtainment of massive amounts of highly pure, standardized *T. cruzi* proteins.(da Silveira *et al.*, 2001)

During the latest three decades, many parasite antigens have been cloned and characterized. The cloned antigens correspond to different parasite stages namely, the trypomastigote sanguineous, the amastigote intracellular and the epimastigote, which is the form found inside the vector bowel and that can be cultured. Several of these antigens were obtained by immunological tracing through expression of cDNA libraries from chagasic patient sera, as well as from immunized animals.(Lafaille *et al.*, 1989;Affranchino *et al.*, 1989;Levin *et al.*, 1989;Cotrim *et al.*, 1990;Gruber & Zingales, 1993) The antigen codifying genes have been identified from cDNA present in the libraries accomplished from epimastigote or trypomastigote forms.(Affranchino *et al.*, 1989;Levin *et al.*, 1989;Gruber & Zingales, 1993;Godsel *et al.*, 1995) Lately, Da Rocha et al. have proposed using amastigote proteins since this is the intracellular parasite form, being these antigens more significant for serodiagnosis.(DaRocha *et al.*, 2002)

The usage of DNA technology brought into light the existence of many parasite antigens with repetitive sequences, a fact that had been previously described when cloning proteins of other parasites.(Hoft *et al.*, 1989) Generally, these are the most immunogenic antigens, and are the mainly selected when performing immunological tracing in cDNA libraries cloned in phages. Therefore, it was initially stated that these were the most valuable antigens for diagnosis.(Frasch & Reyes, 1990) However, it was afterward proved that some non-repetitive antigens have equivalent diagnostic value than repetitive ones. Certainly, a multicenter study evaluated in parallel 4 repetitive recombinants antigens (H49, JL7, B13, JL8) together with 2 non-repetitive ones (A13 y 1F8).(Umezawa *et al.*, 1999) The results demonstrated that both type of antigens were similarly useful for *T. cruzi* infection diagnosis, and the authors suggested that if they were to be used together in a mixture, they could supplemented each other enhancing the sensitivity of the assay. This was afterwards proved by the same group, see Tables 1 A,B and C.(Umezawa *et al.*, 2003)

Once the complete genome sequence of *Trypanosoma cruzi* was annotated, (El Sayed *et al.*, 2005) alternative antigenic candidates have been searched in the parasite genome. The studies have been supported by bioinformatic prediction of putative proteins and antigenicity predictors.(Goto *et al.*, 2008;Cooley *et al.*, 2008;Hernandez *et al.*, 2010) Using these tools, it has been possible to choose antigens which display the lowest homology level with proteins of organisms related to *T. cruzi*.(Hernandez *et al.*, 2010) Moreover, the bioinformatic analysis has allowed describing for the first time a specific antigen to type discrete typing units (DTUs). (Di Noia *et al.*, 2002)

The results published by many different laboratories point towards considering recombinant proteins as the chosen molecules to be used in immunoassays to diagnose *T. cruzi* infection. Moreover, the lack of specificity leading to false-positive results can be overcome by deleting sequence regions encoding for proteins which cross-react when analyzing negative sera,(Aguirre *et al.*, 2006), or using recombinant proteins that are specific for anti-*T. cruzi* antibodies, yet keeping a high sensitivity.(Belluzo *et al.*, 2011;Camussone *et al.*, 2009) Indeed, the largest studies on the diagnosis reveal the convenience of using these antigens, regarding not only specificity but also the possibility of standardizing both, the methodology and the protein production.(Umezawa *et al.*, 1999;Saez-Alquezar *et al.*, 2000;Umezawa *et al.*, 2003)

The following table display the key recombinant antigens discussed in the present chapter, which were evaluated by several authors for *T. cruzi* infection diagnosis. Notice, that many of these antigens particularly named by one author have amino acid sequences, which may be very similar to those obtained by other authors who have named them differently (e.g. FRA, Ag1, JL7, H49). Identical or highly similar antigens were grouped in the same row.

Antigen (grouped by high identity)	Characteristics	Diagnostic use	Described by
CRA Ag30 JL8 TCR27 RP4	Cytoplasmic antigen	Chronic infection	Lafaille *et al.*, 1989 Ibáñez *et al.*, 1988 Levin et al., 1989 Hoft *et al.*, 1989 Camussone *et al.*, 2009
FRA Ag1 JL7 H49 RP1	Cytoskeleton associated protein	Chronic infection	Lafaille *et al.*, 1989 Ibáñez *et al.*, 1988 Levin *et al.*, 1989 Cotrim *et al.*, 1995 Camussone *et al.*, 2009
B13 Ag2 TCR39 PEP-2 RP5	Trypomastigote surface protein	Chronic infection	Gruber *et al.*, 1993 Ibáñez *et al.*, 1988 Hoft *et al.*, 1989 Peralta *et al.*, 1994 Camussone *et al.*, 2009
Ag36 JL9 MAP-like RP3	Microtubule associated protein	Chronic and acute infection. Antibodies against this protein render cross-reactions with mammal cell cytoskeleton.	Ibáñez *et al.*, 1988 Levin *et al.*, 1989 Kerner *et al.*, 1991 Camussone *et al.*, 2009

Table 1A. Relevant repetitive recombinant antigens proposed for diagnostic uses. Abbreviations used: CRA, cytoplasmic repetitive antigen; FRA, flagellar repetitive antigen; MAP, microtubule associated protein. RP1, RP3, RP4 and RP5, repetitive peptide 1, 3, 4 and 5, respectively.

Antigen name	Characteristics	Diagnostic use	Described by
SAPA RP2	Trans-sialidase family	Acute and congenital infections. Chronic infection in leishmaniasis endemic regions	Frasch & Reyes, 1990 Russomando *et al.*, 2010 Breniere et al., 1997 Gil *et al.*, 2011 Camussone *et al.*, 2009
TcLo1.2	Trans-sialidase family	Chronic infection	Houghton *et al.*, 1999
TcD	Trans-sialidase family	Chronic and acute infection	Burns, Jr. *et al.*, 1992
Trans-sialidase catalytic region	Trans-sialidase family	Confirmation of chronic infection	Buchovsky *et al.*, 2001
FL-160 CEA CRP160	Complement regulatory protein from TS-like family	Chronic infection and cure monitoring Chronic infection and cure monitoring Cure monitoring	Cetron *et al.*, 1992 Jazin *et al.*, 1995 Meira *et al.*, 2004
TSSAI	Trypomastigote muscin of TS-like family	*T. cruzi* typing (named lineage Tc I, in the previous nomenclature)	Di Noia *et al.*, 2002
TSSAII	Trypomastigote muscin of TS-like family	*T. cruzi* typing (named lineage Tc II, in the previous nomenclature) DTUII, V and VI in the current nomenclature Confirmatory diagnostic in Chagas and leishmaniasis co-endemic regions	Di Noia *et al.*, 2002 Bhattacharyya *et al.*, 2010 Cimino *et al.*, 2011

Table 1B. Relevant recombinant antigens which belong to tran-sialidase (TS) and TS-like family, proposed for diagnostic uses. Abbreviations used: CEA, chronic exoantigen (160 KDa); CRP, complement regulatory protein; FL-160, surface flagellar protein (160 KDa); RP2, repetitive peptide 2; SAPA, shed-acute phase antigen.

Antigen name	Characteristics	Diagnostic use	Described by
R13	Last 13 amino acids from ribosomal protein.	Specific of cardiac disease	Aznar *et al.*, 1995
		Stages of cardiac disease	Diez *et al.*, 2006
P2β	Full length ribosomal P2β protein	Stages of cardiac disease	Fabbro *et al.*, 2011
		All stages	Breniere *et al.*, 2002
TcE	Ribosomal protein	Chronic infection	Houghton et al., 1999
FcaBP	Flagellar calcium binding protein	Chronic and acute infection	Engman *et al.*, 1989
1F8		Chronic infection	Gonzalez *et al.*, 1985
Tc-24		Cure monitoring patients	Krautz *et al.*, 1995
F29		Cure monitoring patients	Fabbro *et al.*, 2007
Tc-29		Chronic infection	Abate *et al.*, 1993
Calflagin		Chronic infection	Marcipar *et al.*, 2005
cy-hsp70	Heat Shock Proteins	Chronic infection and cure monitoring	Krautz *et al.*, 1998
mt-hsp70			
grp-hsp78			
TcAg29	Alginate regulatory protein	Chronic infection	DaRocha *et al.*, 2002
TcAg48	RNA binding protein	Chronic infection	DaRocha *et al.*, 2002
Tc1	Repetitive proteins obtained by bioinformatic analysis of the genome	Chronic infection	Goto *et al.*, 2008
Tc3	Idem	Chronic infection	Goto *et al.*, 2008
Tc4	Idem	Chronic infection	Goto *et al.*, 2008
Tc9	Idem	Chronic infection	Goto *et al.*, 2008
Tc10	Idem	Chronic infection	Goto *et al.*, 2008
Tc12	Idem	Chronic infection	Goto *et al.*, 2008
Tc15	Idem	Chronic infection	Goto *et al.*, 2008

Table 1C. Other relevant recombinant antigens proposed for diagnostic uses. Abbreviations used: cy-hsp70, cytoplasmic thermal-shock protein; FCaBP, flagellar calcium-binding protein; grp.hsp 78, endoplasmic reticule thermal-shock protein (78 KDa); mt-hsp 70, thermal-shock mitochondrial protein (70 KDA).

4. Recombinant proteins use: Mixtures vs. fusion proteins

The first works dealing with a single recombinant protein for diagnostic purposes reported lack of sensitivity when using only one of those antigens.(Levin *et al.*, 1991;Moncayo & Luquetti, 1990;Peralta *et al.*, 1994) Consequently, most of these proteins have been evaluated not only alone and independently from others, but also together as part of mixtures or as fusion proteins, carrying several recombinant epitopes.(Umezawa *et al.*, 1999;Umezawa *et al.*, 2004;Camussone *et al.*, 2009;Foti *et al.*, 2009) Accordingly, a multicenter study evaluating 6 recombinant proteins separately with a serum panel composed by sera from patients of several countries, described that using the set of results of the 6 proteins together had yield a sensitivity and specificity compatible with the reference assays.(Umezawa *et al.*, 1999) Later, the same group evaluated the mixture of the 6 proteins, supporting the use of the mixture to reach the same sensitivity and specificity.(Umezawa *et al.*, 2003) Soon after, the reactivity of individual antigens vs. antigen mixtures was systematically assessed by ELISA.(Umezawa *et al.*, 2004) This study confirmed that the results obtained with recombinant protein mixtures led to higher media values of optical densities, ODs, than the results produced when using the individual recombinant proteins. Moreover, sera rendering low ODs when examined with individual recombinant proteins produced higher ODs outcomes when using the protein mixtures. Along with this, several commercial ELISA kits with recombinant protein mixtures display equivalent or even higher sensitivities and specificities than those produced by kits with total parasite homogenate.(Gadelha *et al.*, 2003;Pirard *et al.*, 2005;Remesar *et al.*, 2009;Caballero *et al.*, 2007) These works have studied kits using Ag1, Ag2, Ag30, Ag13 together with Ag36 recombinant antigens (Chagatest Rec from Wiener lab, Argentina), and FRA and CRA recombinant antigens (Biomanguinhos, Friocruz, Brazil). However, another study reported that Chagatest Rec v3.0 (Wiener) displayed a rather low 95% sensitivity.(Ramirez *et al.*, 2009)

One of the strategies proposed to enhance reagents production standardization is to obtain multiepitope molecules, designed as a unique construction by fusing several relevant diagnostic antigens.(Houghton *et al.*, 1999;Aguirre *et al.*, 2006;Camussone *et al.*, 2009) It has recently been proved that when using these constructions, the ODs of sera with low reactivity increases, as well as it had been reported for mixtures.(Camussone *et al.*, 2009) Moreover, by this approach the attachment of the antigen turned out to be homogenous and reproducible when using different surfaces such as ELISA plaques, latex particles or bioelectrodes.(Camussone *et al.*, 2009;Gonzalez *et al.*, 2010;Belluzo *et al.*, 2011) It has been proposed that when there is only one molecule exposed to the surface, competition for the active sites is prevented, therefore resulting in a uniform attachment. Furthermore, sensitivity may be increased because a higher number of freely accessible epitopes are available to capture the antibodies present in samples, as depicted in Fig. 1.(Camussone *et al.*, 2009)

A few articles report on the use of this strategy to produce commercial ELISA kits which have demonstrated to be highly satisfying. One of these works, analyzes the performance of the TcF antigen, previously described by Houghton et al in 1999, with which the Biolab Merieux reagent was prepared.(Ferreira *et al.*, 2001) In this case, the recombinant protein used bears the PEP2, TcD, TcE and TcLo1.2 peptides. Recently, Abbot Laboratories have presented a new kit which uses a 4-antigen multiepitope protein containing TcF, FP3 -built up with TcR27 and FcaBP-, FP6 –with TcR39 and FRA- and FP10 -with SAPA and MAP-.(Praast *et al.*, 2011) According to the authors, this kit performed even better than the Biolab Merieux one.

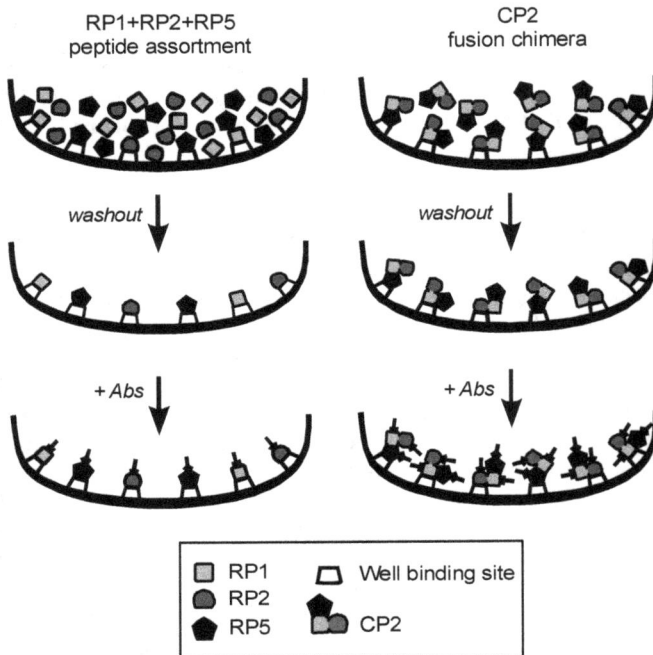

Fig. 1. Illustration of the ELISA plaque sensitizing process and the exposure to the sample: left-hand side, when using a protein mixture of three recombinant peptides RP1+RP2+RP5; right-hand side, when using a multiepitope chimeric protein bearing the same peptides fused in a single protein, CP2. RP: recombinant peptide, CP: chimeric protein obtained by fusion of peptides RP1, RP2 and RP5 together in only one molecule. Reproduction from Camussone et al 2009.

5. Recombinant antigens use for the diagnosis of the different clinical entities

5.1 Acute phase diagnosis

As previously mentioned, during acute infection, serological methods are poorly sensitive. In the case of immunosuppressed individuals, as they do not develop an appropriate humoral immunological response, the direct method or molecular techniques are advisable. Serology is pertinent for in the neonatal congenital diagnostic when microhematocrit repeatedly shows negative results, or when diagnosis has not been made during the first month of life of the newborn. In these cases, it is necessary to serologically monitor congenital infection between 6 to 9 months, no matter if conventional reagents or recombinant ones are used.

Nevertheless, the search for antibodies which are usually triggered during acute phase could enhance results. In the early nineties a shed acute phase antigen (SAPA) was proposed to discriminate between acute and chronic infection.(Reyes et al., 1990) This antigen was described when a panel of recombinant proteins obtained from a cDNA library was used to analyze the reactivity of IgG antibodies occurring in sera of chronic chagasic mothers and their newborns. The recognized IgGs against different *T. cruzi* antigens produced the same signal in sera from newborns and their respective mothers but SAPA antigen was recognized most frequently by antibodies from the infected newborns than it was by antibodies occurring in their mothers serum. Accordingly, the authors proposed it to be used to detect specific anti-*T. cruzi* IgG antibodies in neonates. Other works report that antibodies anti-SAPA allows the discrimination between acute and chronic *T. cruzi* infection because they were not present in the later stage of the infection.(Lorca *et al.*, 1993) Nevertheless, later works described SAPA as reactive when assessed with sera from chronic infected individuals.(Breniere *et al.*, 1997;Camussone *et al.*, 2009) This apparent contradiction could be explained considering the significant differential reactivity of anti-SAPA antibodies generated during the different stages of the infection. Indeed, anti-SAPA antibodies are detected in almost all infected individuals but its reactivity is higher in the acute infection. It has recently been performed a study by following up of 2283 chagasic mothers, from which 209 transmitted the infection to the newborns.(Russomando *et al.*, 2010) This work provides evidence on SAPA utility to serologically diagnose congenital infection before the third month of life, thus turning the protein into a promising inexpensive reagent to reduce the required time to detect the neonatal infection, and proceed to its early treatment.

Although different reactivity patterns have been described in Western Blot assays which use native *T. cruzi* excretion antigens, to discriminate between acute and chronic infection (Umezawa *et al.*, 1996) no other useful recombinant antigen different from SAPA has been described to diagnose the acute phase.

5.2 Chronic infection diagnosis

It has been already mentioned above that, when *T. cruzi* homogenate is used to perform ELISA tests, the assay sensitivity is high leading to a quite reliable result, therefore some authors have suggested that a single assay could be enough to test sera in blood banks. (Sosa Stani *et al.*, 2008; Otani *et al.*, 2009)

Several multicenter studies carried out on samples from blood-banks, report that ELISA tests which use parasite homogenates perform similarly than those which used recombinant proteins.(Remesar *et al.*, 2009; Otani *et al.*, 2009) However, cross-reactivity of antibodies towards antigens from *T. cruzi* and *Leishmania sp* has been frequently informed, and can be explained considering the phylogenic proximity between both parasite species.(Chiller *et al.*, 1990;Vexenat *et al.*, 1996;Chiaramonte *et al.*, 1996;Desquesnes *et al.*, 2007;Aguirre *et al.*, 2006) When sera from patients infected with *Leishmania ssp* parasites are included in the evaluations, specificity of recombinant proteins are higher (Umezawa *et al.*, 1999; Ferreira *et al.*, 2001; Aguirre *et al.*, 2006; Caballero *et al.*, 2007; Camussone *et al.*, 2009)

It has been recently reported that the antigen TSSA2 displays 87.8% sensitivity and 100% specificity to discriminate between chagasic and leishmaniasic patients.(Cimino *et al.*, 2011) TSSA2 is the only reported recombinant antigen, which has displayed specificity to type *T. cruzi* genotypes DTUII, DTUV or DTUVI by specific antibodies from infected patients. (di Noia *et al.*, 2002; Bhattacharyya *et al.*, 2010) As these DTUs are those predominant in South America, the authors proposed using this antigen in confirmatory *T. cruzi* infection diagnostic tests, in regions which are co-endemic for both infections. It was also described that SAPA antigen could be specific and sensitive enough to be used when trying to distinguish between chronic *T. cruzi* and leishmaniasic infections, in regions where both illnesses are co-endemic.(Gil *et al.*, 2011)

It should be considered that it is difficult to discard *T. cruzi* infection in patients suffering from leishmaniasis, because these are co-endemic diseases. That is why antigens cross-reactivity is normally assayed testing sera from patients who live in Chagas' disease non-endemic regions, because this allows ruling out *T. cruzi* infection from an epidemiological point of view. (Hernandez *et al.*, 2010;Caballero *et al.*, 2007;Aguirre *et al.*, 2006)   It therefore follows the need to discuss and define new criteria to study the performance of immunochemical tests at those regions. In this regard, the enhanced sensitivity displayed by PCR techniques should allow overcoming the mentioned drawback.

The lack of cross-reactions of *T. cruzi* recombinant proteins towards samples from *T. rangeli* infected individuals was also described. (Caballero *et al.*, 2007) However, these are only preliminary results, and large evaluations have not been still performed since *T. cruzi* and *T. rangelli* are co-endemic and mixed infections are difficult to exclude with conventional or epidemiologic analysis. The first studies reporting discrimination of both infections using molecular approaches have been published in the last year and will allow to compose a serum panel with samples from patients suffering from either only one or both infections.(Botero *et al.*, 2010)

In spite of the advantages yielded when using recombinant antigens in ELISA, it has also been described that sensitivity varies according to the antigen used to sensitize plaques and the geographical region. Thus, sensitivity obtained when performing tests in Colombia using recombinant antigens related to the predominant strain in South America is different from that obtained when assays are carried out in regions at the South of the continent.(Ramirez *et al.*, 2009) The same holds true when examining samples from Panamá patients, where *T. cruzi* strains are very similar to those from Colombia. (Caballero *et al.*, 2007) These works point out that serum level of antibodies in Panamanian patients were significantly lower than those from Brazilian individuals, from where the recombinant proteins were obtained using parasite genotypes isolated in Brazil. These data are in agreement with the serological differential reactivity produced by experimental infections in a mouse model, when strains representatives of different DTUs are inoculated.(dos Santos *et al.*, 2009).

5.3 Laboratory treatment monitoring

The evaluation of treatment effectiveness is normally carried out through serological analysis. Direct parasitological techniques miss reliability because of the extremely low parasitemia, which after treatment diminishes more, even when total parasite elimination could have not been reached.

Conventional serology turns into negative for more than 80% of the patients treated during the acute phase, once passed about 2 years after treatment. However, this percentage drops to less than 10% for patients who have been treated during the chronic phase, this taking several years.(Cancado, 1999)

The patient status is classified, according to the laboratory tests results. Thus, patients are considered cured when parasitological tests and conventional serology are negative. When parasitological tests are negative and 2 of 3 conventional serological tests are positive, the patient is classified as dissociated. Patients are considered not to be cured when the 3 tests are positive.

The serological test that demonstrated to be especially useful to monitor treatment effectiveness is the assessment of lytic antibodies. This test showed 100% correlation with parasitological cure, when lytic antibodies were evaluated in sera from patients who were confirmed to be cured.(Krettli et al., 1979) The drawback of this test is the need to count with in vivo trypomastigotes culture, thus not being available in clinical diagnostic laboratories. Consequently, several recombinant antigens to evaluate patient's treatment response have been proposed and assessed by ELISA as follows.

The target antigen of lytic antibodies was identified as a 160 KDa molecule, a complement regulatory protein, usually named CRP.(Krettli, 2009) The assessment of antibodies against this protein displayed 100% correlation with that of lytic antibodies, when using both the native protein and the recombinant one.(Meira et al., 2004)

Cruzipain and Tc24 are other recombinant proteins which were also evaluated to monitor patient's treatment, and displayed 70% and 80% correlation with the lytic antibodies method, respectively.(Gazzinelli et al., 1993;Krautz et al., 1995) F29, which is Tc24 homologous, was used to follow up the treatment in children younger than 12 years old, after 48 months of initiated the medication.(Sosa et al., 1998) This work reports that 67% of sera from treated children showed lack of anti-F29 antibodies whereas 100% of untreated children showed positive results for the specific antibodies. Therefore, the authors proposed to confirm the lack of anti-F29 antibodies as a serological marker of children cure. More recently, F29 was again evaluated as antigen of treatment monitoring in adults.(Fabbro et al., 2007) Results showed lack of the specific antibodies in 82.4% of sera from treated patients who still showed positive conventional serology. The same group has recently evaluated the levels of specific antibodies against the ribosomal protein TcP2β, as a cure marker. (Fabbro et al., 2011) Their results showed a significant decrease of specific anti-TcP2β in sera from treated patients, although no negative results occurred, which is a similar behavior than that displayed when performing conventional serology. Therefore, anti-TcP2β does not resemble to be an apparently good candidate to be used as an early marker of the infection cure.

Another interesting study is the one where CRA and FRA antigens were evaluated, and displayed a 67% correlation with the reference technique. This makes CRA and FRA as quite promising antigens to be used for cure monitoring. The results are interesting considering that the Bio-manguinhos, Fiocruz commercial kit, commercialized in Brazil is manufactured with a single mixture of these two recombinant proteins.

5.4 Chronic infection monitoring

In the context of Chagas disease autoimmune hypothesis, during the nineties, it was proposed that different antigens contributed to the generation of autoantibodies, which could be used as illness evolution markers.(Leon & Engman, 2001) Among these antigens we should mention cruzipain, (Giordanengo et al., 2000;Goin et al., 1999;Duschak et al., 2001) sulfo-cerebrosides (Avila et al., 1993) and the ribosomal protein TcP2β.(Levitus et al., 1991) Precursor works had described that this ribosomal antigen that shares the C terminal region with its homologous from humans, generated autoimmune antibodies, whose concentration was increased in patients who had developed chagasic cardiopathy.(Levin et al., 1991;Aznar et al., 1995). Our group evaluated the concentration of antibodies against cruzipain, sulfo-cerebrosides and ribosomal TcP2β in three different groups of patients: those classified as asymptomatic, those who only displayed electrocardiographic alterations and those who had evident cardiopathy.(Diez et al., 2006) In our experience, only those samples from patients with evident cardiopathy had increased specific anti-TcP2β concentration. However, these results have not yet been confirmed analyzing a larger number of patients. In another study, anti-TcP2β concentration was higher in sera from patients at indeterminate stage than in sera from symptomatic individuals.(Breniere *et al.*, 2002) In a longitudinal evaluation of asymptomatic and cardiac groups of patients, we described that only the individuals who evolved to a more severe clinical status increased specific anti-TcP2β concentration in late stages of the infection.(Fabbro *et al.*, 2011) However, the transversal comparison of the sera from patients with and without cardiopathy revealed that anti-TcP2β concentration between both groups was not significantly different. The discrepant results mentioned above show that it is not still clear if anti-TcP2β can be used as a serological marker of myocardic damage.

Also, muscarinic acetylcholine receptor subtype II, in this case a host antigen, has shown to be quite auspicious to monitor the chronic infection.(Goin *et al.*, 1999) Nevertheless, recent studies suggest that it is not apparent that this protein is useful to discriminate between different stages of the illness.(Tovar *et al.*, 2009;Talvani *et al.*, 2006)

The difficulties to establish clear illness evolution markers lead to the present state, where we do not count yet with useful tools to evaluate Chagas' disease prognosis.

6. Future prospects

The number of recombinant proteins assessed and proposed as candidates to be used as tools for *T. cruzi* infection diagnosis is quite high. However, there is no serum panel to be used as international reference. Therefore, the reports on results produced by using these proteins can hardly be compared. Usually, serum panels, previously typified with other validated methods are used to appraise new serology reagents. These already standardized serological reagents have their own sensitivity and specificity, which may lead to a bias when typifying the panel.

Currently, several diagnostic tests have been proposed as the reference one, such as immunofluorescence or different versions of Western blot.(Otani *et al.*, 2009;Caballero *et al.*, 2007) However, no consensus exists among researchers and regulatory agencies on which tests are preferable.

Another inconvenience is that there is evidence on the absence of humoral response in some patients of endemic regions, whose infection was proved by parasitological techniques or by tests evaluating the cellular immune response.(Salomone *et al.*, 2003;Olivera *et al.*, 2010) These reports alert us on a potential overestimation of the sensitivity and specificity underestimation of the immunochemical assays when they are assessed with serum panels typified by conventional serology.

Conventional serology is still a crucial tool to diagnose the different entities studied during the chronic phase of the infection. The main multicenter studies carried out in regions where leishmaniasis is not endemic have shown that ELISAs using both parasite extractive antigens, as well as the recombinant ones, display optimal sensitivity and specificity. Although both kind of antigens perform similarly in those leishmaniasis-free places, when determinations are carried out where Chagas' disease and leishmaniasis are co-endemic, ELISAs using recombinant proteins have demonstrated to be the most useful.

In the same line, presently, several authors who have evaluated ELISA commercial kits with plaques sensitized with parasite homogenate or with recombinant antigens, have shown that it is not mandatory to carry out 2 different tests. Certainly, when performing only one ELISA, it is feasible to diagnose the infection, if the result is positive. This is acknowledged because results obtained with both kinds of ELISA correlate appropriately. (Remesar *et al.*, 2009;Otani *et al.*, 2009) However, considering the poor sensitivity of IHA, this latter one would not be recommended as a second test. (Remesar *et al.*, 2009)

Even though some recombinant proteins have been used to monitor Chagas´ disease treatment, it could not be still demonstrated that these proteins give diagnostic information to evaluate cardiopathy diagnosis and prognosis. During recent years, the description of the whole genome of *T. cruzi* has prompt to systematically analyze new antigens, some of which have been described as putative antigens, but has not yet confirmed. This is being evaluated nowadays by different research groups which, it is expected will suggest new interesting markers that are useful for cure monitoring and cardiopathy prognosis.

Lately, several research works on infection diagnostic tools have reported on the development of latex particle agglutination and amperometric biosensors to diagnose *T. cruzi* infection.(Gonzalez *et al.*, 2010;Belluzo *et al.*, 2011;Ribone *et al.*, 2006) Latex particle vs. conventional agglutination has the advantage of allowing particle sensitization with recombinant proteins, what leads to a more reproducible, standardized reagents production.(Gonzalez *et al.*, 2010) Biosensors technology admits reutilization of the device, potentially yielding to automation, thus facilitating laboratory operation. Moreover, the simplicity of the equipment required, permits the analysis to be performed in the field, which is an important attribute because infected people generally live in the countryside and do not attend health centers.(Belluzo *et al.*, 2011) The electrochemical biosensor technology developed follows the same ELISA format, exchanging the colorimetric signal readout by the amperometric one.(Belluzo *et al.*, 2011) Although no commercial device is yet available, the results of our studies are quite promising. This methodology could allow reducing costs and time of analysis in the near future, keeping the same or even higher standards of sensitivity and specificity than ELISA.(Belluzo *et al.*, 2011)

7. References

Affranchino,J.L.; Ibanez,C.F.; Luquetti,A.O.; Rassi,A.; Reyes,M.B.; Macina,R.A.; Aslund,L.; Pettersson,U. & Frasch,A.C. (1989) Identification of a Trypanosoma cruzi antigen that is shed during the acute phase of Chagas' disease. *Mol. Biochem. Parasitol.* 34(3), 221-228.

Aguirre,S.; Silver,A.M.; Brito,M.E.F.; Ribone,M.E.; Lagier,C.M. & Marcipar,I.S. (2006) Design, Construction and Evaluation of a Specific Chimeric Antigen to Diagnose Chagasic Infection. *J. Clin. Microbiol.* 44, 1043-1046.

Araujo,F.G. (1986) Analysis of *Trypanosoma cruzi* antigens bound by specific antibodies and by antibodies to related trypanosomatids. *Infect. Immun.* 53(1), 179-185.

Avila,J.L.; Rojas,M. & Carrasco,H. (1993) Elevated levels of antibodies against sulphatide are present in all chronic chagasic and dilated cardiomyopathy sera. *Clin. Exp. Immunol.* 92(3), 460-465.

Aznar,C.; Lopez-Bergami,P.; Brandariz,S.; Mariette,C.; Liegeard,P.; Alves,M.D.; Barreiro,E.L.; Carrasco,R.; Lafon,S.; & Kaplan,D. (1995) Prevalence of anti-R-13 antibodies in human *Trypanosoma cruzi* infection. *FEMS Immunol. Med. Microbiol.* 12(3-4), 231-238.

Barfield,C.A.; Barney,R.S.; Crudder,C.H.; Wilmoth,J.L.; Stevens,D.S.; Mora-Garcia,S.; Yanovsky,M.J.; Weigl,B.H. & Yanovsky,J. (2011) A highly sensitive rapid diagnostic test for Chagas disease that utilizes a recombinant Trypanosoma cruzi antigen. *IEEE Trans. Biomed. Eng.* 58(3), 814-817.

Belluzo,M.S.; Ribone,M.E.; Camussone,C.; Marcipar,I.S. & Lagier,C.M. (2011) Favorably orienting recombinant proteins to develop amperometric biosensors to diagnose Chagas' disease. *Anal. Biochem.* 408(1), 86-94.

Bhattacharyya,T.; Brooks,J.; Yeo,M.; Carrasco,H.J.; Lewis,M.D.; Llewellyn,M.S. & Miles,M.A. (2010) Analysis of molecular diversity of the Trypanosoma cruzi trypomastigote small surface antigen reveals novel epitopes, evidence of positive selection and potential implications for lineage-specific serology. *Int. J. Parasitol.* 40(8), 921-928.

Bitran,R.; Martorell,B.; Escobar,L.; Munoz,R. & Glassman,A. (2009) Controlling and eliminating neglected diseases in Latin America and the Caribbean. *Health Aff. (Millwood.).* 28(6), 1707-1719.

Botero,A.; Ortiz,S.; Munoz,S.; Triana,O. & Solari,A. (2010) Differentiation of Trypanosoma cruzi and Trypanosoma rangeli of Colombia using minicircle hybridization tests. *Diagn. Microbiol. Infect. Dis.* 68(3), 265-270.

Bowling,J.; Walter,E.A. (2009) Recognizing and meeting the challenge of Chagas disease in the USA, *Expert Rev. Anti. Infect. Ther.* 7, 1223-1234.

Breniere,S.F.; Yaksic,N.; Telleria,J.; Bosseno,M.F.; Noireau,F.; Wincker,P. & Sanchez,D. (1997) Immune response to Trypanosoma cruzi shed acute phase antigen in children from an endemic area for Chagas' disease in Bolivia. *Mem. Inst. Oswaldo Cruz.* 92(4), 503-507.

Breniere,S.F.; Bosseno,M.F.; Noireau,F.; Yacsik,N.; Liegeard,P.; Aznar,C. & Hontebeyrie,M. (2002) Integrate study of a Bolivian population infected by Trypanosoma cruzi, the agent of Chagas disease. *Mem. Inst. Oswaldo Cruz.* 97(3), 289-295.

Brutus,L.; Schneider,D.; Postigo,J.; Romero,M.; Santalla,J. & Chippaux,J.P. (2008) Congenital Chagas disease: diagnostic and clinical aspects in an area without vectorial transmission, Bermejo, Bolivia. *Acta Trop.* 106(3), 195-199.

Buchovsky,A.S.; Campetella,O.; Russomando,G.; Franco,L.; Oddone,R.; Candia,N.; Luquetti,A.; Gonzalez Cappa,S.M. & Leguizamon,M.S. (2001) trans-sialidase inhibition assay, a highly sensitive and specific diagnostic test for Chagas' disease. *Clin. Diagn. Lab. Immunol.* 8(1), 187-189.

Burns,J.M.; Jr. Shreffler,W.G.; Rosman,D.E.; Sleath,P.R.; March,C.J. & Reed,S.G. (1992) Identification and synthesis of a major conserved antigenic epitope of *Trypanosoma cruzi.* *Proc. Natl. Acad. Sci. U. S. A.* 89(4), 1239-1243.

Caballero,Z.C.; Sousa,O.E.; Marques,W.P.; Saez-Alquezar,A. & Umezawa,E.S. (2007) Evaluation of serological tests to identify Trypanosoma cruzi infection in humans and determine cross-reactivity with Trypanosoma rangeli and Leishmania spp. *Clin. Vaccine Immunol.* 14(8), 1045-1049.

Camussone,C.; Gonzalez,V.; Belluzo,M.S.; Pujato,N.; Ribone,M.E.; Lagier,C.M. & Marcipar,I.S. (2009) Comparison of recombinant Trypanosoma cruzi peptide mixtures versus multiepitope chimeric proteins as sensitizing antigens for immunodiagnosis. *Clin. Vaccine Immunol.* 16(6), 899-905.

Cancado,J.R. (1999) Criteria of Chagas disease cure. *Mem. Inst. Oswaldo Cruz.* 94(1), 331-335.

Carlier,Y. & Torrico,F. (2003) Congenital Infection with Trypanosoma cruzi: From mechanisms of transmission to strategies for diagnosis and control. *Rev. Bras. Med. Trop.* 36(6), 767-771.

Carvalho,M.R.; Krieger,M.A.; Almeida,E.; Oelemann,W.; Shikanai-Yassuda,M.A.; Ferreira,A.; Pereira,J.B.; Saez-Alquezar,A.; Dorlhiac-Llacer,P.E.; Chamone,D.F. &

Goldenberg,S. (1993) Chagas' disease diagnosis: evaluation of several tests in blood bank screening. *Transfusion*. 33, 830-834.

Cetron,M.S.; Hoff,R.; Kahn,S.; Eisen,H. and Van Voorhis,W.C. (1992) Evaluation of recombinant trypomastigote surface antigens of Trypanosoma cruzi in screening sera from a population in rural northeastern Brazil endemic for Chagas' disease. *Acta Trop.* 50(3), 259-266.

Chiaramonte,M.G.; Zwirner,N.W.; Caropresi,S.L.; Taranto,N.J. & Malchiodi,E.L. (1996) Trypanosoma cruzi and Leishmania spp. human mixed infection. *Am. J. Trop. Med. Hyg.* 54(3), 271-273.

Chiari,E.; Dias,J.C.; Lana,M. & Chiari,C.A. (1989) Hemocultures for the parasitological diagnosis of human chronic Chagas' disease. *Rev. Soc. Bras. Med. Trop.* 22(1), 19-23.

Chiller,T.M.; Samudio,M.A. & Zoulek,G. (1990) IgG antibody reactivity with Trypanosoma cruzi and Leishmania antigens in sera of patients with Chagas' disease and leishmaniasis. *Am. J. Trop. Med. Hyg.* 43(6), 650-656.

Cimino,R.O.; Rumi,M.M.; Ragone,P.; Lauthier,J.; Alberti,D.'A.; Quiroga,I.R.; Gil,J.F.; Cajal,S.P.; Acosta,N.; Juarez,M.; Krolewiecki,A.; Orellana,V.; Zacca,R.; Marcipar,I.; Diosque,P. & Nasser,J.R. (2011) Immuno-enzymatic evaluation of the recombinant TSSA-II protein of Trypanosoma cruzi in dogs and human sera: a tool for epidemiological studies. *Parasitology.*; 1-8.

Cooley,G.; Etheridge,R.D.; Boehlke,C.; Bundy,B.; Weatherly,D.B.; Minning,T.; Haney,M.; Postan,M.; Laucella,S. & Tarleton,R.L. (2008) High throughput selection of effective serodiagnostics for Trypanosoma cruzi infection. *PLoS. Negl. Trop. Dis.* 2(10), e316.

Cotrim,P.C.; Paranhos,G.S.; Mortara,R.A.; Wanderley,J.; Rassi,A.; Camargo,M.E. & da Silveira,J.F. (1990) Expression in *Escherichia coli* of a dominant immunogen of *Trypanosoma cruzi* recognized by human chagasic sera. *J. Clin. Microbiol.* 28(3), 519-524.

Cotrim,P.C.; Paranhos-Baccala,G.; Santos,M.R.; Mortensen,C.; Cano,M.I.; Jolivet,M.; Camargo,M.E.; Mortara,R.A. & da Silveira,J.F. (1995) Organization and expression of the gene encoding an immunodominant repetitive antigen associated to the cytoskeleton of Trypanosoma cruzi. *Mol. Biochem. Parasitol.* 71(1), 89-98.

Coura,J.R. (2007) Chagas disease: what is known and what is needed--a background article. *Mem. Inst. Oswaldo Cruz.* 102 Suppl 1, 113-122.

da Silveira,J.F.; Umezawa,E.S. & Luquetti,A.O. (2001) Chagas disease: recombinant *Trypanosoma cruzi* antigens for serological diagnosis. *Trends Parasitol.* 17(6), 286-291.

da Silveira,A.B.; Lemos,E.M.; Adad,S.J.; Correa-Oliveira,R.; Furness,J.B. & D'Avila,R.D. (2007) Megacolon in Chagas disease: a study of inflammatory cells, enteric nerves, and glial cells. *Hum. Pathol.* 38(8), 1256-1264.

DaRocha,W.D.; Bartholomeu,D.C.; Macedo,C.D.; Horta,M.F.; Cunha-Neto,E.; Donelson,J.E. & Teixeira,S.M. (2002) Characterization of cDNA clones encoding ribonucleoprotein antigens expressed in *Trypanosoma cruzi* amastigotes. *Parasitol. Res.* 88(4), 292-300.

de Moraes,M.H.; Guarneri,A.A.; Girardi,F.P.; Rodrigues,J.B.; Eger,I.; Tyler,K.M.; Steindel,M. & Grisard,E.C. (2008) Different serological cross-reactivity of Trypanosoma rangeli forms in Trypanosoma cruzi-infected patients sera. *Parasit. Vectors.* 1(1), 20.

Desquesnes,M.; Bosseno,M.F. & Breniere,S.F. (2007) Detection of Chagas infections using Trypanosoma evansi crude antigen demonstrates high cross-reactions with Trypanosoma cruzi. *Infect. Genet. Evol.* 7(4), 457-462.

Di Noia,J.M.; Buscaglia,C.A.; De Marchi,C.R.; Almeida,I.C. & Frasch,A.C. (2002) A Trypanosoma cruzi small surface molecule provides the first immunological evidence that Chagas' disease is due to a single parasite lineage. *J. Exp. Med.* 195(4), 401-413.

Dias,J.C.; Amato Neto, V.; Luna, E.J. (2011) Alternative transmission mechanisms of *Trypanosoma cruzi* in Brazil and proposals for their prevention. *Rev. Soc. Bras. Med. Trop.* 44(3) 375-9.

Diez,C.N.; Gea,S.; Marcipar,I.S.; Pezzotto,S.M.; Beloscar,J.; Pellizzon,O.; Marcipar,A. & Bottasso,O. (2006) Cardiovascular risk factors in chronic Chagas' disease are associated with a different profile of putative heart-pathogenic antibodies. *FEMS Immunol. Med. Microbiol.* 48(1), 26-33.

Diez,C.N.; Manattini,S.; Zanuttini,J.C.; Bottasso,O. & Marcipar,I.S. (2008) The value of molecular studies for the diagnosis of congenital Chagas disease in northeastern Argentina. *Am. J. Trop. Med. Hyg.* 78(4), 624-627.

dos Santos,D.M.; Talvani,A.; Guedes,P.M.; hado-Coelho,G.L.; de,L.M. & Bahia,M.T. (2009) Trypanosoma cruzi: Genetic diversity influences the profile of immunoglobulins during experimental infection. *Exp. Parasitol.* 121(1), 8-14.

Duschak,V.G.; Riarte,A.; Segura,E.L. & Laucella,S.A. (2001) Humoral immune response to cruzipain and cardiac dysfunction in chronic Chagas disease. *Immunol. Lett.* 78(3), 135-142.

Editorial (2009) Chagas disease: a neglected emergency. *Lancet.* 373(9678), 1820.

El Sayed,N.M.; Myler,P.J.; Bartholomeu,D.C.; Nilsson,D.; Aggarwal,G.; Tran,A.N.; Ghedin,E.; Worthey,E.A.; Delcher,A.L.; Blandin,G.; Westenberger,S.J.; Caler,E.; Cerqueira,G.C.; Branche,C.; Haas,B.; Anupama,A.; Arner,E.; Aslund,L.; Attipoe,P.; Bontempi,E.; Bringaud,F.; Burton,P.; Cadag,E.; Campbell,D.A.; Carrington,M.; Crabtree,J.; Darban,H.; da Silveira,J.F.; de Jong,P.; Edwards,K.; Englund,P.T.; Fazelina,G.; Feldblyum,T.; Ferella,M.; Frasch,A.C.; Gull,K.; Horn,D.; Hou,L.; Huang,Y.; Kindlund,E.; Klingbeil,M.; Kluge,S.; Koo,H.; Lacerda,D.; Levin,M.J.; Lorenzi,H.; Louie,T.; Machado,C.R.; McCulloch,R.; McKenna,A.; Mizuno,Y.; Mottram,J.C.; Nelson,S.; Ochaya,S.; Osoegawa,K.; Pai,G.; Parsons,M.; Pentony,M.; Pettersson,U.; Pop,M.; Ramirez,J.L.; Rinta,J.; Robertson,L.; Salzberg,S.L.; Sanchez,D.O.; Seyler,A.; Sharma,R.; Shetty,J.; Simpson,A.J.; Sisk,E.; Tammi,M.T.; Tarleton,R.; Teixeira,S.; Van Aken,S.; Vogt,C.; Ward,P.N.; Wickstead,B.; Wortman,J.; White,O.; Fraser,C.M.; Stuart,K.D. & Andersson,B. (2005) The genome sequence of *Trypanosoma cruzi*, etiologic agent of Chagas disease. *Science.* 309(5733), 409-415.

Engman,D.M.; Krause,K.H.; Blumin,J.H.; Kim,K.S.; Kirchhoff,L.V. & Donelson,J.E. (1989) A novel flagellar Ca2+-binding protein in trypanosomes. *J. Biol. Chem.* 264(31), 18627-18631.

Fabbro,D.L.; Streiger,M.L.; Arias,E.D.; Bizai,M.L.; del,B.M. & Amicone,N.A. (2007) Trypanocide treatment among adults with chronic Chagas disease living in Santa Fe city (Argentina), over a mean follow-up of 21 years: parasitological, serological and clinical evolution. *Rev. Soc. Bras. Med. Trop.* 40(1), 1-10.

Fabbro,D.L.; Olivera,V.; Bizai,M.L.; Denner,S.; Diez,C.; Marcipar,I.; Streiger,M.; Arias,E.; del,B.M.; Mendicino,D. & Bottasso,O. (2011) Humoral immune response against

P2beta from Trypanosoma cruzi in persons with chronic Chagas disease: its relationship with treatment against parasites and myocardial damage. *Am. J. Trop. Med. Hyg.* 84(4), 575-580.

Ferreira,A.W.; Belem,Z.R.; Lemos,E.A.; Reed,S.G. & Campos-Neto,A. (2001) Enzyme-linked immunosorbent assay for serological diagnosis of Chagas' disease employing a Trypanosoma cruzi recombinant antigen that consists of four different peptides. *J. Clin. Microbiol.* 39(12), 4390-4395.

Foti,L.; Fonseca,B.P.; Nascimento,L.D.; Marques,C.F.; da Silva,E.D.; Duarte,C.A.; Probst,C.M.; Goldenberg,S.; Pinto,A.G. & Krieger,M.A. (2009) Viability study of a multiplex diagnostic platform for Chagas disease. *Mem. Inst. Oswaldo Cruz.* 104 Suppl 1, 136-141.

Frasch,A.C. & Reyes,M.B. (1990) Diagnosis of Chagas disease using recombinant DNA technology. *Parasitol. Today.* 6(4), 137-139.

Freilij,H.; Muller,L. & Gonzalez Cappa,S.M. (1983) Direct micromethod for diagnosis of acute and congenital Chagas' disease. *J. Clin. Microbiol.* 18(2), 327-330.

Freilij,H. & Storino,R. (1994) Diagnóstico de laboratorio. In: *Enfermedad de Chagas,* Storino,R. & Milei,J. (eds.), Mosby-Doyma, Buenos Aires.

Freilij,H. & Altcheh,J. (1995) Congenital Chagas' disease: diagnostic and clinical aspects. *Clin. Infect. Dis.* 21(3), 551-555.

Gadelha,A.A.; Vercosa,A.F.; Lorena,V.M.; Nakazawa,M.; Carvalho,A.B.; Souza,W.V.; Ferreira,A.G.; Silva,E.D.; Krieger,M.A.; Goldenberg,S. & Gomes,Y.M. (2003) Chagas' disease diagnosis: comparative analysis of recombinant ELISA with conventional ELISA and the haemagglutination test. *Vox Sang.* 85(3), 165-170.

Gascon,J.A.; Bern,C.B.; Pinazo,M.J. (2009) Chagas disease in Spain, the United States and other non-endemic countries. *Acta Tropica.* 115 (1-2) 22-27.

Gazzinelli,R.T.; Galvao,L.M.; Krautz,G.; Lima,P.C.; Cancado,J.R.; Scharfstein,J. & Krettli,A.U. (1993) Use of Trypanosoma cruzi purified glycoprotein (GP57/51) or trypomastigote-shed antigens to assess cure for human Chagas' disease. *Am. J. Trop. Med. Hyg.* 49(5), 625-635.

Gil,J.; Cimino,R.; Lopez,Q.; I, Cajal,S.; Acosta,N.; Juarez,M.; Zacca,R.; Orellana,V.; Krolewiecki,A.; Diosque,P. & Nasser,J. (2011) Reactivity of GST-SAPA antigen of Trypanosoma cruzi against sera from patients with Chagas disease and leishmaniasis. *Medicina (B Aires).* 71(2), 113-119.

Giordanengo,L.; Fretes,R.; Diaz,H.; Cano,R.; Bacile,A.; Vottero-Cima,E. & Gea,S. (2000) Cruzipain induces autoimmune response against skeletal muscle and tissue damage in mice. *Muscle Nerve.* 23(9), 1407-1413.

Godsel,L.M.; Tibbetts,R.S.; Olson,C.L.; Chaudoir,B.M. & Engman,D.M. (1995) Utility of recombinant flagellar calcium-binding protein for serodiagnosis of *Trypanosoma cruzi* infection. *J. Clin. Microbiol.* 33(8), 2082-2085.

Goin,J.C.; Sterin-Borda,L.; Bilder,C.R.; Varrica,L.M.; Iantorno,G.; Rios,M.C. & Borda,E. (1999) Functional implications of circulating muscarinic cholinergic receptor autoantibodies in chagasic patients with achalasia. *Gastroenterology.* 117(4), 798-805.

Gomes,Y.M.; Lorena,V.M. & Luquetti,A.O. (2009) Diagnosis of Chagas disease: what has been achieved? What remains to be done with regard to diagnosis and follow up studies? *Mem. Inst. Oswaldo Cruz.* 104 Suppl 1, 115-121.

Gonzalez,A.; Lerner,T.J.; Huecas,M.; Sosa-Pineda,B.; Nogueira,N. & Lizardi,P.M. (1985) Apparent generation of a segmented mRNA from two separate tandem gene families in Trypanosoma cruzi. *Nucleic Acids Res.* 13(16), 5789-5804.

Gonzalez,V.D.; Garcia,V.S.; Vega,J.R.; Marcipar,I.S.; Meira,G.R. & Gugliotta,L.M. (2010) Immunodiagnosis of Chagas disease: Synthesis of three latex-protein complexes containing different antigens of Trypanosoma cruzi. *Colloids Surf. B Biointerfaces.* 77(1), 12-17.

Goto,Y.; Carter,D. & Reed,S.G. (2008) Immunological dominance of *Trypanosoma cruzi* tandem repeat proteins. *Infect. Immun.* 76(9), 3967-3974.

Gruber,A. & Zingales,B. (1993) *Trypanosoma cruzi*: characterization of two recombinant antigens with potential application in the diagnosis of Chagas' disease. *Exp. Parasitol.* 76(1), 1-12.

Hernandez,P.; Heimann,M.; Riera,C.; Solano,M.; Santalla,J.; Luquetti,A.O. & Beck,E. (2010) Highly effective serodiagnosis for Chagas' disease. *Clin. Vaccine Immunol.* 17(10), 1598-1604.

Hoft,D.F.; Kim,K.S.; Otsu,K.; Moser,D.R.; Yost,W.J.; Blumin,J.H.; Donelson,J.E. and Kirchhoff,L.V. (1989) *Trypanosoma cruzi* expresses diverse repetitive protein antigens. *Infect. Immun.* 57(7), 1959-1967.

Houghton,R.L.; Benson,D.R.; Reynolds,L.D.; McNeill,P.D.; Sleath,P.R.; Lodes,M.J.; Skeiky,Y.A.; Leiby,D.A.; Badaro,R. & Reed,S.G. (1999) A multi-epitope synthetic peptide and recombinant protein for the detection of antibodies to *Trypanosoma cruzi* in radioimmunoprecipitation-confirmed and consensus-positive sera. *J. Infect. Dis.* 179(5), 1226-1234.

Ibáñez,C.F.; Affranchino,J.L.; Macina,R.A.; Reys,M.B.; Aslund,U.; Petterson,U. & Frasch,A.A.C. (1988) Multiple *Trypanosoma cruzi* antigens containing tandemly amino acid sequence motif. *Mol. Biochem. Parasitol.* 30, 27-34.

Jazin,E.E.; Bontempi,E.J.; Sanchez,D.O.; Aslund,L.; Henriksson,J.; Frasch,A.C. & Pettersson,U. (1995) Trypanosoma cruzi exoantigen is a member of a 160 kDa gene family. *Parasitology.* 110 (Pt 1), 61-69.

Kerner,N.; Liegeard,P.; Levin,M.J. & Hontebeyrie-Joskowicz,M. (1991) *Trypanosoma cruzi*: antibodies to a MAP-like protein in chronic Chagas' disease cross-react with mammalian cytoskeleton. *Exp. Parasitol.* 73(4), 451-459.

Konishi,E. (1993) Naturally occurring antibodies that react with protozoan parasites. *Parasitol. Today.* 9(10), 361-364.

Krautz,G.M.; Galvao,L.M.; Cancado,J.R.; Guevara-Espinoza,A.; Ouaissi,A. & Krettli,A.U. (1995) Use of a 24-kilodalton *Trypanosoma cruzi* recombinant protein to monitor cure of human Chagas' disease. *J. Clin. Microbiol.* 33(8), 2086-2090.

Krautz,G.M.; Peterson,J.D.; Godsel,L.M.; Krettli,A.U. & Engman,D.M. (1998) Human antibody responses to Trypanosoma cruzi 70-kD heat-shock proteins. *Am. J. Trop. Med. Hyg.* 58(2), 137-143.

Krettli,A.U.; Weisz-Carrington,P. & Nussenzweig,R.S. (1979) Membrane-bound antibodies to bloodstream Trypanosoma cruzi in mice: strain differences in susceptibility to complement-mediated lysis. *Clin. Exp. Immunol.* 37(3), 416-423.

Krettli,A.U. (2009) The utility of anti-trypomastigote lytic antibodies for determining cure of Trypanosoma cruzi infections in treated patients: an overview and perspectives. *Mem. Inst. Oswaldo Cruz*. 104 Suppl 1, 142-151.

Lafaille,J.J.; Linss,J.; Krieger,M.A.; Souto-Padron,T.; de Souza,W. & Goldenberg,S. (1989) Structure and expression of two *Trypanosoma cruzi* genes encoding antigenic proteins bearing repetitive epitopes. *Mol. Biochem. Parasitol.* 35(2), 127-136.

Leon,J.S. & Engman,D.M. (2001) Autoimmunity in Chagas heart disease. *Int. J. Parasitol.* 31(5-6), 555-561.

Lescure,F.X.; Paris,L.: Elghouzzi,M.H.; Le,L.G.; Develoux,M.; Touafek,F.; Mazier,D.; Pialoux, G. (2009) Experience of targeted screening of Chagas disease in Ile-de-France, *Bull. Soc. Pathol. Exot.* 102, 295-299.

Lescure,F.X.; Le,L.G.; Freilij,H.; Develoux,M.; Paris,L.; Brutus,L. & Pialoux,G. (2010) Chagas disease: changes in knowledge and management. *Lancet Infect. Dis.* 10(8), 556-570.

Levin,M.J.; Mesri,E.; Benarous,R.; Levitus,G.; Schijman,A.; Levy-Yeyati,P.; Chiale,P.A.; Ruiz,A.M.; Kahn,A.; and Rosenbaum,M.B. (1989) Identification of major *Trypanosoma cruzi* antigenic determinants in chronic Chagas' heart disease. *Am. J. Trop. Med. Hyg.* 41(5), 530-538.

Levin,M.J.; da Silveira,J.F.; Frasch,A.C.; Camargo,M.E.; Lafon,S.; Degrave,W.M. & Rangel-Aldao,R. (1991) Recombinant *Trypanosoma cruzi* antigens and Chagas' disease diagnosis: analysis of a workshop. *FEMS Microbiol. Immunol.* 4(1), 11-19.

Levitus,G.; Hontebeyrie-Joskowicz,M.; Van Regenmortel,M.H. & Levin,M.J. (1991) Humoral autoimmune response to ribosomal P proteins in chronic Chagas heart disease. *Clin. Exp. Immunol.* 85(3), 413-417.

Lorca,M.; Gonzalez,A.; Reyes,V.; Veloso,C.; Vergara,U. & Frasch,C. (1993) [The diagnosis of chronic Chagas disease using recombinant antigens of Trypanosoma cruzi]. *Rev. Med. Chil.* 121(4), 363-368.

Luquetti,A.O. & Schmunis,G.A. (2010) Diagnosis of T. cruzi infection. In: *American Trypanosomiasis. Chagas Disease One Hundred Years Of Research,* Telleria,J. & Tibayrenc,M. (eds.), pp. 743-792. Elsevier, Madrid, Spain.

Marin-Neto,J.A.; Rassi,A.; Jr.; Morillo,C.A.; Avezum,A.; Connolly,S.J.; Sosa-Estani,S.; Rosas,F. & Yusuf,S. (2008) Rationale and design of a randomized placebo-controlled trial assessing the effects of etiologic treatment in Chagas' cardiomyopathy: the BENznidazole Evaluation For Interrupting Trypanosomiasis (BENEFIT). *Am. Heart J.* 156(1), 37-43.

Meira,W.S.; Galvao,L.M.; Gontijo,E.D.; hado-Coelho,G.L.; Norris,K.A. & Chiari,E. (2004) Use of the Trypanosoma cruzi recombinant complement regulatory protein to evaluate therapeutic efficacy following treatment of chronic chagasic patients. *J. Clin. Microbiol.* 42(2), 707-712.

Moncayo,A. & Luquetti,A.O. (1990) Multicentre double blind study for evaluation of Trypanosoma cruzi defined antigens as diagnostic reagents. *Mem. Inst. Oswaldo Cruz*. 85(4), 489-495.

Moya,P.; Basso,B. & Moretti,E. (2005) [Congenital Chagas disease in Cordoba, Argentina: epidemiological, clinical, diagnostic, and therapeutic aspects. Experience of 30 years of follow up]. *Rev. Soc. Bras. Med. Trop.* 38 (Suppl 2), 33-40.

Nóbrega,A.A.; Garcia,M.H.; Tatto,E. Obara,M.T.; Costa,E.; Sobel,J.; Araujo,W.N. (2009) Oral Transmission of Chagas Disease by Consumption of Açaí Palm Fruit, Brazil. *Emer. Infect. Dis.* 15 (4) 653-655.

Olivera,G.C.; Albareda,M.C.; Alvarez,M.G.; De Rissio,A.M.; Fichera,L.E.; Cooley,G.; Yachelini,P.; Hrellac,H.A.; Riboldi,H.; Laucella,S.A.; Tarleton,R.L. & Postan,M. (2010) Trypanosoma cruzi-specific immune responses in subjects from endemic areas of Chagas disease of Argentina. *Microbes. Infect.* 12(5), 359-363.

Otani,M.M.; Vinelli,E.; Kirchhoff,L.V.; del,P.A.; Sands,A.; Vercauteren,G. & Sabino,E.C. (2009) WHO comparative evaluation of serologic assays for Chagas disease. *Transfusion.* 49(6), 1076-1082.

Peralta,J.M.; Teixeira,M.G.; Shreffler,W.G.; Pereira,J.B.; Burns Jr,J.M.; Sleath,P.R. & Reed,S.G. (1994) Serodiagnosis of Chagas' disease by enzyme-linked immunosorbent assay using two synthetic peptides as antigens. *J. Clin. Microbiol.* 32(4), 971-974.

Perez-Molina,J.A.; Perez-Ayala,A.; Moreno,S.; Fernandez-Gonzalez,M.C.; Zamora,J. & Lopez-Velez,R. (2009) Use of benznidazole to treat chronic Chagas' disease: a systematic review with a meta-analysis. *J. Antimicrob. Chemother.* 64(6), 1139-1147.

Pinto,A.Y.; Valente,S.A. & Valente,V.C. (2004) Emerging acute Chagas disease in Amazonian Brazil: case reports with serious cardiac involvement. *Braz. J. Infect. Dis.* 8(6), 454-460.

Pirard,M.; Iihoshi,N.; Boelaert,M.; Basanta,P.; Lopez,F. & Van der,S.P. (2005) The validity of serologic tests for Trypanosoma cruzi and the effectiveness of transfusional screening strategies in a hyperendemic region. *Transfusion.* 45(4), 554-561.

Pittella,J.E. (2009) Central nervous system involvement in Chagas disease: a hundred-year-old history. *Trans. R. Soc. Trop. Med. Hyg.* 103(10), 973-978.

Ponce,C.; Ponce,E.; Vinelli,E.; Montoya,A.; de,A.; V, Gonzalez,A.; Zingales,B.; Rangel-Aldao,R.; Levin,M.J.; Esfandiari,J.; Umezawa,E.S.; Luquetti,A.O. & da Silveira,J.F. (2005) Validation of a rapid and reliable test for diagnosis of chagas' disease by detection of Trypanosoma cruzi-specific antibodies in blood of donors and patients in Central America. *J. Clin. Microbiol.* 43(10), 5065-5068.

Praast,G.; Herzogenrath,J.; Bernhardt,S.; Christ,H. & Sickinger,E. (2011) Evaluation of the Abbott ARCHITECT Chagas prototype assay. *Diagn. Microbiol. Infect. Dis.* 69(1), 74-81.

Ramirez,J.D.; Guhl,F.; Umezawa,E.S.; Morillo,C.A.; Rosas,F.; Marin-Neto,J.A. & Restrepo,S. (2009) Evaluation of adult chronic Chagas' heart disease diagnosis by molecular and serological methods. *J. Clin. Microbiol.* 47(12), 3945-3951.

Rassi,A.; Jr.; Rassi,A. & Rassi,S.G. (2007) Predictors of mortality in chronic Chagas disease: a systematic review of observational studies. *Circulation.* 115(9), 1101-1108.

Reiche,E.M.; Inouye,M.M.; Pontello,R.; Morimoto,H.K.; Itow,J.S.; Matsuo,T. & Jankevicius,J.V. (1996) Seropositivity for anti-trypanosoma cruzi antibodies among blood donors of the "Hospital Universitario Regional do Norte do Parana", Londrina, Brazil. *Rev. Inst. Med. Trop. Sao Paulo.* 38(3), 233-240.

Remesar,M.C.; Gamba,C.; Colaianni,I.F.; Puppo,M.; Sartor,P.A.; Murphy,E.L.; Neilands,T.B.; Ridolfi,M.A.; Leguizamon,M.S.; Kuperman,S. & Del Pozo,A.E. (2009) Estimation of sensitivity and specificity of several Trypanosoma cruzi antibody assays in blood donors in Argentina. *Transfusion.* 49(11), 2352-2358.

Reyes,M.B.; Lorca,M.; Munoz,P. & Frasch,A.C. (1990) Fetal IgG specificities against *Trypanosoma cruzi* antigens in infected newborns. *Proc. Natl. Acad. Sci. U. S. A.* 87(7), 2846-2850.

Ribone,M.E.; Belluzo,M.S.; Pagani,D.; Marcipar,I.S. & Lagier,C.M. (2006) Amperometric bioelectrode for specific human immunoglobulin G determination: optimization of the method to diagnose American trypanosomiasis. *Anal. Biochem.* 350(1), 61-70.

Roddy,P.; Goiri,J.; Flevaud,L.; Palma,P.P.; Morote,S.; Lima,N.; Villa,L.; Torrico,F. and bajar-Vinas,P. (2008) Field evaluation of a rapid immunochromatographic assay for detection of Trypanosoma cruzi infection by use of whole blood. *J. Clin. Microbiol.* 46(6), 2022-2027.

Rosenblatt,J.E. (2009) Laboratory diagnosis of infections due to blood and tissue parasites. *Clin. Infect. Dis.* 49(7), 1103-1108.

Russomando,G.; Sanchez,Z.; Meza,G. & de,G.Y. (2010) Shed acute-phase antigen protein in an ELISA system for unequivocal diagnosis of congenital Chagas disease. *Expert. Rev. Mol. Diagn.* 10(6), 705-707.

Saez-Alquezar,A.; Luquetti,A.; Borges-Pereira,J.; Moreira,M.; Gadhaela,M.T.; García Zapata,M.T. & Strugo Arruda,A.H. (1997) Estudo multicéntrico: validação do desempenho de conjuntos diagnósticos de hemaglutinação indirecta disponíveis no Brasil para o diagnóstico serológico da infeção pelo *Trypanosoma cruzi. Rev. Patol. Trop.* 26, 343-374.

Saez-Alquezar,A.; Sabino,E.C.; Salles,N.; Chamone,D.F.; Hulstaert,F.; Pottel,H.; Stoops,E. & Zrein,M. (2000) Serological confirmation of Chagas' disease by a recombinant and peptide antigen line immunoassay: INNO-LIA chagas. *J. Clin. Microbiol.* 38(2), 851-854.

Salles,N.A.; Sabino,E.C.; Cliquet,M.G.; Eluf-Neto,J.; Mayer,A.; Almeida-Neto,C.; Mendonca,M.C.; Dorliach-Llacer,P.; Chamone,D.F. & Saez-Alquezar,A. (1996) Risk of exposure to Chagas' disease among seroreactive Brazilian blood donors. *Transfusion.* 36(11-12), 969-973.

Salomone,O.A.; Basquiera,A.L.; Sembaj,A.; Aguerri,A.M.; Reyes,M.E.; Omelianuk,M.; Fernandez,R.A.; Enders,J.; Palma,A.; Barral,J.M. & Madoery,R.J. (2003) Trypanosoma cruzi in persons without serologic evidence of disease, Argentina. *Emerg. Infect. Dis.* 9(12), 1558-1562.

Silva,E.D.; Pereira,V.R.; Gomes,J.A.; Lorena,V.M.; Cancado,J.R.; Ferreira,A.G.; Krieger,M.A.; Goldenberg,S.; Correa-Oliveira,R. & Gomes,Y.M. (2002) Use of the EIE-recombinant-Chagas-biomanguinhos kit to monitor cure of human Chagas' disease. *J. Clin. Lab Anal.* 16(3), 132-136.

Sosa,E.S.; Segura,E.L.; Ruiz,A.M.; Velazquez,E.; Porcel,B.M. & Yampotis,C. (1998) Efficacy of chemotherapy with benznidazole in children in the indeterminate phase of Chagas' disease. *Am. J. Trop. Med. Hyg.* 59(4), 526-529.

Sosa-Estani,S.; Gamboa-Leon,M.R.; Del Cid-Lemus,J.; Althabe,F.; Alger,J.; Almendares,O.; Cafferata,M.L.; Chippaux,J.P.; Dumonteil,E.; Gibbons,L.; Padilla-Raygoza,N.; Schneider,D.; Belizan,J.M. & Buekens,P. (2008) Use of a rapid test on umbilical cord blood to screen for Trypanosoma cruzi infection in pregnant women in Argentina, Bolivia, Honduras, and Mexico. *Am. J. Trop. Med. Hyg.* 79(5), 755-759.

Sosa-Estani,S. & Segura,E.L. (2006) Etiological treatment in patients infected by Trypanosoma cruzi: experiences in Argentina. *Curr. Opin. Infect. Dis.* 19(6), 583-587.

Soto,M.; Requena,J.M.; Quijada,L. & Alonso,C. (1996) Specific serodiagnosis of human leishmaniasis with recombinant *Leishmania* P2 acidic ribosomal proteins. *Clin. Diagn. Lab. Immunol.* 3(4), 387-391.

Strout,R. (1962) A method for concentrating hemoflagellates. *J. Parasitol.* 48, 100.

Talvani,A.; Rocha,M.O.; Ribeiro,A.L.; Borda,E.; Sterin-Borda,L. & Teixeira,M.M. (2006) Levels of anti-M2 and anti-beta1 autoantibodies do not correlate with the degree of heart dysfunction in Chagas' heart disease. *Microbes. Infect.* 8(9-10), 2459-2464.

Teixeira,A.R.; Nitz,N.; Guimaro,M.C.; Gomes,C. & Santos-Buch,C.A. (2006) Chagas disease. *Postgrad. Med. J.* 82(974), 788-798.

Tovar,N.C.; Echeverry,M.C. & Mora,G. (2009) [Presence of antibodies to cardiac neuroreceptors in patients with Chagas disease]. *Biomedica.* 29(3), 476-494.

Umezawa,E.S.; Nascimento,M.S.; Kesper,N.; Jr.; Coura,J.R.; Borges-Pereira,J.; Junqueira,A.C. & Camargo,M.E. (1996) Immunoblot assay using excreted-secreted antigens of *Trypanosoma cruzi* in serodiagnosis of congenital, acute, and chronic Chagas' disease. *J. Clin. Microbiol.* 34(9), 2143-2147.

Umezawa,E.S.; Bastos,S.F.; Camargo,M.E.; Yamauchi,L.M.; Santos,M.R.; Gonzalez,A.; Zingales,B.; Levin,M.J.; Sousa,O.; Rangel-Aldao,R. & da Silveira,J.F. (1999) Evaluation of recombinant antigens for serodiagnosis of Chagas' disease in South and Central America. *J. Clin. Microbiol.* 37(5), 1554-1560.

Umezawa,E.S.; Bastos,S.F.; Coura,J.R.; Levin,M.J.; Gonzalez,A.; Rangel-Aldao,R.; Zingales,B.; Luquetti,A.O. & da Silveira,J.F. (2003) An improved serodiagnostic test for Chagas' disease employing a mixture of *Trypanosoma cruzi* recombinant antigens. *Transfusion.* 43(1), 91-97.

Umezawa,E.S.; Luquetti,A.O.; Levitus,G.; Ponce,C.; Ponce,E.; Henriquez,D.; Revollo,S.; Espinoza,B.; Sousa,O.; Khan,B. & da Silveira,J.F. (2004) Serodiagnosis of chronic and acute Chagas' disease with *Trypanosoma cruzi* recombinant proteins: results of a collaborative study in six Latin American countries. *J. Clin. Microbiol.* 42(1), 449-452.

Vexenat,A.C.; Santana,J.M. & Teixeira,A.R. (1996) Cross-reactivity of antibodies in human infections by the kinetoplastid protozoa Trypanosoma cruzi, Leishmania chagasi and Leishmania (viannia) braziliensis. *Rev. Inst. Med. Trop. Sao Paulo.* 38(3), 177-185.

Voller,A.; Draper,C.; Bidwell,D.E. & Bartlett,A. (1975) Microplate enzyme-linked immunosorbent assay for chagas' disease. *Lancet.* 1(7904), 426-428.

WHO (2002) Control of Chagas disease. Second report of the WHO Expert Committee. *World Health Organization.* http://whqlibdoc.who.int/trs/WHO_TRS_905.pdf(.

WHO (2003) Chagas disease. Burdens and trends. (2003). *World Health Organization.* http://www.who.int/ctd/chagas/burdens.htm(.

Yadon,Z.E. & Schmunis,G.A. (2009) Congenital Chagas disease: estimating the potential risk in the United States. *Am. J. Trop. Med. Hyg.* 81(6), 927-933.

Zuniga,E.; Motran,C.; Montes,C.L.; Diaz,F.L.; Bocco,J.L. & Gruppi,A. (2000) Trypanosoma cruzi-induced immunosuppression: B cells undergo spontaneous apoptosis and lipopolysaccharide (LPS) arrests their proliferation during acute infection. *Clin. Exp. Immunol.* 119(3), 507-515.

9

Echinococcosis/Hydatidosis

Antoni Soriano Arandes and Frederic Gómez Bertomeu
University Hospital Joan XXIII of Tarragona
Spain

1. Introduction

Echinococcosis is a zoonotic infection caused by adult or larval (metacestode) stages of cestodes belonging to the genus *Echinococcus* and the family *Taeniidae*. Life cycles imply two mammal hosts. Definitive hosts are carnivores containing adult forms in the gut. The infection is acquired by the intermediate hosts and humans after the ingestion of eggs from the feces of carnivorous definitive hosts, which harbour the adult egg-producing stage in the intestine. Eggs ingested by infected human develop into the infective metacestode stage causing various forms of Echinococcosis. The disease in humans and intermediate hosts is called Hydatidosis and is characterized according to the morphologic features of the larval stages: cystic echinococcosis (CE) caused by *Echinococcus granulosus* and related organisms, alveolar echinococcosis (AE) caused by *Echinococcus multilocularis*, and polycystic echinococcosis (PE) caused by *Echinococcus vogeli* or *Echinococcus oligarthrus*.

This disease is becoming an important public health problem in many parts of the world where dogs are used for cattle breeding. Control measures are unable to be implemented everywhere, and where control programs were initiated the success of them have been incomplete generating a re-emergence of the disease. This has also lead to the interruption of control measures excluding Echinococcosis from the list of notifiable diseases. As a consequence of this the incidence and prevalence of CE in Mediterranean countries in humans and animals are not known (Dakkak, 2010). Also, there are a number of factors that contribute to the increase of prevalence and to the spreading of CE in the Mediterranean Region. Cyprus is the only country where an eradication programme has been successfully implemented. However, CE has obtained important developments in the last decade, in the epidemiology, in the diagnosis of canine infection, in strain characterisation and in immune strategies against CE in animals. This scientific progress, together with effective health education programmes, will likely improve control programmes and reduce the time required to achieve significant decreases in prevalence or eradication. Thus, European authorities recognized, through the directive 2003/99/CE, Echinococcosis as a disease to be reported to the European Food Safety Authority (EFSA).

The "WHO/OIE Manual on Echinococcosis in Humans and Animals: a Public Health Problem of Global Concern", published in 2001, has been used as a fundamental issue for the redaction of this chapter.

2. Echinococcosis

The first part of this chapter is dedicated to explain the etiology to know the taxonomy and the life transmission cycles which perpetuate the agent in nature. The biology of the causative agents of various forms of Echinococcosis is faced because it can help to understand the maintaining of these parasites in different geographic areas. Following to this part the epidemiology and clinical presentation forms are assessed. Finally, diagnosis, treatment and prevention are developed and emphasis is given to the identification of species and strains within the genus as an essential prerequisite to the establishment of local control programmes.

2.1 Etiology and life cycles

Echinococcus presents certain unique characteristics that set it apart from the other major genus in the family, *Taenia*. The adult form is only few millimetres long, has no gut and all metabolic interchange takes place across the syncytial outer covering, the tegument. Scolex is the anterior part of the *Echinococcus* becoming an attachment organ with four muscular suckers and two rows of hooks. The body is the strobila and is segmented in a different number of reproductive units called proglottids. The adult worm is hermaphrodite with reproductive ducts opening at a common, lateral, genital pore, the position of which may vary depending on species and strain. The uterus dilates after fertilisation, eventually occupying most of the terminal segment when the eggs are fully developed. The eggs are ovoid, consisting of a hexacanth embryo surrounded by several envelopes and are morphologically indistinguishable to those of other tapeworms of the genus *Taenia*. The metacestode is the second larval stage and consists of a bladder with an outer acellular laminated layer and an inner nucleated germinal layer. Protoscoleces arise from the inner wall of the brood capsules (figure 1). The structure and development of the metacestode differs between the four species of *Echinococcus*.

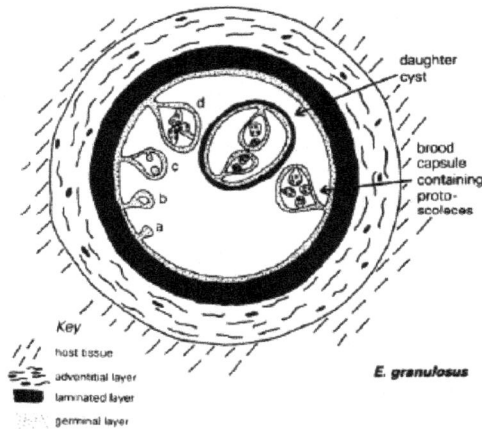

Fig. 1. Representation of the metacestode of *Echinococcus granulosus* (WHO/OIE publication: *Manual on echinococcosis in humans and animals*)

The life cycle of *Echinococcus spp.* requires two mammalian hosts for its completion. Gravid proglottids containing eggs or free eggs are passed in the faeces of the definitive host, a carnivore. These eggs are ingested by an intermediate host, in which the metacestode stage and protoscoleces develop. The cycle is completed if such an intermediate host is eaten by a suitable carnivore. Eggs are highly resistant to the environmental factors being infective for months at lower ranges of temperatures (from +4°C to +15°C). However, they are very sensitive to desiccation and to high temperatures as 60-80°C.

Intermediate hosts are represented by a wide range of mammals which acquire the infection by the ingestion of eggs. The oncosphere is released from the keratinised embryophore in the stomach and small intestine. Bile activates the oncosphere which penetrates the wall due to the hook movements and secretions and arrives to the liver where some of them are retained (figure 2). All mammals (including man) in which metacestodes of *Echinococcus* species develop after infection with eggs may be referred to as 'intermediate hosts'. However, man is an aberrant host because metacestode stages do not become fertile in this host or because does not interact in the transmission cycle. Once the oncosphere has reached its final location, it develops into the metacestode stage. Time of development is variable and it may take several months before protoscoleces are produced (fertile metacestode). There may be several thousand protoscoleces within a single cyst of *E. granulosus* or an aggregation of vesicles of *E. multilocularis*. Each single protoscolex is capable of developing into a sexually mature adult worm. Not all metacestodes produce protoscoleces (sterile metacestode).

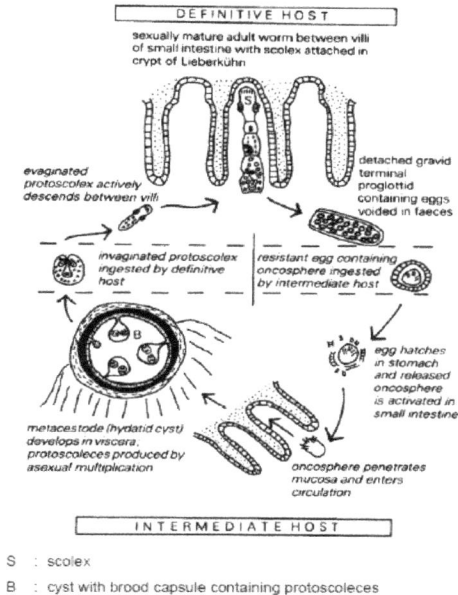

DEFINITIVE HOST

sexually mature adult worm between villi of small intestine with scolex attached in crypt of Lieberkühn

evaginated protoscolex actively descends between villi

detached gravid terminal proglottid containing eggs voided in faeces

invaginated protoscolex ingested by definitive host

resistant egg containing oncosphere ingested by intermediate host

metacestode (hydatid cyst) develops in viscera; protoscoleces produced by asexual multiplication

egg hatches in stomach and released oncosphere is activated in small intestine

oncosphere penetrates mucosa and enters circulation

INTERMEDIATE HOST

S : scolex

B : cyst with brood capsule containing protoscoleces

Fig. 2. Life-cycle of Echinococcus (WHO/OIE publication: Manual on echinococcosis in humans and animals)

Strain identification is possible for all four species of *Echinococcus* using morphological and biological features and/or molecular techniques, such as sequence comparison of a 366 bp-fragment of the mitochondrial cytochrome oxidase subunit 1 DNA (CO1) and a 471 bp-region in the mitochondrial NADH dehydrogenase gene 1 (ND1), by analysis of a ribosomal (r) DNA fragment (1ST2) or by the random amplified polymorphic DNA-PCR (RAPD-PCR). Recent genetic studies have principally confirmed the concept of strain diversity within the species *E. granulosus*, previously based on morphological and biological features. Several molecular techniques are now available which would quite easily allow the identification of certain *E. granulosus* strains using genetic markers. To prepare the identification of the strain using molecular techniques protoscoleces are collected from *E. granulosus* cysts being washed several times in physiological saline solution and preserved in 70% ethanol. The material needs to be examined by an experienced laboratory. The rDNA ITS1 (internal transcribed spacer) region has been shown to be a potentially very useful genetic marker for distinguishing strains and species of *Echinococcus* and small quantities of *Echinococcus* material can be characterised using a PCR-RFLP 'fingerprinting' technique (Bowles & McManus, 1993). Other method is the single strand conformation polymorphism (SSCP) which is technically simple and has high resolution capacity under optimised conditions. The utility of SSCP has been demonstrated for the categorisation of different *Echinococcus* genotypes (Gasser et al., 1998). The different strains of *Echinococcus* have an epidemiological significance for the prognosis in infected patients. Epidemiological studies have evidenced that the sylvatic strain of *E. granulosus* in northern North America is causing a benign infection with low pathogenicity, and affecting the lungs. Also, these epidemiological observations have been demonstrated in the People's Republic of China. In contrast, in parts of Kenya and Libya, it has been suggested that there are local virulent strains of *E. granulosus* (Thompson, 1995). Isoenzyme and molecular studies have confirmed that sheep strain is infective to humans (Bowles & McManus, 1993). Developmental differences between species and strains of *Echinococcus* are likely to be a limiting factor in control programmes which employ regular adult cestocidal treatment of definitive hosts for breaking the cycle of transmission (Thompson, 1995).

2.2 Clinical forms of Echinococcosis
The metacestodes of all four recognised *Echinococcus* species can infect humans and cause various forms of echinococcosis (Table 1). Among these forms cystic and alveolar echinococcosis are of special medical importance.

Forms of Echinococcosis	Causative agent	Disease synonyms
Cystic Echinococcosis	*Echinococcus granulosus*	Hydatid disease, Hydatidosis, *E. granulosus* echinococcosis
Alveolaar Echinococcosis	*Echinococcus multilocularis*	Alveolar hydatid disease, *E. multilocularis* echinococcosis
Polycystic Echinoccosis	*Echinococcus vogeli*	*E.vogeli* echinococcosis
Polycystic Echinococcosis	*Echinococcus oligarthrus*	*E. oligarthrus* echinococcosis

Table 1. Forms of Echinococcosis

Primary echinococcosis is established when metacestodes develop in various sites of the human body from oncospheres liberated from ingested eggs of *Echinococcus* spp. In CE liver and lung are the most frequently affected organs.

Secondary echinococcosis occurs when metacestode material spreads from primary site to adjacent or distant organs and proliferates. Regarding CE this form occurs after release of viable parasite material during invasive treatment procedures.

2.2.1 Cystic echinococcosis (CE)

The causative agent of CE is the metacestode of *Echinococcus granulosus*, becoming a cystic structure filled with a clear fluid. Most of the cysts grow slowly in size and become surrounded by host tissue (pericyst) encompassing the endocyst of metacestode origin. The endocyst consists of the outer laminated layer and the inner cellular germinal layer, which may form brood capsules and protoscoleces. The minimum time required for the development of protoscoleces in cysts in humans is not exactly known, but it is expected to be 10 months or longer after infection (Pawlowski, 1997). Fertile (with protoscoleces) and sterile (without protoscoleces) cysts may coexist in the same patient. Frequently, smaller daughter cysts are formed within a larger mother cyst. If these smaller cysts are growing in close proximity to each other forming clusters the appearance of "polycystic" needs to be distinguished from AE or PE.

The initial phase of primary infection is always asymptomatic remaining as this for many years or permanently. However, the infection may become symptomatic when cysts press adjacent tissues or induce other pathological events. When symptoms appear suddenly a spontaneous or traumatic cyst rupture has to be suspected. Spontaneous cure is possible but improbable, and is due to the collapse and resolution of cysts or due to the cyst rupture into the bile duct or the bronchial tree. The fatality rate is highly dependent on the severity of the infection and on facilities for treatment.

The age of the symptomatic infected patients can vary from below 1 year of age to over 75 years old. In a study from Madrid (Spain), over 1,473 patients admitted to a children's hospital, 2% were <1 year old, 21% between 1 and 4 years and 77% between 5 and 14 years (Utrilla et al., 1991). Many patients (about 40% up to 80%) with CE have a single organ involved and harbour a solitary cyst.

2.2.1.1 Clinical presentation of CE

Clinical symptoms of CE are variable and depend on the organ involved, the size of the cysts, the interaction between the expanding cysts and the adjacent organ structures, and the complications related to the cyst rupture and bacterial infection. CE involving the liver can remain asymptomatic for more than ten years (Frider et al., 1999). Liver and lungs are the two more frequent organ sites involved. Complications affecting the biliary tract are the most common and include the cystic rupture into bile ducts. Other complications are bacterial infection of the cyst, intraperitoneal rupture, and lung involvement.

2.2.1.2 Diagnosis of CE

Diagnosis of CE is done through different steps as follows:
a. Clinical suspect or screening
b. Confirmation by imaging and identification of suspicious cyst structures
c. Confirmation by detection of specific antibodies with immunodiagnostic tests
d. If doubt diagnostic puncture may be considered
e. Material obtained by biopsy puncture or surgery is examined.

Ultrasonography (US) is used for the diagnosis of the cystic structure and portable units are suitable to take into account in field situations. Immunodiagnostic tests for detecting specific antibodies are commonly used for the aetiological confirmation of the findings of imaging examinations.

Protoscoleces or hooks of *E. granulosus* are found in aspirated fluid samples. This technique is not performed frequently because the material can only be available after a surgical intervention, therapeutic puncture (PAIR) or diagnostic puncture. Direct diagnosis can also be made by macroscopic identification of the *E. granulosus* obtained by surgery or biopsy. Other methods include the identification of specific *E. granulosus* antigen (antigen 5) in the fluid from sterile cysts or DNA markers in the cysts fluid or parasite tissue (e.g. by PCR).

Imaging techniques for diagnosis:

- Standard radiology: chest radiography detects uncomplicated cyst structures displaying a homogeneous shadow that indicates a fluid-filled space. Calcification in lung imaging is rare and cysts may be located anywhere as solitary or multiple. For differential diagnosis, cysts filled with clear fluid, with an air shadow or with water-lily sign are pathognomonic. If a rounded parenchymatous opacity is seen, it is necessary to consider tuberculoma, a tumour or pulmonary sequestration. A fluid and air shadow will lead to consideration of a bacterial, fungal or amoebic abscess.

- Ultrasonography (US): an expert committee of the WHO Working Group on echinococcosis presented an internationally agreed classification of US images in hepatic CE in 2001 (WHO, 2001), according to the use of PAIR (Puncture, Aspiration, Injection, Re-aspiration). This technique was proposed in 1986 by the Tunisian team that first used it in a prospective study. PAIR is a minimally invasive therapeutic option for percutaneous drainage of echinococcal cysts located in the abdomen, complementing or replacing surgery in most of the settings. PAIR also helps the use of benzimidazoles (albendazole and mebendazole) for the treatment of CE. The drainage is performed with a fine needle or a catheter, followed by the killing of the protoscolices remaining in the cyst cavity by a protoscolicide agent. If numerous and large daughter cysts are present, an alternative percutaneous technique "Percutaneous Puncture with Drainage and Curettage" (PPDC) may be used.

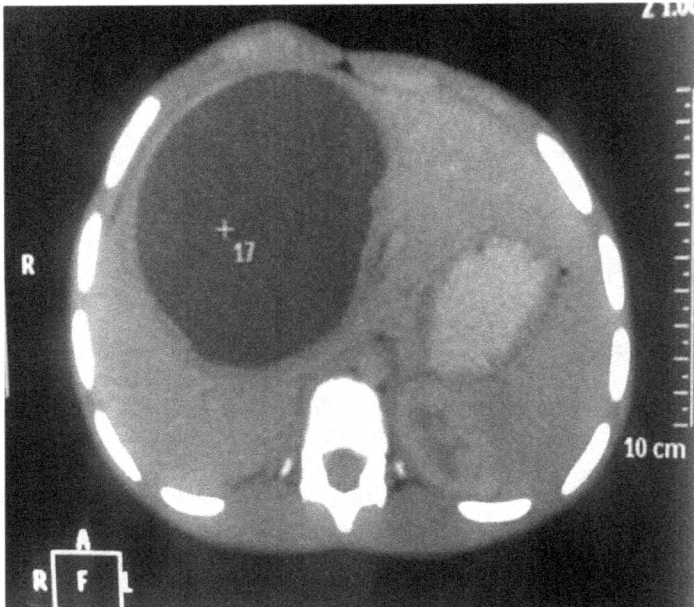

Fig. 3. Image from a computed tomography study of the abdomen of a patient (Soriano Arandes et al., 2010).

- Computed tomography (CT) can detect small cysts, and it also facilitates differential diagnosis of lesions caused by *Echinococcus* metacestodes from non-parasitic lesions (figure 3) (Soriano Arandes et al., 2010). CT is only indicated when US diagnosis is uncertain, mainly in cysts CE4 or CE5. However, CT is the principal method for diagnosis of cerebral cysts showing a spherical cyst with a thin wall, not enhanced after injection of contrast medium, without perilesional oedema the adjacent structures.

2.2.1.3 WHO classification of CE

The WHO classification of CE cysts (WHO, 2001) is done according to the US images:

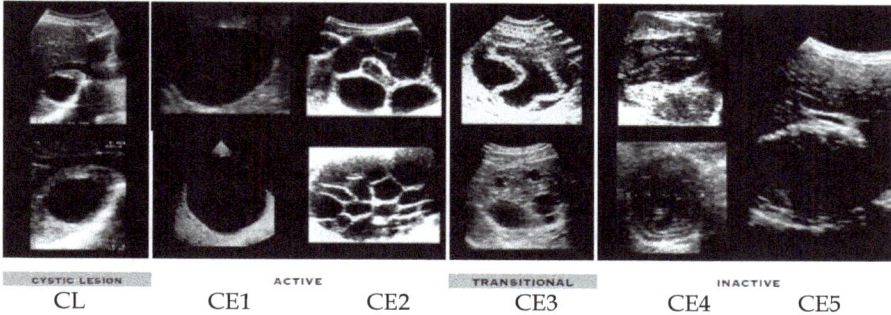

| CYSTIC LESION | ACTIVE | | TRANSITIONAL | INACTIVE | |
| CL | CE1 | CE2 | CE3 | CE4 | CE5 |

Cystic lesion (CL): Unilocular, cystic lesion (s) (CL) with uniform anechoic content, not clearly delimited by a hyperechoic rim (= cyst wall not visible).
- Normally round but may be oval.
- Size: variable but usually small. CLs (< 5.0 cm), CLm (5 – 10 cm), CLl (> 10cm).
- Status: If CE - active.If these cystic lesions are caused by CE at an early stage of development then usually these cysts are not fertile.
- Ultrasound does not detect any pathognomonic signs.
- Differential diagnosis of these cystic lesions requires further diagnostic techniques.

CE1: Unilocular, simple cyst with uniform anechoic content. Cyst may exhibit fine echoes due to shifting of brood capsules which is often called hydatid sand ("snow flake sign") (figure 4).

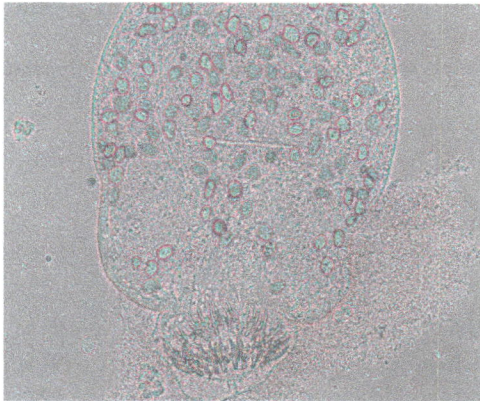

Fig. 4. Hydatid sand containing a protoscolex of *Echinococcus granulosus* seen by light microcopy (Soriano Arandes et al., 2010).

- Cyst wall is visible.
- Normally round or oval.
- Size variable: CE1s (< 5.0 cm), CE1m (5 – 10 cm), CE1l (> 10cm)
- Status: active.
- Usually fertile.
- Pathognomonic signs include visible cyst wall and snow flake sign.

CE2: Multivesicular, multiseptated cysts; cysts septations produce "wheel-like" structures, and presence of daughter cysts is indicated by "rosette-like" or "honeycomb-like" structures. Daughter cysts may partly or completely fill the unilocular mother cyst.

- Cyst wall normally visible.
- Normally round or oval.
- Size variable: CE2s (< 5.0 cm), CE2m (5 – 10 cm), CE2l (> 10cm).
- Status: active.
- Usually fertile.
- Ultrasound features are pathognomonic.

CE3: Unilocular cyst which may contain daughter cysts. Anechoic content with detachment of laminated membrane from the cyst wall is visible as floating membrane or as "water-lily sign" which is indicative of wavy membranes floating on top of remaining cyst fluid.

- Cyst form may be less rounded because of decrease of intra-cystic fluid pressure.
- Size variable: CE3s (< 5.0 cm), CE3m (5 – 10 cm), CE3l (> 10cm).
- Status: transitional.
- Transitional stage. Cyst which may degenerate further or may give rise to daughter cysts.
- Ultrasound features are pathognomonic.

CE4: Heterogenous hypoechoic or hyperechoic degenerative contents. No daughter cysts.

- May show a "ball of wool" sign which is indicative of degenerating membranes.
- Size variable: CE4s (< 5.0 cm), CE4m (5 – 10 cm), CE4l (> 10cm).
- Status: inactive.
- Most cysts of this type are not fertile.
- US features are not pathognomonic and further diagnostic tests are required to ascertain a diagnosis.

CE5: Cysts characterized by thick calcified wall that is arch shaped, producing a cone shaped shadow.

- Degree of calcification varies from partial to complete.
- Size variable: CE5s (< 5.0 cm), CE5m (5 – 10 cm), CE5l (> 10cm).
- Status: inactive.
- Cyst not fertile in most cases.
- Diagnosis is uncertain. Features are not pathognomonic but highly suggestive for *E. granulosus*.

2.2.1.4 Laboratory findings of CE

Routine laboratory tests show non-specific results. Patients with rupture of a cyst into the biliary tree can show transient elevations of GGT or alkaline phosphatase concentrations, often associated with hyperamylasaemia and eosinophilia (>500/µl). When cyst is ruptured eosinophilia achieves higher concentrations.

2.2.1.5 Immunodiagnosis of CE

Immunodiagnosis procedures for serum antibody detection are used for the aetiological confirmation of imaging structures suggestive for CE. Certain proportion of patients with echinococcosis is unable to be diagnosed with highly sensitive diagnostic tests such as IgG-ELISA and false-negative results are obtained. Cysts in the brain or eye and calcified cysts often induce low or no antibody titres. Antibody response may also be low in certain human population groups and in young children. False positive results may also occur, especially in patients with other helminthic diseases. Approaches to the diagnosis of CE using immune methods are specified in table 2.

Fisrt step: Primary antibody test		
Test for serum antibody detection: IgG-ELISA or IgE-ELISA with E. Granulosus antigen		
A combination of two or more primary tests may increase sensitivity		
Subsequent steps		
Seronegative samples +	**Seronegative samples +**	**Seropositive samples +**
No suggestive images for CE	**Suggestive images for CE**	**With or without suggestive images for CE**
	Asymptomatic cases Extended and/or advanced imaging and repeated serological examinations, including differential diagnosis for AE*	
No further serological follow-up or further steps for differential diagnosis	'Wait and observe' approach with repeated serological examinations	**Asymptomatic and symptomatic cases** Secondary antibody test: Arc 5 test IgG4-ELISA Immunoblot for antibodies reactive with subunits of *E. granulosus* antigens
.	**Symptomatic cases** Consideration of cyst puncture Consideration of surgical intervention and/or chemotherapy without further serological examinations	Serological differential diagnosis for AE (ELISA-Em2plus, immunoblot)

Table 2. Approaches for immunodiagnosis of CE

IgG-ELISA is the preferable test used as a primary test for detecting anti-*Echinococcus* serum antibodies. Most of the routine laboratory test systems or commercialized test kits are based on crude or semi-purified preparations of *E. granulosus* antigens. The use of the two major hydatid cyst fluid antigens, antigen 5 (thermolabile) and antigen B (thermostable), is predominantly restricted to scientific applications, and these antigens are not generally available. Secondary tests for antibody detection are used to increase specificity and these are: arc 5, identification of IgG subclasses, and immunoblotting which demonstrates the reactivity of serum antibodies with subunits of *E. granulosus* antigens (Craig, 1997; Di Felice, 1986; Ioppolo, 1996; Leggatt & McManus, 1994; Leggatt, 1992; Ligthowlers & Gottstein, 1995; Profumo, 1994; Sheperd & McManus, 1987; Siracusano & Vuitton, 1997; Wen & Craig, 1994). Generally, these tests are less sensitive, but more specific than primary test systems. Putative hydatid cyst fluid samples obtained by puncture or after surgical intervention can be tested for the presence or absence of *Echinococcus* antigen through binding of enzyme-labelled anti-*Echinococcus* (hydatid cyst fluid) antibodies in an ELISA with a monoclonal antibody against antigen 5 (Ag5) that may be useful in confirmation of the *Echinococcus* nature of the fluid (Paul & Stefaniak, 1997).

2.2.1.6 Treatment of CE

Surgery is still the treatment that has the potential to remove *E. granulosus* cysts and lead to complete cure (WHO, 1996). Up to 90% of the patients can be treated surgically if a cyst does not have a risky localisation or if the disease is not too far advanced. However, surgery may be impractical in patients with multiple cysts localised in several organs and if surgical facilities are inadequate. Chemotherapy and PAIR offer an attractive option for treatment, especially in inoperable patients and for cases with a high surgical risk.

2.2.1.6.1 Surgery

Surgery is indicated for large liver cysts with multiple daughter cysts; single liver cysts, situated superficially that may rupture spontaneously or as a result of trauma; cysts that are infected; cysts communicating with biliary tree and/or exerting pressure on adjacent vital organs; cysts in the lung, brain and kidney, bones and other organs.

Surgery of CE is contraindicated as defined for surgical procedures in general, i.e. patients refusing surgery, patients at the extremes of age, pregnant women, and patients with concomitant severe diseases (i.e. cardiac, renal or hepatic diseases, diabetes and hypertension). Also, surgery is contraindicated in patients with multiple cysts or cysts difficult to access, dead cysts either partly or totally calcified, and in patients with very small cysts.

The protoscolicides appareantly effective are: 70-95% ethanol, 15-20% hypertonic saline solution, and 0.5% cetrimide solution. These substances should be left in the cyst cavity for at least 15 minutes to obtain an optimal efficacy.

The risks of surgical intervention include secondary echinococcosis owing to spillage of viable parasite material during the intervention. Recurrence can be due to incomplete cyst removal or to previously undetected cysts. Anaphylactic reactions represent a further risk on rare occasions. Postoperative fatality is about 2% or less, but may be higher in the second or further operations or if medical facilities are inadequate.

2.2.1.6.2 Puncture, aspiration, injection, re-aspiration (PAIR)

This technique includes the following steps (WHO, 2001):
- percutaneus puncture of cysts under ultrasonic guidance
- aspiration of a substantial amount of cyst fluid
- injection of protoscolicidal substance (preferably 95% ethanol)
- re-aspiration of the fluid cyst content after 15 min to 20 min.

PAIR should be accompanied by a chemotherapeutic coverage to minimise risks of secondary echinococcosis and should be reserved for use by skilled and well experienced physicians with a surgical and intensive care back-up team well prepared to deal immediately with complications. Aspirates of liver cysts must be analysed immediately for traces of bilirubin and protoscoleces or hooks. PAIR should only be performed under chemotherapeutic coverage, except in early pregnant patients (Filice & Brunetti, 1997). The PAIR sequence is (WHO, 2001):

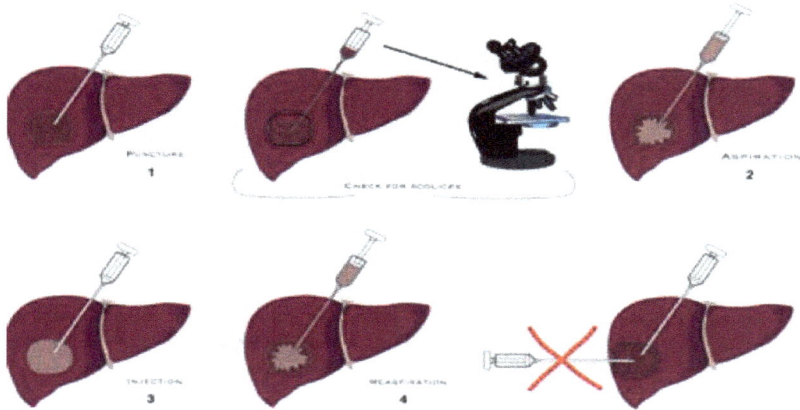

There are some critical points to take into account when proceeding with the PAIR protocol:
- Prophylaxis pre- and post-procedure: albendazole is administered 24 to 4 hours before intervention and 15 days to 30 days after intervention according to the cystic size. No treatment for pregnant women.
- Communication with biliary tree: the minimum requirements are to search for bile in the fluid with fast test.
- Scolicidal agent to be used: hypertonic saline (at least 15% final concentration in cyst) or 95% alcohol.
- Quantity of scolicide injected: at least 1/3 of the aspirated quantity.
- Evaluation of viability: microscopic examination.
- Needle vs. catheter: needle for cysts <5 cm. or in multiloculated cysts. Catheter for cysts >5 cm. (PAIRD)
- Follow-up: every week for the 1st month, then every month for the 1st year, the every year for 10 years.

Indications for PAIR: we use this technique for patients with:
- Non-echoic lesion ≥ 5 cm in diameter (CE1m and I)
- Cysts with daughter cysts (CE2), and/or with detachment of membranes (CE3)
- Multiple cysts if accessible to puncture
- Infected cysts
- Also for pregnant women, children >3 years old, patients who fail to respond to chemotherapy alone, patients in whom surgery is contraindicated, patient who refuse surgery, and patients who relapse after surgery.

Contraindications for PAIR:
- Non-cooperative patients and inaccessible or risky location of the cyst in the liver
- Cyst in spine, brain and/or heart
- Inactive or calcified lesion

- Cysts communicating with the biliary tree
- Cysts open into the abdominal cavity, bronchi and urinary tract.

2.2.1.6.3 Chemotherapy

The documentation of the experience about chemotherapy with benzimidazoles in CE is now extensive. Third part of the patients treated with benzimidazoles is achieving the cure with a complete and definitive disappearing of the cysts, and higher proportion (30-50%) has obtained a considerable reduction of the cyst size and also relieve of their symptoms. However, 20-40% of the cases don't respond as expected. Smaller and isolated cysts (less than 7mm.), surrounded by a minimal adventitial membrane respond better than complicated with multiple separations or with son cysts, or surrounded by a thick or calcified adventitial membrane which are refractory to the treatment. There are two main drugs for chemotherapy: albendazole (10-15 mg/kg/day twice per day; 3- to more than 6 monthly courses with free intervals of 14 days) for treating patients with single or multiple cysts (Gemmell & Roberts, 1995), and mebendazole (40-50 mg/kg/day; everyday in three doses per day during 3-6 months). Albendazole continuous courses have shown equal or improved efficacy for 3 to 6 months or longer without an increase of adverse effects (Franchi et al., 1999). When comparing both drugs, albendazole and mebendazole, some researchers concluded that albendazole was better regarding complete cure rates and relieve of the symptoms (Franchi et al., 1999). Albendazole has a better pharmacokinetic profile than mebendazole facilitating higher intestinal absorption and penetration into the cysts. There are described some adverse reactions (neutropenia, hepatic toxicity, alopecia, and others) in a few number of patients which are reversible when treatment is interrupted. Doses, duration, and follow-up of treatment must be taken individually for each patient. However, it seems that minimum duration has to be for three months. It is difficult to predict the long-term prognosis for every patient; therefore it's necessary to do a long-term follow-up, with US or other imaging methods to be able to evaluate the result of the treatment.

Chemotherapy is also useful as a surgical complement and albendazole has been used as a pre-surgical treatment to facilitate the surgical manipulation of the cysts inactivating the protoscoleces previously, modifying the integrity of the cyst membranes and reducing the consistency of the cysts. Treatment with benzimidazoles is recommended to prevent the relapse of the disease, which is the secondary echinococcosis when the content of the cysts is spread after its spontaneous or accidental rupture. When it occur the best option is to treat with three cycles of albendazole or the continuous administration of mebendazole during 1-3 months.

Praziquantel at doses of 40 mg/kg is a potent protoscolicide and could be used as a preventive drug after the cyst content spillage when the rupture of the cyst or as a protoscolicide when PAIR is applied.

Other drugs as nitazoxamide (at doses of 500mg/12h for 3-24 months) has been evaluated in the effectiveness in disseminated cystic echinococcosis (DCE) that failed to respond to surgical and antiparasitic therapy. Three patients improved: one with muscle involvement (clinico-radiological response), one with lung involvement (radiological response), and another with soft tissue and bony involvement (clinico-radiological response of soft tissue cysts) (Pérez-Molina et al., 2011).

Benzimidazoles are contraindicated in pregnancy because they are teratogenic.

Monitoring of the patients is needed and medical and laboratory examinations for adverse reactions are necessary initially every 2 weeks then monthly (WHO, 1996). Leukocyte counts should be checked at 2-week intervals during the first 3 months because in rare instances severe and not always reversible leukopaenia has been observed in early phases of chemotherapy. Serum drug concentrations (ABZ-sulfoxide or MBZ parent compound) should be monitored after 2 and 4 weeks of chemotherapy, respectively, in order to identify levels too high (possibly toxic) or too low (ineffective). For MBZ, it has been recommended to determine serum or plasma levels 4 h after the morning dose. Oral drug doses can be adapted to individual patients in order to achieve adequate serum levels, but such attempts are not always effective. Unfortunately, only few laboratories have the capability to measure ABZ-sulfoxide or MBZ serum drug levels (see also section on AE). Follow-up examinations, including imaging if needed, should be carried out at intervals of about 3 to 6 months for 1 to 3 years after termination of chemotherapy because of the relatively high rate of relapses.

2.2.1.6.4 Vaccines

A new vaccine against echinococcosis would be highly desirable in order to provide long-term prevention of the disease and to complement control programs. Vaccines against ovine hydatidosis have demonstrated its efficacy when targeting the larval stage of the parasite (Lightowlers, 2001). However, if used in the field we would need to vaccinate all the animals in a herd to achieve good results and this would be very costly to control programs. Otherwise, a vaccine protecting dogs against the adult worm would have to be given to only a few animals to protect the environment, because dogs are less numerous than other animals in the herd. Also, domestic dogs are the key in the transmission to livestock and humans. Therefore, some authors have proposed a recombinant oral vaccine given to the small number of dogs keeping the herd would decrease the number of E. granulosus adult worms and, consequently, the number of infective eggs. This measure would help reduce the contamination risk factors for humans and livestock, would be cost-effective for the owners of the dogs, and could help increase the overall efficacy of control programs in endemic countries (Petavy, 2008).

Some candidates have been used to induce immune response with vaccination. One of those is Eg-95 encoding gene that is expressed in the oncosphere, protoscoleces, and immature and mature adult worms of E. granulosus. EG95 vaccine antigen is a secreted glycosylphosphatydilinositol (GPI)-anchored protein containing a fibronectin type III domain, which is ubiquitous in modular proteins involved in cell adhesion. EG95 protein represents one of the targets of immunity induced by the vaccine because there is a high degree of sequence gene conservation between different isolates (Zhang, 2003). A mixture of different EG95 isoforms increases the ability of E. granulosus to invade different hosts and could possibly maximize vaccine efficacy (Haag, 2009). Other candidates for vaccine are the homologous sequences of two of the S3Pvac peptides, GK1 and KETc1, identified and further characterized in Taenia crassiceps WFU, Taenia solium, Taenia saginata, E. granulosus and E. multilocularis. Comparisons of the nucleotide and amino acid sequences coding for KETc1 and GK1 revealed significant homologies in these species and the results of a study indicate that GK1 and KETc1 may be considered candidates to be included in the formulation of a multivalent and multistage vaccine against these cestodiases because of their enhancing effects on other available vaccine candidates (Rassy, 2010).

2.2.2 Alveolar echinococcosis (AE)

Alveolar echinococcosis (AE) is an infection caused by the metacestode stage of E. multilocularis, which is characterised by a tumour-like, infiltrative and destructive growth with the potential to induce serious disease with a high fatality rate. Metacestodes develop primarily almost exclusively in the liver varying from small foci of a few millimetres in size to large areas of infiltration (15-20 cm.). From the liver, the metacestode tends to spread to both the adjacent and distant organs by infiltration or metastasis formation (Eckert, 1998). Cases of AE are characterized by an initial asymptomatic incubation period of 5-15 years duration and a subsequent chronic course. Fatality rate in untreated or inadequately treated persons is high.

High burden of AE is known to be common in certain rural communities in China whilst it is generally rare and sporadic elsewhere. Recently, a study was carried out to estimate the global incidence of this disease by country (Torgerson, 2010). They undertook a detailed review of published literature and data from other sources suggesting that there are approximately 18,235 (CI 11,900–28,200) new cases of AE per annum globally with 16,629 (91%) occurring in China and 1,606 outside China. Most of these cases are in regions where there is little treatment available and therefore will be fatal cases. They were able to calculate that AE results in a median of 666,434 DALYs per annum (CI 331,000-1.3 million).

2.2.2.1 Clinical presentation of AE

Age at the time of diagnosis of AE is significantly higher than for CE. The primary site of metacestode development is almost exclusively in the liver. The right lobe is predominantly infected, but the liver hilus together with one or two lobes may also be involved. Extra hepatic primarily locations are rare. During the infection, secondary echinococcosis may occur in variety of adjacent or distant organs. Symptoms of AE are primarily cholestatic jaundice (1/3 of cases) and/or epigastric pain (1/3 of the cases). In the remaining third of patients, AE is detected incidentally during medical examination for symptoms such as fatigue, weight loss, hepatomegaly, or abnormal routine laboratory findings.

2.2.2.2 Classification and staging of AE

PNM system for classification of human alveolar echinococcosis
Classification of findings
P: Hepatic localisation of the parasite
PX: Primary lesion cannot be assessed
P0: No detectable lesion in the liver
P1: Peripheral lesions without proximal vascular and/or biliary involvement
P2: Central lesions with proximal vascular and/or biliary involvement of one lobe (a)
P3: Central lesions with hilar vascular and biliary involvement of both lobes and/or with involvement of two hepatic veins
P4: Any liver lesion with extension along the vessels (b) and the biliary tree
N: Extrahepatic involvement of neighbouring organs
Diaphragm, lung, pleura, pericardium, heart, gastric and duodenal wall, adrenal glands, peritoneum, retroperitoneum, parietal wall (muscles, skin, bone), pancreas, regional lymph nodes, liver ligaments, kidney
NX: Not evaluable
N0: No regional involvement (see above)
N1: Regional involvement of contiguous organs or tissues
M: Absence or presence of distant metastases
Lung, distant lymph nodes, spleen, CNS, orbital, bone, skin, muscle, distant peritoneum and retroperitoneum]

MX: Not completely evaluated
M0: No metastasis(c)
M1: Metastasis

a. For classification, the plane projecting between the bed of the gallbladder and the inferior vena cava divides the liver in two lobes
b. Vessels means inferior vena cava, portal vein and arteries
c. Chest X-ray and cerebral CT negative

Source: European Network for Concerted Surveillance of AE: PNM system for the classification of human cases of AE.

Staging of alveolar echinococcosis cases based on PNM classification

Stage of alveolar echinococcosis	PNM classification
Stage I	P1 N0 M0
Stage II	P2 N0 M0
Stage IIIa	P3 N0 M0
Stage IIIb	P1-3 N1 M0
	P4 N0 M0
Stage IV	P4 N1 M0
	Any P Any N M1

Source: European Network for Concerted Surveillance of Alveolar Echinococcosis: PNM system for the classification of human cases of alveolar echinococcosis.

2.2.2.3 Diagnosis of AE

Diagnosis of AE is based on similar findings and criteria as in CE.

Hepatic lesions are characterised in US and CT by heterogenous hypodense masses, often associated with necrotic cavities. The lesion contours are irregular and there is lack of a welldefined wall. Calcifications are often found and exhibit a typical pattern in regard to shape and distribution: clusters of microcalcifications or irregular plaque-like calcified foci are located in the central or peripheral parts of the lesions. Discrepancies between US and CT patterns can be found. Hyperechoic haemangioma-like nodules could represent early forms of AE lesions. Quite frequently an extension of the lesions beyond the liver is found toward diaphragm, lungs, pericardium, retroperitoneum, hepatoduodenal ligament and pancreas.

Magnetic resonance imaging is used to observe compression or obstruction of inferior vena cava, the hepatic veins or the portal branches. Pathognomonic aspects are represented by multicystic honeycomb-like images.

2.2.2.4 Laboratory findings of AE

The routine laboratory tests do not yield specific findings. The blood sedimentation rate is elevated in most of the cases. The numbers of leucocytes and platelets may be depressed in patients with splenomegaly. Lymphopaenia is frequent in advanced cases, and eosinophilia is usually absent. Cholestasis with or without jaundice is observed in patients with intrahepatic bile duct compression or obstruction. Cholangitis and/or liver abscesses, which usually result from bile duct obstruction, are associated with typical alterations of the laboratory parameters. Hypergammaglobulinaemia is present in most of the patients and reflects the specific and polyclonal antibody response. In about one-half of the patients, the presence of specific anti-*E. multilocularis* – IgE can be demonstrated.

2.2.2.5 Immunodiagnosis of AE (table 3)

Fisrt step: Primary antibody test		
Tests with high sensitivity and less specific value		
Subsequent steps		
Seronegative samples + No suggestive images for AE	Seronegative samples + Suggestive images for AE	Seropositive samples + With or without suggestive images for AE
No further serological follow-up. Persons with suspected infection risk may require repeated serological examinations after 3-6 months, and US imaging.	**Asymptomatic cases** Extended and/or advanced imaging and repeated serological examinations. Fine needle biopsy for PCR or immunohistology may be considered in rare cases. If lesions are fully calcified, serological and imaging follow-up after 6 months to confirm parasite abortion. **Symptomatic cases** Consideration of surgical intervention and/or chemotherapy without further serological examinations	**Asymptomatic and symptomatic cases** Secondary antibody test: Em2Plus-ELISA (Gottstein et al., 1993) Em alkaline phosphatise-antigen-ELISA (Sarciron et al., 1997) Immunoblot for specific bands or similar test Serological differential diagnosis for CE

Table 3. Approaches for immunodiagnosis of AE

2.2.2.6 Pathological and histological examination of AE

Metacestode of *E. multilocularis* typically exhibits an alveolar structure composed of numerous irregular cysts with diameters between less than 1 mm and 30 mm. when is examined in a macroscopic section of the liver. Due to necrosis of the lesion, cavities filled with liquid and necrotic material may be formed in the central parts of the parasite (Eckert, 1998). Microscopically, the cysts consist of a relatively thin PAS-positive laminated layer and a delicate germinal layer often with only a few nuclei. Brood capsules and protoscoleces are rarely formed in the human host (Eckert, 1998). The cysts are surrounded by an inner zone of necrotic tissue and outer layers of histiocytes and lymphocytes. In later phases, tissue reactions of chronic inflammation, often with giant cell foreign body reaction, fibrous tissue and calcifications are seen around cysts.

2.2.2.7 Treatment of AE

There are a variety of options to select the adequate treatment for each individual patient. Clinical experience is crucial for AE; therefore patients should be referred to a recognised national or regional reference centre. Early diagnosis of AE is of special importance for successful treatment because the lesion is acting as a malignant tumour. Screening programmes in Japan and Europe have shown that early diagnosis reduces mortality and morbidity due to AE. Some considerations for treatment of AE are generally accepted: the first choice treatment in all operable cases is radical surgical resection of the entire parasitic lesion from the liver and other affected organs, chemotherapy is indicated after radical surgery for a limited period of time, and long-term chemotherapy is mandatory after incomplete resection of the lesions, in inoperable patients and in AE patients after liver transplantation.

Chemotherapy has several indications, as follows:

- Applicable for limited period of time after radical surgery. Since residual parasite tissue may remain undetected at radical surgery, post-operative chemotherapy for at least 2 years should be carried out and patients should be monitored for a minimum of 10 years for possible recurrence
- Long-term chemotherapy for several years is mandatory in inoperable AE patients, in cases following incomplete surgical resection of the parasite lesions and after liver transplantation
- Pre-surgical chemotherapy is not indicated in cases of AE. However, in rare cases that surgery was contraindicated at the time of diagnosis of AE, surgery can be carried out after a prolonged course of chemotherapy.

Benzimidazoles are preferentially used for AE:

Mebendazole (MBZ) is given as 500-mg tablets in daily doses of 40-50 mg/kg bw in three divided doses postprandially. After an initial continuous treatment of 4 weeks, it is advisable to adjust the oral doses in order to obtain plasma drug levels of >250 nmol/l (= 74 ng/ml). The duration of treatment is at least 2 years after radical surgery or continuously for many years in inoperable cases, as well as for patients who have undergone incomplete resection or liver transplantation.

Albendazole (ABZ) is given as 400-mg tablet or as a 4% suspension at daily doses of 10 -15 mg/kg bw (in two divided doses). In practice, a daily dose of 800 mg is given to adults, divided into two doses of 400 mg. Repeated cycles of 28 days treatment should be followed by a 'wash out' phase without chemotherapy of 14 days. However, data from the People's Republic of China (Liu, 1997) and Italy indicate that a continuous ABZ treatment of AE is at least equally or more effective and well tolerated. The duration of necessary chemotherapy has not yet been determined but might well be life-long for most of the patients without complete resection of the AE lesions.

Adverse effects of the chemotherapy with benzimidazoles are neutropaenia, alopecia and liver dysfunction. They are contraindicated in pregnancy due to its potential embryotoxicity and teratogenicity. Monitoring of the AE patients is similar to that in CE patients. A long-term follow-up of more than 10 years is recommended.

Interventional procedures are indicated for AE patients for whom surgery is contraindicated. Some of them are dilation and stent implantation in vessels or bile ducts, and endoscopic sclerosing of oesophageal varices.

Liver transplantation should only be considered in patients with very severe hilar extension, leading to uncontrolled biliary infections, symptomatic secondary biliary cirrhosis with ascites or severe variceal bleeding owing to portal hypertension (Bresson-Hadni, 1997). It requires long-term and continuous postoperative chemotherapy.

2.2.3 Polycystic echinococcosis (PE)

Forms of human polycystic echinococcosis (PE) are caused by *E. vogeli* and *E. oligarthrus*, which are confined in their distribution to Latin American countries.

Metacestode of *E. vogeli* is characterized by its polycystic form filled with liquid with a tendency to form conglomerates with multiples small spaces inside. The most affected organ in the intermediate host is the liver. Metacestode of *E. oligarthrus* is similar to *E. vogeli* but the division in secondary spaces is less frequent and the laminar membrane is significantly thinner.

Wild and domestic dogs as definitive hosts and paca (*Cuniculus paca*) as intermediate host participate in the life-cycle of *E. vogeli*. Polycystic echinococcosis due to *E. vogeli* has been communicated in the majority of the countries belonging to the neotropical region of America; including Panama, Colombia, Argentina, Ecuador, Brasil, Bolivia and Venezuela.

E. oligarthrus is the unique *Echinococcus* specie that uses felids as definitive hosts. Infections naturally acquired have been demonstrated affecting pumas, jaguars, and other wild felids.

2.2.3.1 Polycystic echinococcosis due to *E. vogeli*

Clinical and radiological presentation is very similar to infection with multiple cysts of *E. granulosus*, and differential diagnosis depends on isolation of protoscoleces and morphological hook characteristics (D'Alessandro, 1997). Immunodiagnosis using a purified antigen of *E. vogeli* allowed discrimination between cases of PE and CE, but differentiation between PE and AE was not always possible (Gottstein, 1995). Albendazole with doses of 10 mg/kg/day has been used for chemotherapy in six cases with success of treatment in four and improvement in two (D'Alessandro, 1997).

2.2.3.2 Polycystic echinococcosis due to *E. oligarthrus*

Only three human cases have been reported to date, two orbital in Venezuela and Surinam and one cardiac in Brazil with 2 cysts (1.5 cm diameter) (D'Alessandro, 1997). The diagnosis was based on morphology of protoscolex hooks.

3. Conclusion

Human echinococcosis is a zoonotic larval cestode disease usually caused by *Echinococcus granulosus* or *E. multilocularis*. Infection is chronic taking years for symptoms to develop. The medical impact of the late stages of human cystic or alveolar echinococcosis may be significant though morbidity and mortality are usually grossly under-reported in endemic areas. Because of diagnosis and treatment are difficult and reservoirs of infection are maintained in domestic livestock, dogs or wildlife, the disease is difficult to assess in terms of public health and requires long-term control interventions. Globally, 3.6 million disability-adjusted life-years (DALYs) could be lost due to echinoccocosis, and this disease is included in an important group of neglected non vector-borne zoonotic infections that are currently not sufficiently prioritised (WHO/DFID-AHP, 2006).

Echinococcosis is therefore a neglected disease which is under-reported and requires urgent attention in common with a number of other zoonoses in order to reduce morbidity and to help alleviate poverty in poor pastoral areas of the sub-tropics and temperate zones. It's also difficult to formulate interventions and to apply cost-effective control programmes in this disease.

Human behaviour is crucial in facilitating transmission of this infection between domestic animal hosts as a result of traditional pastoral and husbandry practices (Mcpherson, 2005; Craig, 2007). Dogs are also susceptible to infection with E. multilocularis and E. vogeli (whose intermediate hosts are principally rodents) and therefore dogs may constitute a greater zoonotic reservoir of infection compared to natural wild canid hosts. Peri-domestic transmission may occur and could for example sustain a level of transmission of E. multilocularis in highly endemic communities (Li, 2005), but is probably not responsible for long-term maintenance of these Echinococcus species adapted to small mammals. Therefore, echinococcosis is a disease where humans may acquire infection from wild or domestic animal hosts but the parasite cannot be directly transmitted between humans (Wolfe, 2007), and due to all of these concepts treatment of human echinococcosis cases will have no effect on pathogen transmission. We will need to apply interventions to reduce human exposure or break transmission cycles in order to control the disease. This places echinococcosis in a 'difficult-to-deal-with' category; firstly, unlike the other neglected parasitic diseases humans can not act as a definitive host, and secondly, echinococcosis in livestock (or dogs) is not perceived as an animal health problem.

Clinical symptoms and subsequent diagnosis occur in adults (20-60 years) but infections in children may also become symptomatic (Soriano Arandes et al., 2010), and imaging techniques are the basis for diagnosis preferably accompanied by a specific serological test (Craig et al., 2003). Surgical removal of cysts/cystic masses, cyst drainage or organ resection, are the main form of treatment, often supported by high dose albendazole cover; the latter also has a benefit in medically-only treated cases (WHO, 2001).

The key factors of echinococcosis as a neglected disease are best described in a recent paper (Craig et al., 2007):

- Human echinococcosis is a zoonosis, non vector-borne zoonosis, that is not transmitted between humans. Therefore, it's a disease that is not amenable to vector-based control nor to direct human-treatment-approaches for case prevention.

- Human CE and AE are chronic diseases with very long asymptomatic periods so that endemic communities and health authorities fail to properly recognise the negative health impacts. Prevalence values represent infection events some years previously. CE remains an important health problem in many regions of the world, both where no control measures have been implemented, and where control programs have been incompletely successful with ensuing re-emergence of the disease. In Spain, official data on CE show an increase in the proportion of intermediate hosts with CE during the last few years, and autochthonous pediatric patients have been reported, a sign of active local transmission of disease. However, several crucial aspects related to CE that would help better understand and control the disease have not been tackled appropriately, in particular the emergence of infection in specific geographical areas. The introduction of national registries for CE with online data entry, following the example set by the European Registry for Alveolar Echinococcosis, would help streamline data collection on CE by eliminating the need for evaluating and integrating data from multiple regions, by avoiding duplication of data from patients who access several different health facilities over time, and by providing much needed clinical and epidemiological data that are currently accessible only to clinicians (Rojo-Vazquez et al., 2011).

- Echinococcosis is difficult to detect or diagnose in humans without access to imaging tools (eg. ultrasound, CT scan), furthermore the basis for confirmatory laboratory diagnosis is usually expensive serological tests.

- Treatment is very difficult and not always very effective, relying largely on costly major surgical or percutaneous hospital-based interventions to remove or sterilise cystic lesions. Furthermore, anthelmintic therapy is not ashighly effective as for other helminthic diseases (eg. gastro-intestinal helminthiases, schistosomiasis or onchocerciasis), and is based on long-term high dose albendazole usually re- quiring a minimum 6 months daily course, for which follow-up is very difficult especially in poor-resource areas. In this regard echinococcosis treatment more closely resembles tumour treatments or TB therapy, than that for a parasitic disease.

- Medical records are usually not very explicit/specific, may involve complex follow-up notes, and may be dispersed across several specialities within/between hospitals/clinics and therefore data is not usually properly collated.

- In under-developed regions, human echinococcosis generally occurs in poor, often remote marginalised pastoral societies that may be ethnically/socio-culturally isolated from the general population. Consequently they are not usually very well prioritised by the predominant agricultural-based community district health authorities, and so access to affordable health care is also poor and/or difficult.

- The burden of echinococcosis disease is therefore difficult to quantify, and official hospital or district records often inaccurate, and in any case represent gross under-estimates of the real burden in an endemic area.

- CE is a chronic, asymptomatic infection in domestic animals and is therefore also not recognised by livestock owners as an animal health or economic problem.

- Dogs are the main carrier and spreader of the parasite, but are asymptomatic. In contrast to livestock numbers, official accurate estimates of dog population sizes (owned and stray) are almost never kept/known by municipal, veterinary or agricultural authorities. Canine echinococcosis is treatable with the anthelmintic praziquantel but requires frequent dosing. Unlike for rabies, there is currently no dog vaccine against canine echinococcosis.

- Control of echinococcosis is difficult and exacerbated by the requirement of cooperation between agricultural/veterinary services and medical authorities.

4. Acknowledgment

To my family, and especially to my wife Marta and my sons Marc and Toni for their support everywhere and every moment of my life.

5. References

Bowles, J. & McManus, D.P. (1993). Molecular variation in *Echinococcus*. *Acta trop.*, 53, 291-305.

Bowles, J. & McManus, D.P. (1993). Rapid discrimination of *Echinococcus* species and strains using a polymerase chain reaction-based RFLP method. *Molec. biochem. Parasitol.,* 57, 231-239.

Bresson-Hadni, S., Koch, S., Beutron, L., Vuitton, DA., Bartholomot, B., Hrusovsky, S., Heyd, B., Lenys, D., Minello, A., Becker, MC., Vanlemmens, C., Mantion, GA. & Miguet, JP. (1997). Primary disease recurrence after liver transplantation for alveolar echinococcosis: long-term evaluation in 15 patients. *Hepatology,* 30, 857-863.

Craig, PS. (1997). Immunodiagnosis of *Echinococcus granulosus* and a comparison of techniques for diagnosis of canine echinococcosis, *In:* Compendium on cystic echinococcosis in Africa and Middle Eastern Countries with special reference to Morocco (F.L. Andersen, H. Ouhelli & M. Kachani, eds). Brigham Young University, Print Services, Provo, 85-118.

Craig, PS., Budke, CM., Schantz, PM., Li, T., Qiu, J., Yang, Y., Zeyhle, E., Rogan, MT., and Ito, A. (2007). Human echinococcosis: a neglected disease?, *Trop. Med. Int. Health,* 35(4), 283-292.

Craig, PS., McManus, DP., Lightowlers, MW., Chabalgoity, JA., Garcia, HH., Gavidia, CM., Gilman, RH., Gonzalez, AE., Lorca, M., Naquira, C., Schantz, PM. (2007). Prevention and control of cystic echinococcosis. *Lancet Inf Dis.,* 7, 385-394.

Craig, PS., Rogan, MT., Campos-Ponce, M. (2003). Echinococcosis: disease, detection and transmission. *Parasitology,* 127, S5-S20.

Dakkak, A. (2010). Echinococcosis/hydatidosis: a severe threat in Mediterranean countries. *Vet Parasitol.* 174(1-2), 2-11.

D'Alessandro, A. (1997). Polycystic echinococcosis in tropical America: *Echinococcus vogeli* and *E. oligarthrus. Acta trop.,* 67 (1-2), 43-65.

Di Felice, G., Pini, C., Afferni, C. & Vicari, G. (1986). Purification and partial characterization of the major antigen of *E. granulosus* (antigen 5) with monoclonal antibodies. *Molec. biochem. Parasitol.,* 20, 133-142.

Eckert, J. (1998). Alveolar echinococcosis (*Echinococcus multilocularis*) and other forms of echinococcosis (*Echinococcus oligarthrus* and *Echinococcus vogeli*), *In:* Zoonoses (S.R. Palmer, E.J.L. Soulsby & D.I.H. Simpson, eds). Oxford University Press, Oxford, 689-716.

Filice, C. & Brunetti, E. (1997). Use of PAIR in human cystic echinococcosis. *Acta trop.,* 64, 95-107.

Franchi, C., Di Vico, B. & Teggi, A. (1999). Long-term evaluation of patients with hydatidosis treated with benzimidazole carbamates. *Clin. infect Dis.,* 29, 304-309.

Frider, B., Larrieu, E. & Odriozola, M. (1999). Long-term outcome of asymptomatic liver hydatidosis. *J. Hepatol.,* 30, 228-231.

Gasser, RB., Zhu, XQ. & McManus, DP. (1998). Display of sequence variation in PCR-amplified mitochondrial DNA regions of *Echinococcus* by single-strand conformation polymorphism. *Acta trop.,* 71, 107-115.

Gemmell, M.A. & Roberts, M.G. (1995). Modelling *Echinococcus* life cycles, *In: Echinococcus* and hydatid disease (R.C.A. Thompson & A.L. Lymbery, eds). CAB International, Wallingford, Oxon, 333-354.

Gottstein, B., D'Alessandro, A. & Rausch, R.L. (1995). Immunodiagnosis of polycystic hydatid disease/polycystic echinococcosis due to *Echinococcus vogeli*. *Am. J. trop. Med. Hyg.*, 53, 558-563.

Gottstein, B., Jacquier, P., Bresson-Hadni, S. & Eckert, J. (1993). Improved primary immunodiagnosis of alveolar echinococcosis in humans by an enzyme-linked immunosorbent assay using the Em2plus-antigen. *J. clin. Microbiol.*, 31, 373-376.

Haag, KL., Gottstein, B., Ayala, FJ. (2009). The EG95 Antigen of Echinococcus spp. Contains Positively Selected Amino Acids, which May Influence Host Specificity and Vaccine Efficacy. *PLoS ONE* 4(4): e5362. doi:10.1371/journal.pone.0005362.

Ioppolo, S., Notargiacomo, S., Profumo, E., Franchi, C., Ortona, E., Rigano, R. & Siracusano, A. (1996). Immunological responses to antigen B from *Echinococcus granulosus* cyst fluid in hydatid patients. *Parasite Immunol.*, 18, 571-578.

Leggatt, GR. & McManus, DP. (1994). Identification and diagnostic value of a major antibody epitope on the 12 kDa antigen from *Echinococcus granulosus* (hydatid disease) cyst fluid. *Parasite Immunol.*, 16, 87-96.

Leggatt, GR., Yang, W. & McManus, DP. (1992). Serological evaluation of the 12 kDa subunit of antigen B in *Echinococcus granulosus* cyst fluid by immunoblot analysis. *Trans. roy. Soc. trop. Med. Hyg.*, 86, 189-192.

Li, T., Qiu, J., Yang, W., Craig, PS., Chen, X., Xiao, N., Ito, A., Giraudoux, P., Wulamu, M., Yu, W., Schantz, PM. (2005). Echinococcosis in Tibetan populations, western Sichuan Province, China. *Emerg Inf Dis.*, 11, 1866-1873.

Lightowlers MW & Gauci CG (2001). Vaccines against cysticercosis and hydatidosis. *Vet Parasitol* 101: 337–352.

Ligthowlers, MW. & Gottstein, B. (1995). Echinococcosis/hydatidosis: antigens, immunological and molecular diagnosis, *In: Echinococcus* and hydatid disease (R.C.A. Thompson & A.J. Lymbery, eds). CAB International, Oxon, 355-410.

Liu, YH. (1997). Continuous or intermittent treatment with albendazole? *Arch. int. Hidatid*, 32, 171-173.

Macpherson, CNL. (2005). Human behaviour and the epidemiology of parasitic zoonoses. *Int J Parasito.l*, 35, 1319-1331.

Paul, M. & Stefaniak, J. (1997). Detection of specific *Echinococcus granulosus* antigen 5 in liver cyst bioptate from human patients. *Acta trop.*, 64, 65-77.

Pawłowski, ZS. (1997). Critical points in the clinical management of cystic echinococcosis: a revised review, *In*: Compendium on cystic echinococcosis in Africa and in Middle Eastern Countries with special reference to Morocco (F.L. Andersen, H. Ouhelli & M. Kachani, eds). Brigham Young University, Print Services, Provo, Utah, 119-135.

Pérez-Molina, JA., Díaz-Menéndez, M, Gallego, JI, et al. (2011). Evaluation of nitazoxanide for the treatment of disseminated cystic echinococcosis: report of five cases and literature review. *Am. J. Trop. Med. Hyg.*, 84(2), 351-6.

Petavy A-F, Hormaeche C, Lahmar S, Ouhelli H, Chabalgoity A, et al. (2008). An Oral Recombinant Vaccine in Dogs against Echinococcus granulosus, the Causative Agent of Human Hydatid Disease: A Pilot Study. *PLoS Negl Trop Dis* 2(1): e125.

Profumo, E., Ortona, E., Rigano, R., Gioia, I., Notargiacomo, S., Ioppolo, S. & Siracusano, A. (1994). Cellular and humoral responses to antigenic subunits of *Echinococcus granulosus* cyst fluid in hydatid patients. *Parasite Immunol.*, 16, 393-398.

Rassy, D., Bobes, RJ., Rosas, G., Anaya, VH., Brehm, K., et al. (2010). Characterization of S3Pvac Anti-Cysticercosis Vaccine Components: Implications for the Development of an Anti-Cestodiasis Vaccine. *PLoS ONE* 5(6): e11287.

Rojo-Vazquez, FA., Pardo-Lledias, J., Francos-Von Hunefeld, M., et al. (2011). Cystic echinococcosis in Spain: current situation and relevance for other endemic areas in Europe. *PLoS neglected tropical diseases.*, 5 (1): e893.

Sarciron, EM., Bresson-Hadni, S., Mercier, M., Lawton, P., Duranton, C., Lenys, D., Petavy, AF. & Vuitton, DA. (1997). Antibodies against *Echinococcus multilocularis* alkaline phosphatase as markers for the specific diagnosis and the serological monitoring of alveolar echinococcosis. *Parasite Immunol.*, 19, 61-68.

Sheperd, A. & McManus, D.P. (1987). Specific and cross reactive antigens of *Echinococcus granulosus* cyst fluid. *Molec. biochem. Parasitol.*, 25, 143-154.

Siracusano, A. & Vuitton, D. (1997). Immunology and immunopathology of *Echinococcus granulosus* and *Echinococcus multilocularis* infections. *Arch. int. Hidatid.*, 32, 132-135.

Soriano Arandes, A., Gómez Bertomeu, F., and Maldonado Artero, J. (2010). Microscopic Image of the Protoscolex of *Echinococcus granulosus* on the "Hydatid Sand". *Am. J. Trop. Med. Hyg.*, 82(6), 980.

Thompson, RCA. (1995). Biology and systematics of *Echinococcus, In: Echinococcus* and hydatid disease (R.C.A. Thompson & A.J. Lymbery, eds). CAB International, Wallingford, 1-50.

Torgerson, PR., Keller, K., Magnotta, M., Ragland, N. (2010). The Global Burden of Alveolar Echinococcosis. *PLoS Negl Trop Dis* 4(6): e722.

Utrilla, JG., Eyre, FP., Muguerza, R., Alami, H. & Bueno, J. (1991). Hidatidosis en la infancia. *Arch. Hidatid.*, 30, 721-730.

Wen, H. & Craig, PS. (1994). Immunoglobulin G subclass responses in human cystic and alveolar echinococcosis. *Am. J. trop. Med. Hyg.*, 51, 741-748.

Wolfe, ND., Dunavan, CP., Diamond, J. (2007). Origins of major human infectious diseases. *Nature.*, 447, 279-283.

World Health Organization (WHO) (1996). Guidelines for treatment of cystic and alveolar echinococcosis. WHO Informal Working Group on Echinococcosis. *Bull. WHO*, 74, 231-242.

World Health Organization (WHO) (2001). International classification of ultrasound images in cystic echinoccosis for application in clinical and field epidemiological settings., *In:* PAIR, an option for the treatment of cystic echinococcosis. WHO, Geneva.

World Health Organization (WHO) (2001). WHO/OIE Manual on Echinococcosis in Humans and Animals: a Public Health Problem of Global Concern. WHO, Geneva.

WHO/DFID-AHP (2006). The Control of Neglected Zoonotic Diseases-A Route to Poverty Alleviation.World Health Organization, Dept of Food Safety, Zoonoses, and Food-borne Diseases, Geneva.

Zhang, W., Li, J., You, H., Zhang, Z., Turson, G., Loukas, A. & McManus, DP. (2003). Short report: *Echinococcus granulosus* from Xinjiang, PR China: CDNAs encoding the EG95 vaccine antigen are expressed in different cycle stages and are conserved in the oncosphere. *Am. J. Trop. Med. Hyg.*, 68, 40–43.

10

Antischistosomal Natural Compounds: Present Challenges for New Drug Screens

Josué de Moraes
Supervisão de Vigilância em Saúde, SUVIS Casa Verde,
Secretaria de Saúde da Cidade de São Paulo,
Rua Ferreira de Almeida, São Paulo, SP
Brazil

1. Introduction

Schistosomiasis, or bilharzias, is a neglected disease that remains a considerable public health problem in tropical and subtropical regions. This parasitic disease is the most important human helminth infection in terms of morbidity and mortality and is a growing concern worldwide. It is estimated that more than 200 million people have been infected and that 779 million are at risk of infection, resulting in 280,000 deaths annually (van der Werf et al., 2003; Steinmann et al., 2006). Schistosomiasis is caused by blood-dwelling fluke worms of the genus *Schistosoma* and is endemic in African, Asian and South American countries. The main disease-causing species are *S. mansoni*, *S. haematobium*, and *S. japonicum*. *S. mansoni* is the most widely distributed, affecting people in Africa, the Middle East, South America, and the Caribbean, while *S. japonicum* is confined to China, Indonesia, and the Philippines. *S. haematobium* is found in Africa and the Middle East. The adult worms colonise the veins of either the portal system (*S. mansoni* and *S. japonicum*) or the urinary bladder plexus (*S. haematobium*) and can live for years or even decades in human hosts; thus, the disease runs a chronic and debilitating course. Egg production is responsible for both the transmission of the parasite and the aetiology of the disease. Schistosomal species are distinguished by differences in their morphology, both in their parasite stages and in their eggs; further species distinction is made by the species of intermediate host snails that support transmission of the parasite (Gryseels et al., 2006).

The global strategy for the control of schistosomiasis is by chemotherapy. Systematic searching for chemotherapeutic drugs began almost a century ago, and the development of praziquantel (PZQ) in 1970 was essential for a reduction in morbidity and mortality due to schistosomiasis. Currently, treatment is still based on the use of PZQ, but the long-term application of PZQ results in decreased efficiency and serious concerns regarding the onset of resistance. In addition, PZQ has no prophylactic properties and is ineffective against larval stages of parasites (schistosomula), meaning that for effective treatment and sustainable control, PZQ must be given on a regular basis. Thus, it is prudent to search for novel therapeutics, and recent discussions have focused on reawakening the need to search for alternatives to PZQ (Caffrey, 2007; Doenhoff et al., 2008; Fenwick et al., 2003; Hagan et al., 2004; Keiser & Utzinger, 2007).

Natural products, mainly plants, have been the source of medicines for thousands of years. The discovery of pure compounds as active principles in plants was first described at the beginning of the 19th century, and the art of exploiting natural products has become part of the molecular sciences (Kayser et al., 2003). Several extracts or bioactive constituents from living organisms have been used in many communities worldwide against parasitic diseases, including schistosomiasis, and in the past decades, natural products have attracted renewed interest (Kayser et al., 2003; Mølgaard et al., 2001; Ndamba et al., 1994; Sanderson et al., 2002; Tagboto & Townson, 2001).

In vitro screening systems are useful and affordable ways to discover potential anthelmintic candidates for *in vivo* tests (Keiser, 2010; Ramirez et al., 2007; Yousif et al., 2007). Because a molecular-target approach is still rarely employed in schistosomicidal drug discovery, a more common strategy has been the complementary approach of whole-organism phenotypic screening *in vitro* to measure compound efficacy (Keiser, 2010; Ramirez et al., 2007; Yousif et al., 2007). In this context, screening for natural products that are active against schistosome is important in the establishment of future strategies for new antischistosomal drug discovery to control schistosomiasis (Yousif et al., 2007).

Considerable efforts are ongoing to develop novel schistosomicidal agents. As a result, many natural compounds with promising antischistosomal properties have been identified (Braguine et al., 2009; de Moraes et al., 2011; Magalhães et al., 2009, 2010; Moraes et al., 2011; Mølgaard et al., 2001; Parreira et al., 2010; Sanderson et al., 2002). The efficacy of these new compounds against schistosome is defined using three strategies: a) curative, by killing the adult worm; b) prophylactic, by killing schistosomula; and c) suppressive, by inhibiting worm egg-laying. Thus, several parameters, such as motor activity, tegumental changes, and oviposition, are often evaluated as indicators of biological activity and toxicity in studies with schistosome species.

This chapter reviews the present state of *in vitro* drug screening strategies used to discover new compounds active against *S. mansoni*, the most important species infecting humans, with an emphasis on natural products. Also highlighted are the best practices and challenges for drug screenings. Furthermore, information is provided about toxicity, susceptible *Schistosoma* stages, and other interesting laboratory studies on potential antischistosomal compounds, both natural products and natural product-derived compounds.

2. Antischistosomal drugs

For the control of schistosomiasis, which at present is dependent on chemotherapy, it is not satisfactory to have only one single effective treatment (Caffrey, 2007; Doenhoff et al., 2008; Fenwick et al., 2003). Ideally, other antischistosomal drugs would be available so that the classical strategy of alternating treatments to avoid the development of resistance could be used. Unfortunately, the other drugs used before the advent of PZQ, oxamniquine and metrifonate, are restricted in their use. Metrifonate, a drug that exhibits activity against *S. haematobium*, has recently been withdrawn from the market because of medical, operational, and economic criteria (Reich & Fenwick, 2001; Utzinger et al., 2003). Oxamniquine is the only alternative antischistosomal drug, but it is effective only against *S. mansoni*. In the 1970s, oxamniquine was used for individual and mass treatment of schistosomiasis, with satisfactory results regarding efficacy and tolerance. However, its use is currently declining and is being replaced by praziquantel (Cioli, 2000; Reich & Fenwick, 2001; Utzinger et al.,

2001, 2003). As there is currently no available vaccine for this disease in people (Bergquist et al., 2008), chemotherapy may now be at a crucial point.

Chemotherapy against schistosomiasis was reviewed extensively by Cioli et al. (1995), with an emphasis on compounds that were used in the past. Additionally, Cioli (1998) summarised some interesting laboratory studies on potential antischistosomal compounds and the possible emergence of praziquantel-resistant schistosomes. More recently, Ribeiro-dos-Santos et al. (2006) reviewed results from a comprehensive search of the scientific literature for substances and compounds tested for schistosomiasis therapy over the past century. The authors gathered information on the therapeutic action in humans or animal models and the mechanisms of action of over 40 drugs.

Briefly, antimonial compounds were introduced in 1918, and this group of drugs has been the major point of schistosome chemotherapy for approximately 50 years. However, they cause numerous side effects, such as nausea, vomiting, diarrhoea, anorexia, and cardiovascular, hepatic, and dermatological disturbances. Lethality from cardiac syncope and anaphylactic shock was also reported. Emetine, a drug used to treat amoebiasis, was employed in the second decade of the past century, but the doses required against schistosomiasis were at the very limit of toxicity. The introduction of 2,3-dehydroemetine reduced the toxicity of the parent compound, but patients had to be hospitalised over a month for treatment. Thus, the use of 2,3-dehydroemetine as an antischistosomal agent was abandoned (Cioli et al., 1995). Only in the 1960s was there a breakthrough in the treatment of schistosomiasis, with the rise of metrifonate, nitrofurans, lucanthone, niridazole, hycanthone, and, finally, oxamniquine. In the 1970s, several schistosomicidal drugs emerged, such as tubercidin, amoscanate, PZQ and its benzodiazepine derivative Ro11-3128, and oltipraz. Nevertheless, the therapeutic doses of most of these drugs were found to cause major side effects. PZQ, an isoquinoline-pyrazine derivative, immediately proved to be superior to any other schistosomicidal drug and quickly became the drug of choice in most endemic areas (Cioli et al., 1995; Fenwick & Webster, 2006). Because of the reliance on a single drug for the treatment and control of schistosomiasis and the considerable concern regarding the development of PZQ resistance, it is timely to review potential alternatives, with an emphasis on natural products.

2.1 Antischistosomals: Natural product and natural product-derived compounds

The use of natural products for curative and therapeutic purposes has a long history, and compounds derived from natural products have made a big impact on the pharmaceutical industry (Newman, 2003; Newman & Cragg, 2007). In addition to microbes and plants, there has been growing interest in other living organisms, such as arthropods and amphibians, as important sources of biologically active compounds (Kayser et al., 2003). However, the potential for using living beings as sources of new antischistosomal drugs is still poorly explored. In recent decades, there has been a growing interest in the scientific community to search for extracts and pure compounds, especially those derived from plants, that exhibit potential schistosomicidal properties, as one alternative method to the conventional chemical control.

Plants have been traditionally used in the treatment of different diseases, including schistosomiasis, especially in Africa and Asia (Ndamba et al., 1994). In general, medicinal plants are prepared by traditional healers, who have empirical knowledge and cultural communities throughout the world. For example, in Zimbabwe, Ndamba et al. (1994) investigated the herbal remedies used in the treatment of schistosomiasis. Based on interviews with 286 traditional healers, they composed a list of 47 plant species most widely used to treat urinary schistosomiasis. Based on this survey, the seven most commonly used plants, *Abrus precatorius* (Leguminosae) *Ozoroa insignis* (Anacardiaceae), *Dicoma anomala* (Cornpositae), *Ximenia caffra* (Oleaceae), *Lannea edulis* (Anacardiaceae), *Elephantorrhiza goetzei* (Leguminosae) and *Pterocarpus angolensis* (Leguminosae), were collected, prepared as described by the traditional healers, their efficacy was evaluated using laboratory animals previously exposed to *S. haematobium* cercariae, and the activity from the extract of *P. angolensis* bark was almost comparable to that of praziquantel. Later, Mølgaard et al. (2001) screened extracts of 23 plant species, popularly used against schistosomiasis in Zimbabwe, for their anthelmintic effect against schistosomula of *S. mansoni*, and the best results against larval forms were obtained with stem and root extracts from *Abrus precatorius* (Fabaceae) and stem bark from *Elephantorrhiza goetzei* (Mimosaceae). All families and names of the plants that are used by traditional healers to treat urinary schistosomiasis in Zimbabwe are described by Ndamba et al. (1994).

Some of the most interesting antischistosomal compounds are derivatives of artemisinin, such as artemether and artesunate (Utzinger et al., 2001; Xiao et al., 2002). They are highly effective in the treatment of malaria and have also been shown to exhibit antischistosomal properties. Artemisinin is a sesquiterpene lactone with an endoperoxide group, which was isolated from the leaves of *Artemisia annua* L. This plant has been used for centuries in Chinese traditional medicine as antidote to many different ailments (Lee, 2007; Utzinger et al., 2001). Artemisinin has been used as an antimalarial since the early 1970s, and its antischistosomal activity was discovered in 1980 by a group of Chinese scientists. In 1982, antischistosomal properties were confirmed for artemether, the methyl ether derivative of artemisinin. Interestingly, artemether has been shown to be active against immature schistosome in experimentally infected animals, but it is less effective against adult worms (Utzinger et al., 2001). Significant progress has been made with artemether and its potential for the control of schistosomiasis, which has been reviewed by Utzinger et al. (2001). The mechanism of action of artemisinin and its derivatives appears to involve an interaction with heme, which cleaves the endoperoxide bridge of the drug to produce carbon-centred free radicals that then alkylate parasite proteins (Golenser et al., 2006). In addition, scanning electron microscopy showed that artemether caused extensive and severe damage to the tegument in 21-day-old *S. mansoni* harboured in mice (Xiao et al., 2000). Considering that artemether and praziquantel exhibit the highest activity against schistosomula and adult worms, respectively, combined treatment has been proposed to enhance the reduction in worm burden (Utzinger et al., 2003). Currently, new trials to use artemisinin and its synthetic derivatives as lead molecules for drug discovery against schistosomiasis and various other diseases are rapidly growing, and the studies are ongoing (Lee, 2007; Utzinger et al., 2003, 2007; Xiao et al., 2002). Likewise, research on other natural products and natural product-derived compounds against schistosome has been performed by many groups. Accordingly, several plants with antischistosomal properties have been described in the literature (Braguine et al., 2009; de Moraes et al., 2011; Magalhães et al., 2009, 2010; Moraes et al., 2011; Mohamed et al., 2005; Mølgaard et al., 2001; Parreira et al., 2010; Sanderson et al., 2002).

Here, data on natural products and related natural product-derived compounds are reviewed, especially those from recent years or that have received considerable attention due to their antischistosomal properties (Table 1).

Date *	Extract/ Compound and Biological Source	Relevant notes
1980	Artemisinin, active principle from the plant *Artemisia annua* L. (Asteraceae)	Artemisinin derivatives: artemether (1982) and artenusate (1983); effective against immature schistosome in experimentally infected animals; morphological alteration on the tegument (Utzinger et al., 2001)
1989	Extracts from the plant *Pavetta owariensis* P. Beauv (Rubiaceae) contain proanthocyanins	Effective in mice infected with *S. mansoni* (Baldé et al., 1989)
1997	Goyazensolide isolated from the plant *Eremanthus goyazensis* (Gardner) Sch. Bip. (Compositae)	*In vitro* activity on *Schistosoma* adult worms; inhibitory effect on egg-laying; female more susceptible than male; not tested on schistosomula (Barth et al., 1997)
2000	Extract of leaf from the plant *Vernonia amygdalina* Del (Compositae)	Active against *S. mansoni* in mice (Ogboli, 2000)
2001	Mirazid myrrh, an oleo-gumresin from the stem of the plant *Commiphora molmol* (Burseraceae)	There is a great debate about the efficacy and effectiveness of myrrh in the treatment of schistosome infections, both in laboratory and clinical settings (Abdul-Ghani et al., 2009; Badria et al., 2001; Botros et al., 2004, 2005; Sheir et al., 2001)
2002	Oil from the plant *Nigella sativa* L. (Ranunculaceae)	Active on *S. mansoni*-infected mice; crushed seed also has *in vitro* effects against *S. mansoni* miracidia, cercariae, and adult worms, and an inhibitory effect on egg-laying; not tested on schistosomula (Mahmoud et al., 2002; Mohamed et al., 2005)
2002	Extract of the seeds and isoflavonoids from the plant *Millettia thonningii* (Schum. et Thonn.) Baker (Leguminosae)	*In vitro* against *S. mansoni* adult worms; no egg production was observed for experimental worms; not tested on schistosomula. Schistosomicidal activity against *S. mansoni* cercariae and miracidia has been previously described (Lyddiard et al., 2002)

* Dates of introduction or publication are only approximate.

Table 1. *In vitro* and *in vivo* antischistosomal characteristics of natural products.

Date *	Extract/ Compound and Biological Source	Relevant notes
2005	Extract of rhizomes from the plant *Zingiber officinale* Roscoe (Zingiberaceae)	*In vitro* male worms seemed more susceptible than female; reduction in egg output; activity against *S. mansoni* in mice was conflicting between Mostafa et al. (2011) and Sanderson et al. (2005); morphological alteration on the tegument; not tested on schistosomula
2007	Extract from plant *Curcuma longa* L. (Zingiberaceae)	Effective on *S. mansoni*-infected mice (El-Ansary et al., 2007; El-Banhawey et al., 2007); the *in vitro* schistosomicidal activity of curcumin, the major constituent in the rhizome, and reduction in egg production has been reported (Magalhães et al., 2009)
2007	Extract from garlic *Allium sativum* L. (Liliaceae)	Active against *S. mansoni* in mice (50 mg/kg) and not effective in high dose (100 mg/kg); affects the development and maturity of *S. mansoni* eggs in mice and seems to be an agent in protecting hepatic tissue against oxidative damage due to *S. mansoni* infection. *In vitro* allicin (2011), the main constituent of garlic, causes alterations on the tegument of male worm in high doses (10 to 20 µg/ml), but toxicity not assessed; not tested on schistosomula (El Shenawy et al., 2008; Lima et al., 2011; Riad et al., 2007)
2009	Extract from the plant *Clerodendrum umbellatum* Poir (Verbenaceae)	Effective in *S. mansoni* mice model (Jatsa et al., 2009)
2009	Extract from the plant *Zanthoxylum naranjillo* Griseb (Rutaceae) and its isolated compounds	*In vitro* against *S. mansoni* adult worms; reduction in egg-laying; not tested on schistosomula; not toxic in mammalian cells (Braguine et al., 2009)
2010	Phloroglucinol compounds from plants of the *Dryopteris* genus (Dryopteridaceae)	*In vitro* against *S. mansoni* adult worms; reduction in egg-laying; not tested on schistosomula; not toxic in mammalian cells (Magalhães et al., 2010)
2010	Essential oil from the plant of *Baccharis dracunculifolia* DC. (Asteraceae)	*In vitro* against *S. mansoni* adult worms; reduction in egg-laying; not tested on schistosomula; not toxic in mammalian cell (Parreira et al., 2010)
2011	Essential oil from plant *Ageratum conyzoides* L. (Asteraceae)	*In vitro* against *S. mansoni* adult worms; reduction in egg-laying; not tested on schistosomula; not toxic in mammalian cells (de Melo et al., 2011)

Table 1. Continued

Date *	Extract/ Compound and Biological Source	Relevant notes
2011	Sulfated polysaccharide α-D-glucan extracted from lichen *Ramalina celastri* (Spreng.) Krog. & Swinsc	Effective in *S. mansoni*-infected mice (Araújo et al., 2011)
2011	Piplartine, an amide isolated from plant *Piper tuberculatum* Jacq. (Piperaceae)	*In vitro* against *S. mansoni* adult worms; reduction in egg-laying; causes alterations on the tegument of worms; not tested on schistosomula; not toxic in mammalian cells (Moraes et al., 2011)
2011	Dermaseptin 01, an antimicrobial peptide found in the skin of frog of the genus *Phyllomedusa* (Hylidae)	*In vitro* against *S. mansoni* adult worms; reduction in egg-laying; causes alterations on the tegument of worms; not tested on schistosomula; not toxic in mammalian cells (de Moraes et al., 2011)
2011	Epiisopiloturin, an alkaloid isolated from plant *Pilocarpus microphyllus* Stapf ex Holm (Rutaceae)	*In vitro* against *S. mansoni* adult worms; causes alterations on the tegument of worm; not tested on schistosomula; not toxic in mammalian cells (Leite et al., 2011)
2011	Extract from plants of the *Artemisia* genus (Asteraceae)	*In vitro* against *S. mansoni* adult worms; not tested on schistosomula (Ferreira et al., 2011)

Table 1. Continued

As shown in Table 1, several *in vitro* studies have been conducted to search for new natural substances with schistosomicidal activity. These natural products and natural product-derived compounds mostly come from plants. Extensive phytochemical investigations of many species have revealed the presence of a large number of novel compounds belonging to different classes (Kayser et al., 2003; Kato & Furlan, 2007; Parmar et al., 1997; Prassad et al., 2005). For example, various secondary metabolites have been isolated from the family Piperaceae, and these plants have generated great interest as a result of their biologically active metabolites, such as pyrones, terpenes, lactones, chromenes, chalcones, lignoids, amides, and alkaloids (Kato & Furlan, 2007; Parmar et al., 1997). Regarding the variety of biological properties in particular, Moraes et al. (2011) demonstrated the *in vitro* schistosomicidal activity of piplartine, an amide found in several *Piper* species. The authors showed that at low concentrations (9.5 µM) this amide can kill *S. mansoni* adult worms (male and female coupled) and that the sub-lethal concentration of piplartine (6.3 µM) caused a 75% reduction in egg production. Additionally, piplartine was not cytotoxic against mammalian cells when given at concentrations up to three times higher than what is needed for a schistosomicidal effect (31.5 µM). Furthermore, *Piper* species are widely distributed in tropical and subtropical regions of the world, and they are among the most important medicinal plants used in various systems of medicine (Jaramillo & Manos, 2001; Parmar et al., 1997). In addition to the wide geographical distribution and their use in folk medicine, the interest in these compounds and plant extracts is based on the fact that it is easy to isolate secondary metabolites and to propagate the plant, which has a short reproductive cycle. Thus, considering the *in vitro* schistosomicidal activity of the amide piplartine, the importance of more research on the biological activity of the natural compounds isolated from the family Piperaceae and other plants is apparent.

3. *Schistosoma mansoni* life cycle and maintenance in the laboratory

Schistosome species are dioecious (having male and female reproductive organs in separate individuals) platyhelminthes and have complex life cycles comprising multiple morphologically distinct phenotypes in definitive mammalian and intermediate snail hosts. *S. mansoni* is one of the most common etiological agents of human schistosomiasis and is the most widely used schistosome model for chemotherapeutic studies.Schistosome infection of humans (or another definitive host) occurs by direct contact with freshwater containing free-swimming larval forms of the parasite, known as cercariae. Cercariae penetrate the intact human skin and transform into schistosomula, which reside in the skin for up to 72 hours before entering a blood vessel. Within the vascular system, schistosomula migrate via complex routes to their final venous destination, where they mature into male and female adults. The mature flukes dwell in the human portal vasculature, depositing eggs in the intestinal wall that either pass to the gut lumen and are expelled in the faeces or travel to the liver and trigger immune-mediated granuloma formation and peri-portal fibrosis. Egg production commences 5 to 6 weeks after infection and continues for the life of the worm. The life cycle is completed when the eggs passed in the faeces hatch in the water, releasing the larval form miracidia, which then infect freshwater snails of the *Biomphalaria* spp. The infected snails, bearing schistosomal sporocysts, release cercariae into the water, which in turn penetrate the skin of their definitive host (Gryseels et al., 2006).

To complete a life cycle in the laboratory, *S. mansoni* is commonly maintained using rodents, ranging from hamsters to mice, as the definitive hosts and *Biomphalaria glabrata* as the intermediate host snail species (Figure 1). Infections of rodents of the same gender, 3 to 4 weeks of age and weighing 18 to 25 g, with *S. mansoni* are commonly initiated by subcutaneous injection of 100 to 150 cercariae (infective larvae). At 42, 49 or 56 days postinfection, animals are sacrificed with CO_2, dissected, and miracidia are hatched from *S. mansoni* eggs taken from animal livers. Each intermediate host snail is exposed to approximately 10 miracidia. All animals should be handled in strict accordance with good animal practice adhering to the institutional guidelines for animal husbandry. Thus, all studies should have a statement from their ethics committee or institutional review board indicating the approval of the research.

The use of *in vivo* animal models in drug discovery and the techniques used for these studies in the laboratory have recently been described in detail elsewhere by Keiser (2010) and Ramirez et al. (2007). This chapter will focus on the techniques used for *in vitro* studies. Many methods have been described that aim to determine the antischistosomal activity of drugs *in vitro*. The assessment of the viability of different stages of schistosome, tegumental changes, oviposition, toxicity in mammalian cells and other parameters are important in the search for antischistosomal substances. The techniques detailed here will be the key to better assess the methodology employed during screening tests.

4. Parasite culture system

In vitro studies with schistosomula, juvenile and adult worms of *S. mansoni* are frequently used in screening strategies for the discovery of new antischistosomal drugs (Abdulla et al., 2009; Keiser, 2010; Mølgaard et al., 2001; Peak et al., 2010; Ramirez et al., 2007; Smout et al., 2010; Yousif et al., 2007). Parasites at different stages might show differences with regard to drug sensitivity. The *in vitro* methods currently utilised have recently been reviewed, and following the establishment of the *S. mansoni* life cycle in the laboratory, *in vitro* parasite culture techniques were developed (Keiser, 2010; Ramirez et al., 2007). For *in vitro* trials, parasites of different ages are used, such as 3-h-old and 1-, 3-, 5- and 7-day-old schistosomula, 21 day-old juveniles, and 42- to 56-day-old adults. Figure 1 shows the life cycle of *S. mansoni* in the laboratory, illustrating the collection points for *in vitro* chemotherapeutic studies.

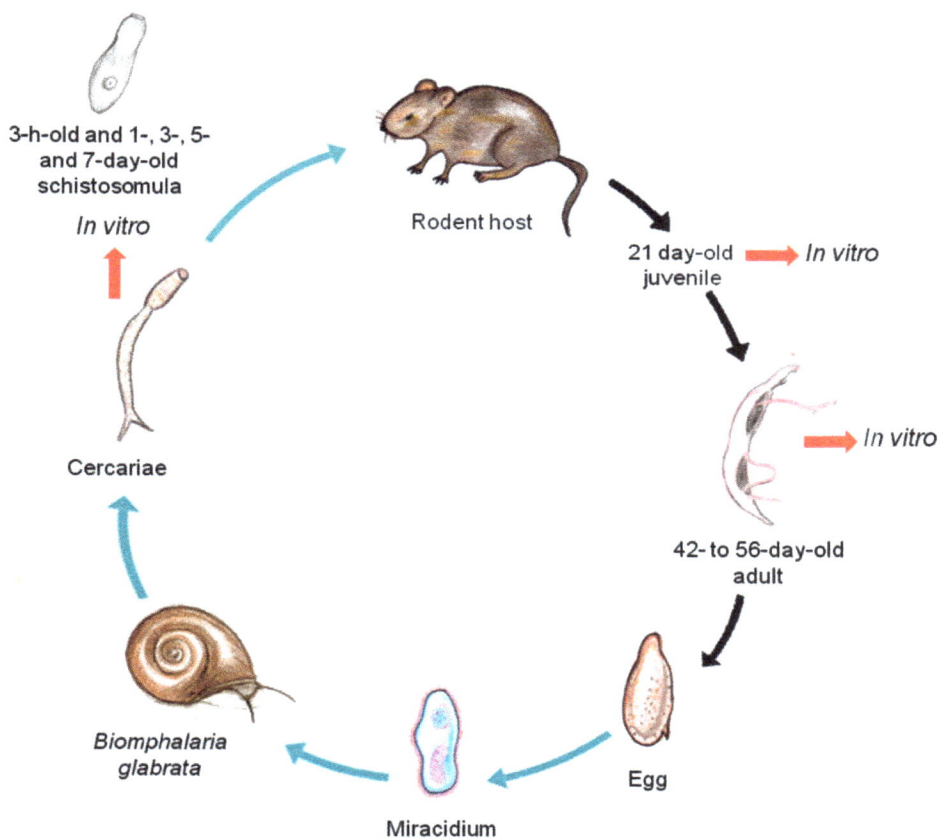

Fig. 1. Life cycle of *S. mansoni,* illustrating the collection points for *in vitro* chemotherapeutic studies. Black arrow: maturation of parasite within final host. Blue arrow: aquatic phase

4.1 Juvenile and adult schistosomes

Adult worms have been more commonly used for antischistosome drug discovery. Today, *in vitro* chemotherapeutic studies using juvenile worms are also highly recommended. For these assays, each rodent is commonly infected with either 100-150 or 400-500 cercariae. Rodents exposed to 400-500 cercariae are sacrificed 21 days after infection for juvenile recovery, while mice exposed to 100-150 cercariae are sacrificed 42 to 56 days after infection for adult recovery. Juveniles or adults are collected using a perfusion technique with Hanks' balanced salt solution (HBSS), Dulbecco's Modified Eagle's Medium (DMEM), or Roswell Memorial Park Institute (RPMI) 1640 medium, containing an anticoagulant such as heparin at a concentration range of 5-20 U/ml (Smithers & Terry, 1965). The worms are washed in RPMI 1640 medium, kept at pH 7.5 with 25 mM N-2-hydroxyethylpiperazine-N'-2-ethanesulfonic acid (HEPES) containing 200 U/ml penicillin, 200 μg/ml streptomycin, and 0.25 μg/ml amphotericin B. After washing, ten to fifteen juveniles or one pair of adult worms (male and female coupled) are transferred to each well of a 24-well culture plate containing 2 ml of the same medium supplemented with 10% bovine foetal serum and incubated at 37 °C in a humid atmosphere containing 5% CO_2. Only viable, contractile worms showing total tegument integrity as assessed by light microscopy should be included in the different investigations (Figure 2).

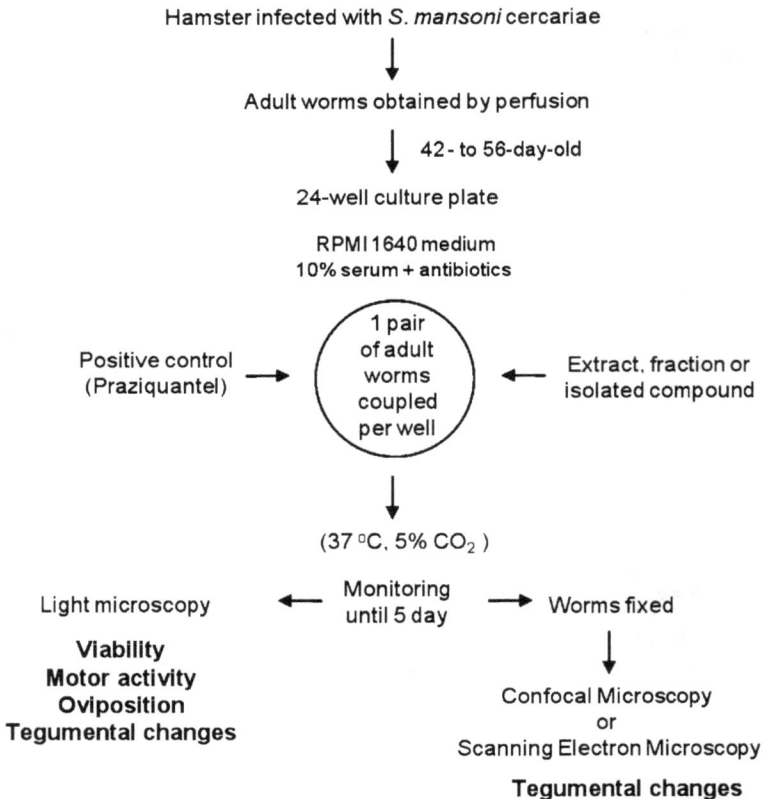

Fig. 2. *In vitro* assay models with *Schistosoma mansoni* adult worms.

4.2 Schistosomula

Obtaining sufficient quantities of schistosomula directly from skin or lung tissue for most research purposes is time consuming and involves working with mammalian hosts. These difficulties led to the development of techniques for transforming cercariae and maintaining schistosomula. In fact, schistosomula can be obtained by transforming cercariae using simple techniques, such as centrifugation, vortexing, repeated aspiration through a syringe needle, or chemical stimulation, and these schistosomula are easily maintained *in vitro* for several days (Basch, 1981). These *in vitro* strategies are advantageous because they confer uniformity in parasite maturation, which cannot be achieved *in vivo* due to the variation in the time required for individual parasites to penetrate the host skin and enter the vasculature. In addition, the use of mechanically obtained schistosomula is an alternative method that reduces, refines and replaces the use of animals in laboratory research in accordance with animal protection principles (Broadhead & Bottrill, 1997).

Among the techniques available for the production of schistosomula, the current methods most commonly used for the removal of tails from cercariae are the repeated aspiration through a syringe needle, based on Colley and Wikel (1974), and the use of a Vortex mixer, based on Ramalho-Pinto et al. (1974). In our laboratory, for example, schistosomula are mechanically transformed according to Ramalho-Pinto et al. (1974) and cultured *in vitro* in 169 medium, as described by Bash (1981). This method is recommended over the syringe-passage technique, which severely stresses and damages the parasites. In addition, the mechanical transformation procedure in a Vortex mixer is simpler than the passage of the parasites under pressure many times through a needle. Briefly, to obtain cercariae, *B. glabrata* snails infected with miracidia are exposed to incandescent light for 2 h, and then cercariae are collected, concentrated in glass conical centrifuge tubes and cooled in a ice bath for 10 minutes to reduce the motility of the worms. The ice-cold cercarial suspension is centrifuged, resuspended in RPMI 1640 medium with 25 mM HEPES, 200 UI/ml penicillin, 200 µg/ml streptomycin, and 0.25 µg/ml amphotericin B, and vortexed for 2 minutes to trigger tail loss. The resulting cercarial bodies are isolated from free tails by centrifugation through a 60% Percoll gradient (Lazdins et el., 1982) or decantation (Ramalho-Pinto et al., 1974). Microscope examination is used to assess the quantity and quality of purified schistosomula. Finally, schistosomula are cultivated in 169 medium containing antibiotics and supplemented with 10% bovine foetal serum at 37 °C in a 5% CO_2 atmosphere. Schistosomula are cultured until day 7, which corresponds to the lung-stage worm. For *in vitro* drug screening assays, schistosomula are transferred into 96-well culture microplates, with approximately 50 parasites per well, and maintained in 200 µl 169 medium under the conditions described above.

After penetrating the definitive host, significant morphological, physiological, and biochemical changes occur in the developing schistosomula (Gobert et al., 2007; Skelly & Alan Wilson, 2006). Although mechanically transformed schistosomula are different from the schistosomula that have penetrated the skin, these larval cultures have been maintained in *vitro* for different amounts of time to produce all the mammalian host stages, including skin- and lung-stage schistosomula and paired, mature adult males and females (Basch, 1981). Mechanically transformed schistosomula are now commonly used in studies of behaviour, development, metabolic activity, biochemistry, molecular biology, immunology, and in vaccine development and drug screening protocols (Abdulla et al., 2009; Gobert et al., 2007; Harrop & Wilson, 1993; Peak et al., 2010). There is evidence that mechanically transformed schistosomula are structurally similar to their lung schistosomula counterparts (Chai et al., 2006), and after 7 days in culture, the larvae have the morphological features of lung worms and are capable of maturation when introduced into the portal vein of mice (Harrop & Wilson, 1993). Furthermore, mechanically transformed schistosomula are able to develop steadily until adult worm pairing (Basch, 1981). Because of these reasons, drug-screening assays in our laboratory are based on mechanically transformed schistosomula of different ages *in vitro* (3-h-, 1-, 3-, 5- and 7-day-olds). It takes roughly 3 h for the cercariae to secrete the contents of their acetabular glands; the 1- to 7-day-olds correspond to the skin- and lung-stage schistosomula.

5. Operating procedures for antischistosomal drug screening and the techniques employed

In recent years, the search for new anthelmintics has intensified, but little significant progress has been made in developing new techniques. The *in vitro* drug screening approaches must take into account some specific concerns, particularly to be simple and inexpensive. Important methodologies can objectively and rapidly distinguish helminth viability or phenotype. *In vitro* screening could identify novel anthelmintics and could eventually translate into practical applications. Herein, a general overview is given of the most common methodologies used for screening antischistosomal compounds and their effects on the whole organism.

5.1 Compound storage and handling

To test new compounds, including synthetic or natural products and crude extracts or fractions of a natural source, it is necessary to consider factors such as solubility and stability. The compounds are usually stored in hermetically sealed glass containers, covered with aluminium foil to protect the contents from light, and kept refrigerated at 8 °C or at ambient temperature until used. The compounds are commonly dissolved in dimethyl sulfoxide (DMSO), which should not exceed a final concentration of 2% in the culture medium containing parasites. Control schistosomes are incubated in the presence of the highest concentration of solvent used.

For *in vitro* screening assays, there is not a set maximum concentration to evaluate the activity of compounds on schistosomes, as long as no toxicity occurs on mammalian cells. However, in our laboratory, *in vitro* screenings are performed at final maximum concentrations of up to 500 μg/ml for crude extracts or fractions and 1,000 μM for isolated compounds. The reference drug praziquantel is used as a positive control at final concentrations ranging from 5 to 10 μM (Figure 2).

5.2 Assessment of parasite viability

The effects of compounds on *S. mansoni* are commonly assessed by phenotypic changes. The parasites are kept for 5 days as described above, and monitored at different time points (e.g., 24, 48, 72, 96, and 120 h) to evaluate their general condition, using parameters such as motor activity, morphological changes, and mortality rate (Figure 2).

Current methods utilised to assess schistosomal viability have recently been reviewed, and most of these methods involve microscopic techniques (Keiser, 2010; Ramirez et al., 2007). The phenotypic changes are scored by using a viability scale. For example, a scale of 0 - 4, where 4= normally active, 3= slowed activity, 2= minimal activity, 1= absence of motility apart from gut movements, and 0= total absence of mobility, is based on standard procedures for compound screening at the Special Programme for Research and Training in Tropical Diseases, World Health Organization, WHO-TDR (Ramirez et al., 2007). Alternatively, as described by Manneck et al. (2010, 2011), drug activity is defined as 3= totally vital, normally active, and no morphological changes; 2= slowed activity, primary morphological changes and visible granularity; 1= minimal activity, severe morphological changes and granularity; 0= all worms dead, severe morphological changes and granularity; the granularity is characterised only for schistosomula. The regular movement of both larval and adult schistosomes has proven to be a valuable trait in assessing schistosome viability *in vitro* because lack of movement is a good indicator of death. Worm death is usually defined as no movement observed for at least 2 min of examination (Manneck et al., 2010). In this context, the viability of worm during the culture period is also assessed by motor activity reduction, and it is defined as "slight " or "significant". This subjective criterion is commonly used by several research groups (Braguine et al., 2009; de Melo et al., 2011; de Moraes et al., 2011; Magalhães et al., 2009, 2010; Moraes et al., 2011, Parreira et al., 2010; Pereira et al., 2011; Xiao et al., 2007). Size measurements of parasites are also employed to study phenotypic changes.

In addition to the phenotypic approaches, another *in vitro* drug-screening assay method is based on microcalorimetry. Manneck et al. (2011) analysed the effects of drugs on the metabolic activity of schistosomula and adult *S. mansoni* by comparing their heat flow. In this study, a multi-channel isothermal microcalorimeter equipped with 48 measuring channels was used to monitor the heat production by schistosomes as a result of their metabolism over time. The results show that microcalorimetry can be a valuable tool to study antischistosomal drugs, and the microcalorimetric measurements confirmed, in part, the results of the phenotypic evaluation. However, the level of agreement between microscopy and microcalorimetry data requires further investigation (Manneck et al., 2011). In the following section, other methods are described that are used to determine the effect of drugs on schistosomula and adult *S. mansoni*.

Phenotypic changes are determined as mentioned above. However, because of the lack of standardisation between laboratories, the replication of results obtained by microscopic means is not always possible. In an effort to avoid the subjective nature of quantifying schistosome viability from the microscopic examination of phenotype alone, further adaptations have been developed and are based on the differentiating potential of some colorimetric vital dyes. Diamidinophenylindole (DAPI) has been used as a differential stain of dead schistosomula during microscopy; in addition, the low DAPI concentration (1 µg/ml) in the medium proved not to be toxic to the schistosomula, nor did it cause any background fluorescence (Van Der Linden & Deelder, 1984). Trypan blue has also been shown to be a reliable dye for differentially staining dead schistosomula (Harrop & Wilson, 1993) and by means of a methylene blue dye exclusion test (Gold, 1997). The tetrazolium salt 3-(4,5-dimethylthiazol-2-yl)-2,5-diphenyltetrazolium bromide (MTT) is also a vital dye that has been successfully used to assess the viability of worms. The use of this assay on helminths was pioneered by Comley et al. (1989), and several nematode species have been assessed. Nare et al. (1991) used the MTT marker to evaluate the viability of adult schistosomes; currently, some *in vitro* bioassays used to study the effects of drugs have demonstrated the ability of MTT to assess the viability of adult worms (Braguine et al., 2009; de Melo et al., 2011; Magalhães et al., 2009, 2010; Parreira et al., 2010; Pereira et al., 2011).

Recently, Peak et al. (2010) validated a high-throughput system for detecting the viability of schistosomula using a microtiter plate-based method. In this study, the authors combined the use of propidium iodide with fluorescein diacetate to allow the easy assessment of the percent of viable schistosomula present in a sample. This helminth fluorescent bioassay was developed into a method of wide-scale application because it is sensitive, relevant to industrial high-throughput (384-well microtiter plate compatibility, 200 schistosomula/well) and academic (96-well microtiter plate compatibility, 1000 schistosomula/well) settings, translatable to drug screening assays, does not require a priori knowledge of schistosome biology or extensive training in parasite morphology, and is objective and quantitative.

The development of high-content screening systems is an important step for the assessment of parasite viability in a high-throughput format. A novel assay for anthelmintic drug screening by real-time monitoring of parasite motility was developed by Smout et al. (2010). This technological advance is based on the detection of changing electrical currents running through mini gold electrodes on the bottom of tissue culture plates. In this assay, the authors assessed the motility of *S. mansoni* using an xCELLigence system (Real Time Cell Assay, RTCA SP instrument), which monitors cellular events in real time without the incorporation of labels by measuring the electrical impedance across interdigitated micro-electrodes integrated on the bottom of tissue culture plates. This technology was applied to adult schistosome using one pair (one coupled male and female worm) in 200 µl per well of an E-plate, which is a 96-well plate for cell-based assays on the RTCA instruments. Because the real-time system measures changes in worm motility with the high level of precision necessary for high-throughput studies, it is widely applicable to a range of helminth species and developmental stages (Smout et al., 2010). This motility assay may provide a superior methodology to microscopy by removing the subjectivity from helminth phenotype characterisation and making available a technology that could allow the direct comparison of results from different laboratories. However, the initial cost of this RTCA system and E-plates may restrict its use, especially in an academic laboratory.

5.3 Assessment of changes in the tegument of parasites

The tegument is the major interface between the schistosome and its external environment. In addition to providing protection, the tegument is an important site of the uptake of nutrients and other molecules. Moreover, the tegument is extremely important for infection success and survival in the host, and it has been a major target for the development of antischistosomal drugs (Skelly & Wilson, 2006; Van Hellemond et al., 2006). Therefore, most of the drugs currently used against schistosome act by damaging the worm tegument (Doenhoff et al., 2008; Fenwick et al., 2003; El Ridi et al., 2010; Keiser, 2010; Manneck et al., 2010, 2011; Mostafa et al., 2011; Xiao et al., 2000).

The schistosome tegument is often approached as a drug target in schistosomiasis and is associated with the subjective assessment of parasite viability described here. The morphological alterations of the tegument of *S. mansoni* are also assessed by methods that involve microscopic analysis. Indeed, during the assay, the parasite is manipulated *in vitro*, and the effect of such manipulation is assessed by bright-field examination of the morphology of the parasite (Figure 2). The criteria used to assess morphological changes induced by a drug require visual scoring by skilled operators and is assessed subjectively. Morphological changes are usually defined qualitatively as "partial" or "extensive" (Braguine et al., 2009; de Melo et al., 2011; de Moraes et al., 2011; Magalhães et al., 2009, 2010; Moraes et al., 2011; Parreira et al., 2010; Pereira et al., 2011; Xiao et al., 2007). Therefore, the effect of anthelmintic drugs on the tegument of schistosome cannot be evaluated in a dose-dependent manner. In addition, a question remains: is the death of the parasite is associated with damage to the coat?

The inherent subjectivity of this qualitative analysis led Moraes et al. (2011) and de Moraes et al. (2011) to develop a quantitative method for evaluating the effect of drugs on the tegument of *S. mansoni* using confocal microscopy. In this quantitative analysis, areas of the tegument of male worms are assessed, and the numbers of tubercles are counted. Briefly, the parasites are fixed in Formalin-Acetic-Alcohol solution (FAA) and analysed under a confocal microscope at 488 nm (excitation) and 505 nm (emission), as described by Moraes et al. (2011) and de Moraes et al. (2011). During the microscopic analysis of the three-dimensional images captured using LSM Image Browser software (Zeiss), areas of the tegument of parasite are assessed, and the numbers of tubercles on the dorsal surface of male helminths are counted in a 20,000 μm^2 area, which is calculated using the same software image capture. Importantly, the area chosen is in the dorsal region of the male adult worm, close to the ventral sucker (acetabulum) region, because there is no significant variation in the number of tubercles in this region. Furthermore, schistosome and others trematodes are self-fluorescent (Moraes et al., 2009), and this fluorescence is increased when the parasites are in the FAA solution. This is advantageous because it allows images to be captured without using a fluorescent fluorophore. The FAA solution consists of a 2:9:30:59 mixture of acetic acid, formaldehyde, ethanol (95%) and distilled water. This methodology is summarised in Figure 3.

As previously mentioned, drug effects are currently assessed by observing morphological changes in parasites using light microscopy methods. However, these techniques do not allow the microscopic analysis of the tegument in detail. The quantitative analysis described by Moraes et al. (2011) and de Moraes (2011) must be performed with high-resolution microscopy, such as confocal or scanning electron microscopy. Therefore, the drug effects assessed by phenotypic changes, such as tegumental alterations, cannot be trusted. For example, Moraes et al. (2011) used confocal microscopy to evaluate the *in vitro* schistosomicidal activity of piplartine, an amide isolated from *Piper tuberculatum*, and demonstrated that the tegumental damage occurs after incubation with doses higher than the lethal concentrations, suggesting that worm death is caused by different mechanisms. Thus, tegumental damage may not always result in death, and a quantitative assessment technique is needed to understand the mechanisms of action of newly discovered antischistosomal drugs. In addition, the advent of screening methods that allow high-throughput, scalable, automated, and objective assays for helminth viability, combined with knowledge of the molecular biology of the schistosome to identify possible new drug targets, will make drug development for schistosomiasis easier.

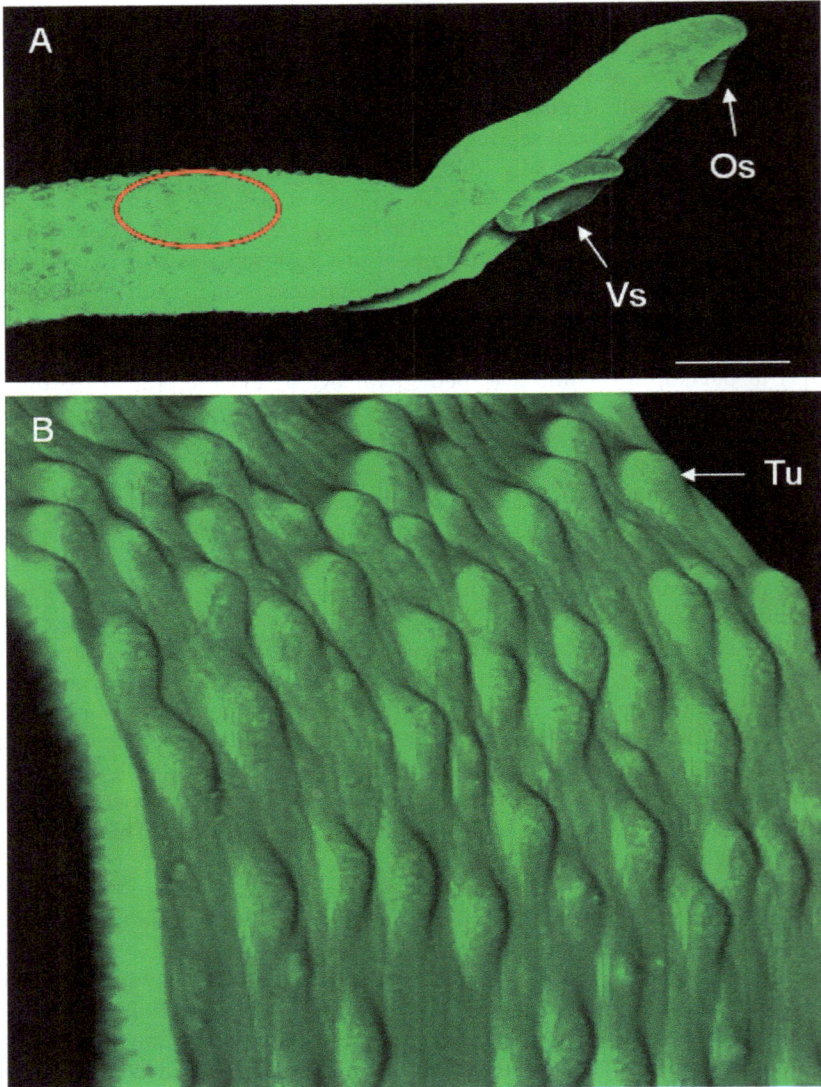

Fig. 3. Dorsal region of a *Schistosoma mansoni* adult male worm, on which the effect of antischistosomal compounds on the tegument is evaluated quantitatively. The parasite was fixed in FAA solution, and fluorescent images were obtained using a confocal microscope. A: General view of the anterior helminth region showing, in red, the location where tubercles were counted. Bar = 500 µm. B: View of an area of 20,000 µm², calculated with the Zeiss LSM Image Browser software, showing the tubercles. This image is a higher magnification of the dorsal region of the *S. mansoni* adult worm marked in red in panel A. X and Y: three-dimensional images obtained from laser scanning confocal microscopy. Os: oral sucker; Vs: ventral sucker; Tu: tubercles

5.4 In vitro assessment of the reproductive fitness of adult worms

The effects of natural or synthetic products on the reproductive fitness of *S. mansoni* have been previously reported in several studies (Braguine et al., 2009; de Moraes et al., 2011; Magalhães et al., 2009, 2010; Mohamed et al., 2005; Moraes et al., 2011; Sanderson et al., 2002). To evaluate drug effects on schistosome during *in vitro* screening drug assays, cultures are continually monitored to assess the sexual fitness of worms treated with sub-lethal concentrations of drug. In this case, the following parameters are assessed: (1) changes in the pairing, an indicator of the mating process; (2) egg production, an indicator of egg output per worm; and (3) egg development.

In the experiments, adult worm pairs (male and female coupled) are incubated in a 24-well culture plate, as previously described here, and parasites are monitored on daily basis for 5 days using an inverted microscope and a stereomicroscope (Figure 2). Therefore, it is important that, after collection by the perfusion technique, the parasites are carefully washed to prevent the separation of the worm pairs.

Schistosome egg output *in vitro* is usually determined by counting the number of eggs. Egg development can be analysed quantitatively and scored as developed or undeveloped on the basis of the presence or absence of the miracidium (de Melo et al., 2011; Magalhães et al., 2009, 2010). This is a simple and recommended method because conventional light microscopy is able to distinguish morphologic differences in eggs. However, the characterisation of the viability of immature eggs is very difficult. Alternatively, the analysis of egg viability, distinguishing live immature eggs from dead immature ones, can be performed using a fluorescent label, as described by Sarvel et al. (2006). In this assay, the eggs obtained in culture are stained with the Hoescht 33258 probe and observed with fluorescent microscopy. The authors evaluated fluorescent labels and vital dyes, aiming at differentiating live and dead eggs, and showed the only the fluorescent Hoechst 33258 can be considered a useful tool to differentiate between dead and live eggs.

5.5 Cytotoxicity assays

Finding a new compound capable of killing a parasite is not difficult. However, it is difficult to find a substance that can kill the parasite without affecting the host. Therefore, early *in vitro* studies of new compounds must include comparative cytotoxicity data from human or animal cells in tissue culture to establish that the compound has selective antischistosomal activity and may be a realistic prospect for future clinical use in humans. In our operating procedures for antischistosomal drug screening, mammalian cells are exposed to concentrations of at least two times higher than what is needed to elicit a schistosomicidal effect. Thus, the *in vitro* schistosomicidal activity of compounds cannot be associated with cytotoxic effects.

General toxicity tests can be conducted in many cell types (e.g., fibroblasts and epithelial and hepatoma cells). Peripheral blood mononuclear cells and erythrocytes are widely used in *in vitro* studies to detect cytotoxicity or cell viability following exposure to antischistosomal compounds. Vero mammalian cells (African green monkey kidney fibroblasts) are also commonly used to examine whether natural or synthetic antiparasitic compounds are tolerated by mammalian cells (da Silva Filho et al., 2009; Moraes et al., 2011; Parreira et al., 2010).

The crystal violet staining method and the neutral red and MTT assays are the most common methodologies used to detect cytotoxicity or cell viability following exposure to toxic substances. In our *in vitro* cytotoxicity assays with cultured cells, the crystal violet staining method is routinely used because it is rapid and inexpensive. This method measures the effects of compounds on cell growth through the colorimetric evaluation of fixed cells stained with crystal violet. Briefly, cells maintained in culture medium are seeded into 96-well culture microplates in the presence of different concentrations of extracts, fractions or isolated compounds. After different timepoints of incubation (e.g., 2, 24, 48, 72, and 96 h), the supernatants are removed and the remaining live cells are assessed by fixing and staining them with crystal violet (0.2% in 20% methanol). Viable cells attach to the bottom of the well plate, and the absorbance is measured by reading each well at 595 nm in a microplate reader (Moraes et al., 2011).

Neutral red is another cell viability assay often used to determine cytotoxicity following exposure to toxic substances (Borenfreund & Puerner, 1985). It has been used as an indicator of cytotoxicity in cultures of primary hepatocytes and other cell lines (Fautz et al., 1991; (Fotakis & Timbrell, 2006; Morgan et al., 1991). Living cells take up the neutral red, which is concentrated within the lysosomes of cells.

The MTT assay is also used to measure cell viability. MTT is a water-soluble tetrazolium salt, which is converted to an insoluble purple formazan upon the cleavage of the tetrazolium ring by succinate dehydrogenase within the mitochondria. The formazan product is impermeable to the cell membranes, and therefore, it accumulates in healthy cells. The MTT assay has been tested for its validity in various cell lines (Fotakis & Timbrell, 2006; Mossmann, 1983).

Alternatively, the lactate dehydrogenase (LDH) leakage assay and protein assay are also used to detect cytotoxicity, despite the fact that they have low sensitivity when compared to the methods already described. The LDH leakage assay is based on the measurement of LDH activity in the extracellular medium. The loss of intracellular LDH and its release into the culture medium is an indicator of irreversible cell death due to cell membrane damage (Decker & Lohmann-Matthes, 1988; Fotakis & Timbrell, 2006). The protein assay is an indirect measurement of cell viability because it measures the protein content of viable cells. Despite the existence of several protocols to establish total protein concentration (e.g., biuret, bicinchoninic acid, Lowry and Bradford protocols), the two most commonly used methods for protein quantification are the Lowry and Bradford assays (Bradford et al., 1976; Lowry et al., 1951).

Finally, tritiated thymidine-based methods, which act through the incorporation of tritium into the DNA of cells, have also been used currently to detect cytotoxicity, especially in immune cells (Pechhold et al., 2002).

6. Conclusions

Schistosomiasis is a neglected disease that is one of the most common chronic infections among the poorest people in the world. Most chemotherapeutic-based programs attempting to eradicate schistosomiasis in the developing world rely on the effectiveness of a single drug, praziquantel; therefore, there is an urgent need to identify new parasite targets and effective antischistosomal compounds. Secondary plant metabolites have attracted the attention of many researchers over the years as a result of the variety of their chemical structures and their broad range of biological activities that may provide lead structures for the development of new drugs. Recently, marine organisms have also been recognised as an attractive source of antiparasitic compounds, and it can be expected that other living organisms, such as insects and amphibians, will emerge as additional sources in the future.

Discovering untapped natural sources of new anthelmintic compounds remains a major challenge and a source of novelty in the era of combinatorial chemistry and genomics. To find new anthelmintics, all sources of natural, synthetic and semi-synthetic lead compounds must be investigated. *In vitro* bioassays using parasitic worms have played a central role in the early pre-clinical stages of most research on potential natural anthelmintics. The identification of the antiplasmodial and antischistosomal activity of the sesquiterpene lactone artemisinin has stimulated interest in natural products, and soon, promising leads will be identified with new chemical types and active agents against schistosomiasis. Therefore, bioprospecting programmes related to the isolation of bioactive compounds must be rewarded, and the screening *in vitro* of chemical constituents belonging to different classes must be evaluated on the blood fluke *S. mansoni*.

The literature regarding antischistosomal compounds contains a large number of natural products screened for their schistosomicidal properties. However, only a few of these may be promising drug leads in the development of a therapeutic reserve for schistosomiasis. Therefore, it is important to continue to identify new drugs and to explore alternative strategies to improve screening efficacy. Most of the extracts or natural compounds were only evaluated with *in vitro* studies; it is expected that they will be evaluated using *in vivo* experimental models. Further, it must be mentioned that the results of *in vitro* assays with many drugs do not correspond to what is observed *in vivo*; however, *in vitro* screening could identify novel anthelmintics that could eventually translate into practical applications. Thus, while *in vitro* tests are recommended initially, the assessment of therapeutic activity using *in vivo* models should be performed.

The analysis of the *S. mansoni* genome and transcriptome offers great possibilities for identifying possible new drug targets and will facilitate further exploration of differences between host and parasite metabolic pathways. In addition to the isolation and structural determination of new drugs from natural products and information from the originating plant, the integration of the pharmacological properties of natural products with the functional genomic and proteomic studies in schistosome and *in vitro* screening methods with improved automatic high-content screening will be important tools to identify possible new drugs in the future and shed light on the approaches of helminth chemotherapy. Attempting new combinations of natural or synthetic drugs will be also important in discovering alternative drugs to replace the use of praziquantel.

7. Acknowledgments

I thank Dr. Eliana Nakano and Mr. Alexsander S. Souza (Laboratório de Parasitologia, Instituto Butantan, São Paulo, SP, Brazil) for assistance with confocal microscopy. I also thank Ms. Edinéia C. Moraes for drawing the lifecycle diagram and Ms. Aline A. L. Carvalho for comments and suggestions.

8. References

Abdul-Ghani, R.A.; Loutfy, N. & Hassan, A. (2009). Myrrh and trematodoses in Egypt: an overview of safety, efficacy and effectiveness profiles. *Parasitology International*, Vol.58, pp. 210-214, ISSN 1383-5769

Abdulla, M.H.; Ruelas, D.S.; Wolff, B.; Snedecor, J.; Lim, K.C.; Xu, F.; Renslo, A.R.; Williams, J.; Mckerrow, J.H. & Caffrey, CR. (2009). Drug discovery for schistosomiasis: hit and lead compounds identified in a library of known drugs by medium-throughput phenotypic screening. *PLoS Neglected Tropical Disease*, Vol.3, pp. e478, ISSN 1935-2735

Araújo, R.V.; Melo-Júnior, M.R.; Beltrão, E.I.; Mello, L.A.; Iacomini, M.; Carneiro-Leão, A.M.; Carvalho, L.B. Jr & Santos-Magalhães, N.S. (2011). Evaluation of the antischistosomal activity of sulfated α-D-glucan from the lichen *Ramalina celastri* free and encapsulated into liposomes. *Brazilian Journal of Medical and Biological Research*, Vol.44, pp. 311-318, ISSN 0100-879X

Badria, F.; Abou Mohamed, G.; El-Mowafy, A.; Massoud, A. & Salama, O. (2001). Mirazid: a new schistosomicidal drug, *Pharmaceutical Biology*, Vol.39, pp. 127–131. ISSN 1388-0209

Baldé, A.M.; Van Marck, E.A.; Kestens, L.; Gigase, P.L. & Vlietinck, A.J. (1989). Schistosomicidal effects of *Pavetta owariensis* and *Harrisonia abyssinica* in mice infected with *Schistosoma mansoni*. *Planta Medica*, Vol.55, pp. 41-43, ISSN 0032-0943

Barth, L.R.; Fernandes, A.P.; Ribeiro-Paes, J.T. & Rodrigues, V. (1997). Effects of goyazensolide during *in vitro* cultivation of *Schistosoma mansoni*. *Memórias do Instituto Oswaldo Cruz*, Vol.92, pp. 427–429, ISSN 0074-0276

Bergquist, R.; Utzinger, J. & McManus, D.P. (2008). Trick or treat: the role of vaccines in integrated schistosomiasis control, *PLoS Neglected Tropical Disease*, Vol.2, pp. e244, ISSN 1935-2735

Basch, P.F. (1981) Cultivation of *Schistosoma mansoni in vitro*. I. Establishment of cultures from cercariae and development until pairing. *The Journal of Parasitology*, Vol.67, p. 179-185, ISSN 0022-3395

Borenfreund, E. & Puerner, J. (1985). Toxicity determined *in vitro* morphological alterations and neutral red absorption. *Toxicology letters*, Vol.24, pp. 119-124, ISSN 0378-4274

Botros, S.; Sayed, H.; El-Dusoki, H.; Sabry, H.; Rabie, I.; El-Ghannam, M.; Hassanein, M.; El-Wahab, Y.A. & Engels, D. (2005). Efficacy of mirazid in comparison with praziquantel in Egyptian *Schistosoma mansoni*-infected school children and households. *The American Journal of Tropical Medicine and Hygiene*, Vol.72, pp. 119-123, ISSN 0002-9637

Botros, S.; William, S.; Ebeid, F.; Cioli, D.; Katz, N.; Day, T.A.; Bennett, J.L. (2004). Lack of evidence for an antischistosomal activity of myrrh in experimental animals. *The American Journal of Tropical Medicine and Hygiene*, Vol.71, pp. 206-210, ISSN 0002-9637

Bradford, M.M. (1976). A rapid and sensitive method for the quantitation of microgram quantities of protein utilizing the principle of protein dye binding. *Analytical Biochemistry*, Vol.72, pp. 248–254, ISSN 0003-2697

Braguine, C.G.; Costa, E.S.; Magalhães, L.G.; Rodrigues, V.; da Silva Filho, A.A.; Bastos, J. K.; Silva, M.L.; Cunha, W.R.; Januário, A.H. & Pauletti, P.M. (2009). Schistosomicidal evaluation of *Zanthoxylum naranjillo* and its isolated compounds against *Schistosoma mansoni* adult worms. *Zeitschrift für Naturforschung. C, Journal of biosciences*, Vol.64, pp. 793-797, ISSN 0939-5075

Broadhead, C.L. & Bottrill, K. (1997). Strategies for replacing animals in biomedical research. *Molecular Medicine Today*, Vol.3, pp. 483-487, ISSN 1357-4310

Caffrey, C.R. (2007). Chemotherapy of schistosomiasis: present and future. *Current Opinion in Chemical Biology*, Vol.11, pp. 433–439, ISSN 1367-5931

Chai, M.; McManus, D.P.; McInnes, R.; Moertel, L.; Tran, M.; Loukas, A.; Jonesa, M.K. & Gobert, G.N. (2006) Transcriptome profiling of lung schistosomula,in vitro cultured schistosomula and adult *Schistosoma japonicum. Cellular and Molecular Life Sciences,* Vol.63, pp. 919-929, ISSN 1420-682X

Cioli, D. (2000). Praziquantel: is there real resistance and are there alternatives? *Current Opinion in Infectious Diseases,* Vol.13, pp. 659-663, ISSN 0951-7375

Cioli, D.; Pica-Mattoccia, L. & Archer, S. (1995). Antischistosomal drugs: past, present ... and future?. *Pharmacology & therapeutics,* Vol.68, pp. 35-85, ISSN 0163-7258

Cioli, D. (1998). Chemotherapy of schistosomiasis: an update. *Parasitology Today,* Vol.14, pp. 418-422, ISSN 0169-4758

Colley, D.G. & Wikel, S.K. (1974). *Schistosoma mansoni:* simplified method for the production of schistosomules. *Experimental Parasitology,* Vol.35, pp. 44-51, ISSN 0014-4894

Comley, J.C.W.; Rees, M.J.; Turner, C.H. & Jenkins, D.C. (1989). Colorimetric quantitation of filarial viability. *International Journal for Parasitology,* Vol.19, pp. 77–83, ISSN 0020-7519

de Melo, N.I.; Magalhaes, L.G.; de Carvalho, C.E.; Wakabayashi, K.A.; de P Aguiar, G.; Ramos, R.C.; Mantovani, A.L.; Turatti, I.C.; Rodrigues, V.; Groppo, M.; Cunha, W.R.; Veneziani, R.C. & Crotti. A.E. (2011). Schistosomicidal activity of the essential oil of *Ageratum conyzoides* L. (Asteraceae) against adult *Schistosoma mansoni* worms. *Molecules,* Vol.16, pp. 762-773, ISSN 1420-3049

de Moraes, J.; Nascimento, C.; Miura, L.M.; Leite, J.R. ; Nakano, E. & Kawano, T. (2011). Evaluation of the *in vitro* activity of dermaseptin 01, a cationic antimicrobial peptide, against *Schistosoma mansoni. Chemistry & Biodiversity,* Vol.8, pp. 548-558, ISSN 1612-1872

da Silva Filho, A.A.; Resende, D.O.; Fukui, M.J.; Santos, F.F.; Pauletti, P.M.; Cunha, W.R.; Silva, M.L.; Gregório, L.E.; Bastos, J.K. & Nanayakkara, N.P. (2009). *In vitro* antileishmanial, antiplasmodial and cytotoxic activities of phenolics and triterpenoids from *Baccharis dracunculifolia* D. C. (Asteraceae). *Fitoterapia,* Vol.80, pp. 478–482, ISSN 0367-326X

Decker, T.; Lohmann-Matthes, M.L. (1988). A quick and simple method for the quantitation of lactate dehydrogenase release in measurements of cellular cytotoxicity and tumor necrosis factor (TNF) activity. *Journal of Immunological Methods,* Vol.115, pp.61-69, ISSN 0022-1759

Doenhoff, M.; Cioli, D. & Utzinger, J. (2008). Praziquantel: mechanisms of action, resistance and new derivatives for schistosomiasis. *Current Opinion in Infectious Diseases,* Vol.21, pp. 659–667, ISSN 0951-7375

El-Ansary, A.K. Ahmed, S.A. & Aly, S.A. (2007). Antischistosomal and liver protective effects of *Curcuma longa* extract in *Schistosoma mansoni* infected mice. *Indian Journal of Experimental Biology,* Vol.45, pp. 791–801, ISSN 0019-5189

El-Banhawey, M.A.; Ashry, M.A.; El-Ansary, A.K. & Aly, S.A. (2007). Effect of *Curcuma longa* or praziquantel on *Schistosoma mansoni* infected mice liver — histological and histochemical study. *Indian Journal of Experimental Biology,* Vol.45, pp. 877–889 ISSN 0019-5189

El Ridi, R.; Aboueldahab, M.; Tallima, H.; Salah, M.; Mahana, N.; Fawzi, S.; Mohamed, S.H.; Fahmy, O.M. (2010). *In vitro* and *in vivo* activities of arachidonic acid against *Schistosoma mansoni* and *Schistosoma haematobium. Antimicrobial Agents and Chemotherapy,* Vol.54, pp. 3383-3389, ISSN 0066-4804

El Shenawy, N.S.; Soliman, M.F. & Reyad, S.I. (2008). The effect of antioxidant properties of aqueous garlic extract and *Nigella sativa* as antischistosomiasis agents in mice. *Revista do Instituto de Medicina Tropical de São Paulo*, Vol.50, pp. 29-36 ISSN 0036-4665

Fautz, R.; Husein, B. & Hechenberger, C. (1991). Application of the neutral red assay (NR assay) to monolayer cultures of primary hepatocytes: rapid colorimetric viability determination for the unscheduled DNA synthesis test (UDS). *Mutation Research*, Vol.253, pp. 173-179, ISSN 0027-5107

Fenwick, A.; Savioli, L.; Engels, D.; Robert Bergquist, N. & Todd, M.H. (2003). Drugs for the control of parasitic diseases: current status and development in schistosomiasis. *Trends in Parasitology*, Vol.19, pp.509-515, ISSN 1471-4922

Fenwick, A. & Webster, J.P. (2006). Schistosomiasis: challenges for control, treatment and drug resistance. *Current Opinion in Infectious Diseases*, Vol.19, pp. 577–582, ISSN 0951-7375

Ferreira, J.F.; Peaden, P. & Keiser, J. (2011). *In vitro* trematocidal effects of crude alcoholic extracts of *Artemisia annua*, *A. absinthium*, *Asimina triloba*, and *Fumaria officinalis*: Trematocidal plant alcoholic extracts. *Parasitology Research*, ISSN 0932-0113, doi: 10.1007/s00436-011-2418-0

Fotakis, G. & Timbrell, J.A. (2006). *In vitro* cytotoxicity assays: comparison of LDH, neutral red, MTT and protein assay in hepatoma cell lines following exposure to cadmium chloride. *Toxicology Letters*, Vol.160, pp. 171-177, ISSN 0378-4274

Gobert, G.N.; Chai, M. & McManus, D.P. (2007). Biology of the schistosome lung-stage schistosomulum. *Parasitology*, Vol.134, pp. 453-460, ISSN 0031-1820

Gold, D. (1997). Assessment of the viability of *Schistosoma mansoni* schistosomula by comparative uptake of various vital dyes. *Parasitology Research*, Vol.83, pp. 163-169, ISSN 0932-0113

Golenser, J.; Waknine, J.H.; Krugliak, M.; Hunt, N.H. & Grau, G.E (2006). Current perspectives on the mechanism of action of artemisinins. *International Journal for Parasitology*, Vol.36, pp. 1427-1441, ISSN 0020-7519

Gryseels, B.; Polman, K.; Clerinx, J. & Kestens, L. (2006). Human schistosomiasis. *Lancet*, Vol.368, pp. 1106–1118, ISSN 0140-6736

Hagan, P.; Appleton, C.C.; Coles, G.C.; Kusel, J.R. & Tchuem-Tchuenté, L.A. (2004). Schistosomiasis control: keep taking the tablets. *Trends in Parasitology*, Vol.20, pp. 92–97, ISSN 1471-4922

Harrop, R. & Wilson, R.A. (1993). Protein synthesis and release by cultured schistosomula of *Schistosoma mansoni*. *Parasitology*, Vol.107, pp. 265-274, ISSN 0031-1820

Jaramillo, M.A. & Manos, P.S. (2001). Phylogeny and patterns of floral diversity in the genus *Piper* (Piperaceae). *American Journal of Botany*, Vol.88, pp. 706–716, ISSN 0002-9122

Jatsa, H.B.; Ngo Sock, E.T.; Tchuem Tchuente, L.A. & Kamtchouing, P. (2009). Evaluation of the *in vivo* activity of different concentrations of *Clerodendrum umbellatum* Poir against *Schistosoma mansoni* infection in mice. *African Journal of Traditional, Complementary, and Alternative Medicines*, Vol.6, pp. 216-221, ISSN 0189-6016

Kato, M.J. & Furlan, M. (2007). Chemistry and evolution of the Piperaceae. *Pure and Applied Chemistry*, Vol.79, pp. 529–538, ISSN 0033-4545

Kayser, O.; Kiderlen, A.F.; Croft, S.L. (2003). Natural products as antiparasitic drugs. Parasitology Research, Vol.90 (Suppl 2), pp. S55-S62, ISSN 0932-0113

Keiser, J. (2010). *In vitro* and *in vivo* trematode models for chemotherapeutic studies. *Parasitology*, Vol.137, pp. 589-603, ISSN 0031-1820

Keiser, J. & Utzinger, J. (2007). Advances in the discovery and development of trematocidal drugs. *Expert Opinion on Drug Discovery*, Vol.2 (Suppl 1), pp. S9–23, ISSN 1746-0441

Lazdins, J.K.; Stein, M.J.; David, J.R. & Sher, A. (1982). *Schistosoma mansoni*: rapid isolation and purification of schistosomula of different developmental stages by centrifugation on discontinuous density gradients of Percoll. *Experimental Parasitology*, Vol.53, pp. 39-44, ISSN 0014-4894

Lee, S. (2007). Artemisinin, promising lead natural product for various drug developments. *Mini Reviews in Medicinal Chemistry*, Vol.7, pp. 411-422, ISSN 1389-5575

Leite, J.R.S.A.; Miura, L.M.C.V.; Lima, D.F. Carneiro, S.M.P.; Carvalho, F.A.A.; Moraes, J. & Batista, M.C.S. (2011). Processo de obtenção da epiisopiloturina e sua aplicação no combate à infecções parasitárias. PI 0904110-9 A2 *Revista de Propriedade Industrial, Instituto Nacional de Prodiedade Industrial*, No 2108, pp. 132

Lima, C.M. ; Freitas, F.I.; Morais, L.C.; Cavalcanti, M.G.; Silva, L.F.; Padilha, R.J.; Barbosa C.G.; Santos, F.A.; Alves, L.C. & Diniz, M.D. (2011). Ultrastructural study on the morphological changes to male worms of *Schistosoma mansoni* after *in vitro* exposure to allicin. *Revista da Sociedade Brasileira de Medicina Tropical*, ISSN 0037-8682, doi: 10.1590/S0037-86822011005000023

Lowry, O.H.; Rosebrough, N.J.; Farr, A.L. & Randall, R.J. (1951). Protein measurement with the Folin phenol reagent. *The Journal of Biological Chemistry*, Vol.193, pp. 265-275, ISSN 0021-9258

Lyddiard, J.R.; Whitfield, P.J. & Bartlett, A. (2002). Antischistosomal bioactivity of isoflavonoids from *Millettia thonningii* (Leguminosae). *The Journal of Parasitology*, Vol.88, pp. 163-170. ISSN 0022-3395

Magalhães, L.G.; Kapadia, G.J.; da Silva Tonuci, L.R.; Caixeta, S.C.; Parreira, N.A.; Rodrigues, V. & Da Silva Filho (2010). *In vitro* schistosomicidal effects of some phloroglucinol derivatives from *Dryopteris* species against *Schistosoma mansoni* adult worms. *Parasitology Research*, Vol.106, pp. 395-401, ISSN 0932-0113

Magalhães, L.G.; Machado, C.B.; Morais, E.R.; Moreira, E.B.; Soares, C.S.; da Silva, S.H.; Da Silva Filho, A.A.; Rodrigues, V. (2009). *In vitro* schistosomicidal activity of curcumin against *Schistosoma mansoni* adult worms. *Parasitology Research*, Vol. 104, pp. 1197-1201, ISSN 0932-0113

Mahmoud, M.R.; El-Abhar, H.S. & Saleh, S. (2002). The effect of *Nigella sativa* oil against the liver damage induced by *Schistosoma mansoni* infection in mice. *Journal of Ethnopharmacology*, Vol.79, pp. 1-11, ISSN 0378-8741

Manneck, T.; Haggenmüller, Y. & Keiser, J. (2010). Morphological effects and tegumental alterations induced by mefloquine on schistosomula and adult. *Parasitology*, Vol.137, pp. 85-98, ISSN 0031-1820

Manneck, T.; Braissant, O.; Ellis, W. & Keiser J. (2011). *Schistosoma mansoni*: antischistosomal activity of the four optical isomers and the two racemates of mefloquine on schistosomula and adult worms *in vitro* and *in vivo*. *Experimental Parasitology*, Vol.127, pp. 260-269, ISSN 0014-4894

Mohamed, A.M.; Metwally, N.M.; Mahmoud, S.S. (2005). Sativa seeds against *Schistosoma mansoni* different stages, *Memórias do Instituto Oswaldo Cruz*, Vol.100, pp. 205-211, ISSN 0074-0276

Mølgaard,P.; Nielsen, S.B.; Rasmussen, D.E.; Drummond, R.B.; Makaza, N.; & Andreassen, J. (2001). Anthelmintic screening of Zimbabwean plants traditionally used against schistosomiasis. *Journal of Ethnopharmacology*, Vol. 74, pp. 257-264, ISSN 0378-8741

Moraes, J.; Nascimento, C.; Lopes, P.O.; Nakano, E.; Yamaguchi, L.F.; Kato, M.J. & Kawano T. (2011). *Schistosoma mansoni: In vitro* schistosomicidal activity of piplartine. *Experimental Parasitology*, Vol.127, pp. 357-364, ISSN 0014-4894

Moraes, J.; Silva, M.P.; Ohlweiler, F.P. & Kawano, T (2009). *Schistosoma mansoni* and other larval trematodes in *Biomphalaria tenagophila* (Planorbidae) from Guarulhos, São Paulo State, Brazil. *Revista do Instituto de Medicina Tropical de São Paulo*, Vol.51, pp. 77-82, ISSN 0036-4665

Morgan, D.C.; Mills, C.K.; Lefkowitz, L.D. & Lefkowitz, S.S. (1991). An improved colorimetric assay for tumor necrosis factor using WEHI 164 cells cultured on novel microtiter plates. *Journal of Immunological Methods*. Vol.145, pp. 259-262, ISSN 0022-1759

Mossmann, T. (1983). Rapid colorimetric assay for cellular growth and survival: application to proliferation and cytotoxicity assays. *Journal of Immunological Methods*. Vol.65, pp. 55-63, ISSN 0022-1759

Mostafa, O.M.; Eid, R.A. & Adly, M.A. (2011). Antischistosomal activity of ginger (*Zingiber officinale*) against *Schistosoma mansoni* harbored in C57 mice. Parasitology Research, ISSN 0932-0113 doi 10.1007/s00436-011-2267-x

Nare, B.; Smith, J.M. & Prichard, R.K. (1991). Differential effects of oltipraz and its oxy-analogue on the viability of *Schistosoma mansoni* and the activity of glutathione S-transferase. *Biochemical Pharmacology*, Vol.42, pp. 1287-1292, ISSN 0006-2952

Ndamba, J.; Nyazema, N.; Makaza, N.; Anderson, C. & Kaondera, K.C (1994). Traditional herbal remedies used for the treatment of urinary schistosomiasis in Zimbabwe. *Journal of Ethnopharmacology*, Vol.42, pp. 125-132, ISSN 0378-8741

Newman, D.J. & Cragg, G.M. (2007). Natural products as sources of new drugs over the last 25 years *Journal of Natural Products*, Vol.70, pp. 461-477, ISSN 0163-3864

Newman, D.J.; Cragg, G.M. & Snader, K.M. (2003). Natural products as sources of new drugs over the period 1981-2002. *Journal of Natural Products*, Vol.66, pp. 1022-1037, ISSN 0163-3864

Ogboli, A. (2000) Medicinal application of *Vernonia amygdalina* del leaf extracts in the treatment of schistosomiasis in mice. *Nigerian Journal of Natural Products and Medicine*, Vol.4, pp. 73-75, ISSN 1118-6267

Parmar, V.S.; Jain, S.C.; Bisht, K.S.; Jain, R.; Taneja, P.; Jha, A.; Tyagi, O.M.; Prasad, A.K.; Wengel, J.; Olsen, C.E. & Boll, P.M. (1997). Phytochemistry of the genus *Piper*. *Phytochemistry*, Vol.46, pp. 597-673, ISSN 0031-9422

Parreira, N.A.; Magalhães, L.G.; Morais, D.R.; Caixeta, S.C.; de Sousa, J.P.; Bastos, J.K.; Cunha, W.R.; Silva, M.L.; Nanayakkara, N.P.; Rodrigues, V. & da Silva Filho A.A. (2010). Antiprotozoal, schistosomicidal, and antimicrobial activities of the essential oil from the leaves of *Baccharis dracunculifolia*. *Chemistry & Biodiversity*, Vol.7, pp. 993-1001, ISSN 1612-1872

Pereira, A.C.; Magalhães, L.G.; Gonçalves, U.O.; Luz, P.P.; Moraes. A.C.; Rodrigues, V.; da Matta Guedes, P.M.; da Silva Filho, A.A.; Cunha, W.R.; Bastos, J.K.; Nanayakkara, N.P. & E Silva, M.L. (2011). Schistosomicidal and trypanocidal structure-activity relationships for (±)-licarin A and its (-)- and (+)-enantiomers. *Phytochemistry*, Vol.72, pp. 1424-1430, ISSN 0031-9422

Peak, E. Chalmers, I.W. & Hoffmann, K.F. (2010). Development and validation of a quantitative, high-throughput, fluorescent-based bioassay to detect schistosoma viability, *PLoS Neglected Tropical Disease*, Vol.4, pp. e759, ISSN 1935-2735

Pechhold, K.; Craighead, N.; Wesch, D. & Kabelitz, D. (2002). Measurement of cellular proliferation. *Methods in Microbiology*, Vol.32, pp. 77-97, ISSN 0580-9517

Prasad, A. K.; Kumar, V.; Arya, P.; Kumar, S.; Dabur, R.; Singh, N.; Chhillar, A. K.; Sharma, G.; Ghosh, B.; Wengel, J.; Olsen, C. E. & Parmar, V. S. (2005). Investigations toward new lead compounds from medicinally important plants. *Pure and Applied Chemistry*, Vol.77, pp. 25-40, ISSN 0033-4545

Ramalho-Pinto, F.J.; Gazzinelli, G.; Howells, R.E.; Mota-Santos, T.A.; Figueiredo, E.A. & Pellegrino, J. (1974). *Schistosoma mansoni*: defined system for stepwise transformation of cercaria to schistosomule *in vitro*. *Experimental Parasitology*, Vol.36, pp. 360-372, ISSN 0014-4894

Ramirez, B.; Bickle, Q.; Yousif, F.; Fakorede, F.; Mouries, M.A. & Nwaka, S (2007). Schistosomes: Challenges in compound screening. *Expert Opinion on Drug Discovery*, Vol.2, pp. 53-61, ISSN 1746-0441

Reich, M.R. & Fenwick, A. (2001). *Schistosoma haematobium*. *The New England Journal of Medicine*, Vol.344, pp. 1170, ISSN 0028-4793

Riad, N.H.; Fares, N.H.; Mostafa, O.M.; Mahmoud, Y.I. (2007). The effect of garlic on some parasitological parameters and on hepatic tissues reaction in experimental schistosomiasis mansoni. *Journal of Applied Sciences Research*, Vol.3, pp. 949-960, ISSN 1819-544X

Ribeiro-dos-Santos. G.; Verjovski-Almeida, S. & Leite, L.C. (2006). Schistosomiasis – a century searching for chemotherapeutic drugs. *Parasitology Research*, Vol.99, pp. 505-521, ISSN 0932-0113

Sanderson, L.; Bartlett, A. & Whitfield, P.J. (2002). *In vitro* and *in vivo* studies on the bioactivity of a ginger (*Zingiber officinale*) extract towards adult schistosomes and their egg production. *Journal of Helminthology*, Vol.76, pp. 241–247, ISSN 0022-149X

Sarvel, A.K.; Kusel, J.R.; Araujo, N.; Coelho, P.M.Z. & Katz, N. (2006). Comparison between morphological and staining characteristics of live and dead eggs of *Schistosoma mansoni*. *Memórias do Instituto Oswaldo Cruz*, Vol.101, Suppl. I, pp. 289-292, ISSN 0074-0276

Sheir, Z.; Nasr, A.A.; Massoud, A.; Salama, O.; Badra, G.A.; El-Shennawy, H.; Hassan, N. & Hammad, S.M. (2001). A safe, effective, herbal antischistosomal therapy derived from myrrh. *The American Journal of Tropical Medicine and Hygiene*, Vol.65, pp. 700-704, ISSN 0002-9637

Skelly, P.J. & Alan Wilson, R. (2006). Making sense of the schistosome surface, *Advances in Parasitology*, Vol.63, pp. 185-284, ISSN 0065-308X

Smithers, S.R. & Terry, R.J. (1965). The infection of laboratory hosts with cercariae of *Schistosoma mansoni* and the recovery of adults worms. *Parasitology*, Vol.55, pp. 695-700, ISSN 0031-1820

Smout, M.J.; Kotze, A.C.; McCarthy, J.S. & Loukas, A. (2010). A novel high throughput assay for anthelmintic drug screening and resistance diagnosis by real-time monitoring of parasite motility. *PLoS Neglected Tropical Disease*, Vol.4, pp. e885, ISSN 1935-2735

Steinmann, P.; Keiser, J.; Bos, R.; Tanner, M. & Utzinger, J. (2006). Schistosomiasis and water resources development: systematic review, meta-analysis, and estimates of people at risk. *The Lancet Infectious Diseases*, Vol.6, pp. 411–425, ISSN 1473-3099

Tagboto, S. & Townson, S. (2001). Antiparasitic properties of medicinal plants and other naturally occurring products. *Advances in Parasitology*, Vol.50, pp. 199-295, ISSN 0065-308X

Utzinger, J.; Keiser, J.; Shuhua, X.; Tanner, M. & Singer, B.H. (2003). Combination chemotherapy of schistosomiasis in laboratory studies and clinical trials. *Antimicrobial Agents and Chemotherapy*, Vol.47, pp. 1487-1495, ISSN 0066-4804

Utzinger, J.; Xiao, S. N'Goran, E.K.; Bergquist, R. & Tanner, M (2001). The potential of artemether for the control of schistosomiasis. *International Journal for Parasitology*, Vol.31, pp. 1549-1562, ISSN 0020-7519

Utzinger J, Xiao, S.H.; Tanner, M. & Keiser, J. (2007). Artemisinins for schistosomiasis and beyond. *Current Opinion in Investigational Drugs*, Vol.8, pp. 105-116, ISSN 1472-4472

Van der Linden, P.W. & Deelder, A.M. (1984). *Schistosoma mansoni*: a diamidinophenylindole probe for *in vitro* death of schistosomula. *Experimental Parasitology*, Vol.57, pp.125-131, ISSN 0014-4894

van der Werf, M.J.; de Vlas, S.J.; Brooker, S.; Looman, C.W.; Nagelkerke, N.J.; Habbema, J.D. & Engels, D. (2003). Quantification of clinical morbidity associated with schistosome infection in sub-Saharan Africa. *Acta Tropica*, Vol.86, pp. 125-139, ISSN 0001-706X

Van Hellemon, J.J.; Retra, K.; Brouwers, J.F.; van Balkom, B.W.; Yazdanbakhsh, M.; Shoemaker, C.B. & Tielens, A.G. (2006). Functions of the tegument of schistosomes: clues from the proteome and lipidome. *International Journal for Parasitology*, Vol.36, pp. 691-699, ISSN 0014-4894

Xiao, S.; Tanner, M.; N'Goran, E.K.; Utzinger, J.; Chollet, J.; Bergquist, R.; Chen, M. & Zheng, J. (2002). Recent investigations of artemether, a novel agent for the prevention of schistosomiasis japonica, mansoni and haematobia. *Acta Tropica*, Vol.82, pp. 175-181, ISSN 0001-706X

Xiao, S.H.; Keiser, J.; Chollet, J.; Utzinger, J.; Dong, Y.; Endriss, Y.; Vennerstrom, J.L. & Tanner, M. (2007). *In vitro* and *in vivo* activities of synthetic trioxolanes against major human schistosome species. *Antimicrobial Agents and Chemotherapy*, Vol.51, pp. 1440–1445 ISSN 0066-4804

Xiao, S.H.; Binggui, S.; Chollet, J. & Tanner, M. (2000). Tegumental changes in 21-day-old *Schistosoma mansoni* harboured in mice treated with artemether. *Acta Tropica*, Vol.75, pp. 341–348, ISSN 0001-706X

Yousif, F.; Hifnawy, M.S.; Soliman, G.; Boulos, L.; Labib, T.; Mahmoud, S.; Ramzy, F.; Yousif M.; Hassan, I.; Mahmoud, K.; El-Hallouty, S.M.; El-Gendy, M.; Gohar, L.; El-Manawaty, M.; Fayyad, W. & El-Menshawi, B.S. (2007). Large-scale *in vitro* screening of Egyptian native and cultivated plants for schistosomicidal activity. *Pharmaceutical Biology*, Vol. 45, pp. 501–510, ISSN 1388-0209

11

A Programme to Control Taeniosis-Cysticercolsis (*Taenia solium*) in Mexico

Aline S. de Aluja[1], Julio Morales Soto[2] and Edda Sciutto[3]

[1]*Departamento de Patología, Facultad de Medicina Veterinaria y Zootecnia,*
Universidad Nacional Autónoma de México, Ciudad Universitaria, D. F.,
[2]*Lab. MVZ. Aline S. de Aluja, Facultad de Medicina Veterinaria y Zootecnia,*
Universidad Nacional Autónoma de México, Ciudad Universitaria, D. F.
[3]*Lab. de Inmunología, Instituto de Investigaciones Biomédicas,*
Universidad Nacional Autónoma de México, Ciudad Universitaria, D. F.
Mexico

1. Introduction

Taenia solium cysticercosis is a zoonosis which affects animals, mainly pigs, and human beings.

In pigs the cysticerci are found both in muscles and in the brain, in human beings predominantly in the form of neurocysticercosis (Escobar,1983; Fleury et al., 2003, 2006, 2010) but muscular, subcutaneous and ocular forms have also been reported. (Larralde & Aluja, 2006)

The disease is found mainly in countries where poverty prevails, hygiene is lacking and people live in close contact with pigs.

In Mexico the disease is present in marginated rural areas of the southern states, (Guerrero, Oaxaca, Puebla, Veracruz, Tabasco, Yucatan, parts of Morelos and others) where the above mentioned conditions exist and the parasite encounters a favorable environment for its survival. Many of the inhabitants of these areas are extremely poor, their dwellings are made of reed, wood or other cheap materials available in their region. Their number is calculated to be 47,190,000 million (INEGI 2009; CEPAL 2010). Few hamlets or villages have piped water and get their supply from wells that may dry up during the hot season or from ponds where rain water accumulates. Donkeys frequently bring water to isolated dwellings in 20 liter containers of which they carry four. There are villages where water is rationed during the very dry months and people get one bucket per day.

Roads are rarely paved, and many become impassable during the rainy season. Children often have to walk long distances to get to school and depending on the weather and road conditions do not go, some barely learn how to read and write. In many of these remote areas the inhabitants speak their indigenous languages, have difficulties understanding Spanish, and an interpreter is needed to communicate with them.

People usually own a few animals and some land, where they grow corn, the harvest being barely enough to feed their family. Their animals, a few cattle, pigs and chicken receive very little care, and in particular the pigs roam about freely searching for food (Copado et al, 2004).

Some peasants keep their pigs confined, tying them to a tree or in primitive enclosures during the time when the corn grows.

In some of the bigger villages, health centers may be found, where people get rudimentary medical care but in the smaller ones where none is available, they mostly rely on their ancestral remedies, among them herbs and medicinal plants.

Hygiene is understandably one of the big problems for people who live under these conditions of extreme poverty and scarcity of water. Toilets do not exist in many villages and hamlets and people defecate in the open. The health authorities have made efforts to improve hygiene and have introduced latrines, but this has not been accompanied by the necessary control and follow up interventions, with the result that they are not used and are transformed into store rooms, or are built on inadequate grounds and spill over with the torrential rains.

The pigs, being copropaghes, roaming about freely in villages and fields to find their food, and receiving very little attention from their owners, ingest the human feces, which constitute an important addition to their diet (Aluja et al. 1987; Acevedo, 1989; Aluja & Villalobos, 2000; Copado et al., 2004). If the owner keeps his pigs confined in yards next to his dwellings, the animals may have direct access to the outlet of a latrine and consume the feces. If the feces come from a *Taenia solium* carrier, the pig becomes infected and develops cysticerci in its tissues, predominantly skeletal muscles and brain. Occasionally people also ingest eggs which may come from contaminated food or by way of autoinfection if they themselves are the *T. solium* carrier, in which case they develop cysticercosis, mostly in the form of neurocysticercosis. (Escobar 1983; Villagran & Olvera, 1988; Larralde &Aluja, 2006, Aluja 2008)

If human beings eat insufficiently cooked meat of a pig with cysticerci they develop *Taenia solium* in their intestine. (Quiroz 2002; Larralde & Aluja 2006)

Another problem and the reason for the continuation of the Taeniosis-cysticercosis cycle in these remote areas, is that slaughter houses where meat inspection is carried out do not exist. There may be places where animals for meat are being killed, but the methods and the hygiene are unacceptable and meat is not inspected. Animals are mostly slaughtered by their owners for family or other festivities and are consumed without any inspection.

The prerequisites for the continuation of the *Taenia solium* cycle thus are:
-    People who live in conditions of poverty,
-    Lack of toilets or latrines,
-    Scarcity of water,
-    Lack of education,
-    Rambling pigs.
-    Taenia solium carriers.
-    Absence of meat inspection.

These conditions still can be found in many of the developing countries, among them Mexico. (Molinari et al, 1983; Sarti et al. 1988; 1992; Larralde et al 1992; Martinez et al. 1997; Aluja et al 1998; Morales et al. 2006; 2008)

The Ministries of Health and Agriculture in Mexico issue monthly reports with information on the diseases in human beings and animals that are diagnosed in the country. Cysticercosis in pigs and human beings and taeniosis in people are nowadays rarely reported, which has led to the believe that they are practically extinct in the country (Flisser et al. 2010). The explanation for this is that, as has been described, because of the absence of medical and veterinary personal in the areas where it occurs, it is not notified. Pigs are not

slaughtered in official establishments, and health care for the inhabitants does either not exist or is rudimentary with the result that neither enters the official surveillance system.
Nine million four hundred thousand of the total pig population (15´107,785 (SIAP-SAGARPA, 2009; Rodriguez Licea & del Moral Barrera, 2010) in México belong to highly technified and controlled farms where *Taenia solium* carriers and cysticercosis are not found. The meat of these animals proceeds from strictly controlled federal slaughterhouses and cases of pig cysticercosis are almost never seen. These are the animals that enter the official statistics. The rest, 5´600,000 pigs belong to semitechnified farms and to the free roaming group, the latter being estimated around 3´000,000 pigs. (Rodriguez Licea & del Moral Barrera 2010).
By doing serological tests (ELISA) both in humans and in pigs, it was found that the prevalence of positive reactors is rather high in those states of Mexico where the above conditions are found, both in human beings (Larralde et al. 1992) and in pigs (Sosa, 2010; Sciutto [in process]).
Tongue inspection of rural pigs confirm the presence of cysticercosis in marginated areas. In a remote region of the state of Morelos, the prevalence of porcine cysticercosis ranges between 4 and 33%.(Morales et al. 2002). In the state of Guerrero it has also been shown in some villages that the frequency is high (Molinari et al.1983; Keilbach et al., 1989; Martinez et al. 1997; 2000) and in recent unpublished data it was found to range between 0 and 13,5%.
Official data on the frequencies of neurocysticercosis and teniosis in human beings in the country have not been published. As has been pointed out, methods to diagnose cysticercosis in the population are not available in isolated regions. During conversations with people in villages, one may hear of a relative who gets epileptic fits or another one who suffers from intense headaches, both among the symptoms of neurocisticercosis (Ortiz et al. 2006). However, in the absence of diagnostic tools and in view of the fact that the financial means to travel to the city are lacking, these cases remain undiagnosed. In a recent study Fleury, using computerized tomography found that in a rural community of the state of Morelos the frequency of neurocysticercosis was 9,6% (Fleury et al. 2006) and the same author reports that in hospitalized patients in a neurological institution it has remained unchanged during the last 10 years (Fleury et al. 2010).
Evaluating all these factors, a group of Veterinarians, Immunologists and Neurologists of the National Autonomous University of Mexico (UNAM) and of the Institute of Neurology of the Ministry of Health considered that, *T. solium* teniosis-cysticercosis, still being an important disease in parts of Mexico, a programme to control it is needed. One of the reasons that justifies this is that neurocysticercosis is being reported again in the United States of America (USA) and that most cases are traced back to Mexican or other Latin American immigrants (Sorvillo et al. 2007; 2011).
Isolated interventions to control the zoonosis have been carried out in Mexico and elsewhere, but to our knowledge none of them considered follow up activities (Sanchez et al. 1999; Keilbach et al. 1989; Sarti et al. 1997; Boa et al. 2003; Eddi et al. 2003; Engels et al. 2003; Martinez et al. 2003; Pawlowski et al. 2005).
Among the methods to control teniosis-cysticercosis, several strategies have been proposed, like improving infrastructure for sanitation, confinement of pigs, the obligatory installation of latrines, regular antihelmintic treatment of the population, treatment with albendazol of infected pigs, obligatory meat inspection, health education and quite sophisticated measures like meat irradiation (Larralde & Aluja, 2006; Flores et al. 2006).

Most of these proposals cannot be introduced on a short term basis under the conditions that still prevail in those areas where the disease exists. The health authorities offer antihelminthic treatment to adults and children, however the doses they prescribe may not suffice to eliminate taeniae. The suggestion to treat infected pigs is not practical, as it is not possible to inspect all free roaming animals to find the ones with cysticerci and besides, owners would have to wait at least 3 to 4 months before they can sell them for slaughter, in order to eliminate the remnants of the larvae from the muscles.

Integrated into our control programme we decided to use vaccination of pigs.

Vaccines against cysticercosis, both pig, cattle and sheep have been employed in other countries and in México (Johnson et al. 1989; Plancarte et al. 1999; Huerta et al. 2001; Flisser et al. 2004; Sciutto et al. 2007; Harrison et al. 2005; Gonzalez et al. 2005; Assana et al. 2010). The vaccine S3Pvac that we use in our control programme is produced in the Institute for Biomedical Research of UNAM. It contains 3 protective peptides: KETc12 of 8 aminoacids, KETc1 of 12 and KETc7 of 110. (Manoutcharian et al. 1996; Manoutcharian reference 2004; Rosas et al. 1998; Toledo et al. 1999; 2001) In the peptide KETc7 2 protective epitopes GK1 and PT1 of 18 and 10 aminoacids respectively were identified (Manoutcharian et al. 1999). These peptides belong to different developmental stages of *Taenia crassiceps* and *Taenia solium* (Toledo et al. 1999; 2001; Rosas et al. 1998, 2002; Sciutto et al. 1995, 2007, 2008) and are found in different anatomical structures of the cysticerci, in the eggs and in the adult taeniae. Their sequences are detected in both cestodes with minimal differences in certain aminoacids which do not modify their tridimensional structure nor their protective capacity (Rassy et al. 2010).

The first version of the vaccine, S3Pvac, was evaluated in an endemic area in the state of Puebla (Huerta et al. 2001).It reduced the number of infected animals 50% and 98% the number of vesicular and colloidal cysticerci that are capable of developing into the adult worm.

The second version was the recombinant vaccine S3Pvac-phage, which consists of the SP3vac peptides which are expressed in filamentous phages. It was evaluated in communities in the state of Morelos and reduced 54% the prevalence of porcine cysticercosis and 89% the number of established cysticerci. (Morales et al. 2008)

In order to plan a programme with possibilities of success one has to consider all the factors that contribute to the persistence of the zoonosis and which have been enumerated above.

We selected communities in the state of Guerrero, where we had detected a high prevalence in the marginated areas, to start our activities.

The first task was to inform and convince federal and local authorities of the need to include the control of this zoonosis in their official health programmes. This was achieved by underscoring that the disease continues to be a health issue in areas where poverty prevails and that due to migrant workers it has spread to other countries.

The project was well received and the authorities collaborated by facilitating funds to purchase a vehicle to transport the members of the teams and to pay for their travels and salaries. They also authorized funds to purchase ultrasonographs for the diagnosis of porcine cysticercosis. This method has proven to be reliable and easier for both veterinarians and pigs, because it eliminates the often cruel handling of pigs and the strenuous efforts of veterinarians and assistants to immobilize them. (Herrera G. S.C. et al 2007)

Before we started with the activities the village authorities, teachers and peasants had to be informed of the programme, by explaining the cycle of the parasitosis, the consequences of getting neurocysticercosis, and the loss of income if their pigs acquire cysticercosis.

Teams are formed of at least one veterinarian who is responsible for the activitities of the group, last year veterinary students who vaccinate and volunteers, usually veterinary students who want to help and learn. People of the village are employed on a daily basis to help find, catch and hold the animals.

Other teams are trained to educate people. They give talks, whenever possible with audiovisual aids, to inform children, teachers, parents and the population in general on the disease, its consequences and how to avoid becoming infected, how to keep their pigs and the importance of using latrines and how.

The strategy we follow in our programme to control the disease is twofold:
1.   Vaccination of pigs
2.   Education of the population

2. Vaccination of pigs

After having agreed upon the day of vaccination, the owners keep their pigs confined and their tongues are examined by members of the team and each animal is registered in a data base, appointing the name of the owner, his or her address, age and sex of the animal, and where it was borne. All pigs are then vaccinated. If cysticerci were detected in the tongue, the pig is carefully examined with ultrasonography and if found positive, we try to purchase it from the owner. An attempt has been made to exchange it for a better bred animal, but this has not been very successful as these newly introduced piglets do not resist the hardship of their new lives and often die. The vaccine is applied subcutaneously, and repeated 3 times, with 3 months interval between each.

3. Education

The teams make appointments with the village authorities, with teachers, schools, parents, medical staff and nurses in order to explain how to improve their hygiene, how to keep their pigs, the importance of using latrines and other topics that may arise during the discussions. The importance of detecting a *T. solium* carrier is of course stressed and people are advised to get treatment for intestinal parasites, which the government offers free of charge in the health centers, whenever possible.

In order to determine how much people know about the disease and also what their living conditions are, before the programme gets under way, a questionnaire is distributed and people who know how to read and write are asked to answer it. The team members help those who cannot to fill it out. The same questionnaire will be distributed at the end of the project and compared with the initial one, which will show whether the educational campaign was successful. At present (August 2011) we have finished with vaccination and 3 months after the last application we shall start to examine all pigs in the communities and compare the frequency of infected animals with the one registered at the beginning.

During our work we have found the attitude of the people very positive. They are grateful for the dedication of the teams, and for the time they spend with them to show how they can improve their pig breeding methods and their own hygienic habits. The children are thrilled with the audiovisual presentations offered in their schools and go home to explain to their family what they have learnt. It is our conviction that to invest time to teach children is most rewarding, as they are more open to new knowledge than the older generations, who often resist change arguing that "their ancestors have done it this way and why should they do it differently".

Problems may arise identifying pigs. We ask the owners not to introduce new ones into their group during the vaccination period and not to sell or kill animals without letting us know, but this has proven to be almost impossible as some get lost or die according to the owners and others that have been added to the group. We try to identify each animal by their special colors or markings, but inevitably there are failures with this system and to mark all pigs with microchips would be too costly. The possibility thus exists that not all pigs get the 3 planned vaccinations but we hope to be able to cover the majority.

By vaccinating as many pigs as possible, we hope to interrupt the cycle of the zoonosis and by educating the population we are confident that people   will acquire the habit of using correct latrines, of washing their hands whenever possible before preparing food and of abstaining from ingesting meat with cysticerci, also of building correct stalls for their pigs.

4. Acknowledgement

We thank SENASICA-SAGARPA for their interest in the programme and for their financial support. Ms Isabel Aguilar for her competent secretarial help and all the authorities, peasants and their families and all other inhabitants of the communities for their collaboration. We are grateful to all members of the working teams, most particularly to Juanita Pérez, Antonio Celis, Arturo López, Alfredo Figueroa and Raul Suárez for their dedication.

5. References

Acevedo H. (1989). Epidemiología de la cisticercosis porcina. En: Cisticercosis Humana y Porcina, pp 251-253. (Editor. Flisser A, Malagón F) Limusa, Noriega. México, D.F

Aluja A. S. de, et al. (1987). *Cisticercosis: una recopilación actualizada de los conocimientos básicos para el manejo y control de Taenia solium*. Biblioteca de la Salud. ISP and Fondo de Cultura Económica, México, D. F.

Aluja A.S. de. (2008). Cysticercosis in pigs. Curr Top Med Chem. 8(5):368-74.

Aluja A. S. de, Villalobos N. (2000). Cisticercosis por *Taenia solium* en cerdos de México. *Veterinaria México*. 31(3):239-244

Aluja, A. S. de,M. J.Martínez y A. N.Villalobos (1998). Cysticercosis in young pigs: Age at first Infection and histological characteristics", *Veterinary Parasitology* 76:71-79.

Assana E, Kyngdon CT, Gauci CG, Geerts S, Dorny P, De Deken R, Anderson GA, Zoli AP, Lightowlers MW. (2010). Elimination of *Taenia solium* transmission to pigs in a field trial of the HP6-TSOL18 vaccine in Cameroon. Int J Parasitol. 40(5):515-9.

Boa M, Mukaratirwa S, Willingham AL, Johansen MV. (2003).Regional action plan for combating *Taenia solium* cysticercosis/taeniosis in Eastern and Southern Africa. Acta Trop. 87(1):183-6.

Comisión Económica Para América Latina – CEPAL- 2010. América Latina: evolución de la pobreza y la indigencia, 1980-2010.

Copado, B. F., A. S. de Aluja, L.Mayagoitia y F. Galindo (2004). The behaviour of free ranging pigs in the Mexican tropics and its relationships with human faeces consumption. Applied Animal Behaviour Science 88:243-252.

Eddi C, Nari A, Amanfu W. (2003). *Taenia solium* cysticercosis/taeniosis: potential linkage with FAO activities; FAO support possibilities. Acta Trop. 87(1): 145-8.

Engels, D., Urbani, C., Beloto, A., Meslin, F., Savioli, L. (2003). The control of human (neuro) cysticercosis: which way forward? Acta Trop., 87:177-82.

Escobar A. (1983). The Pathology of Neuro-cysticercosis. In: E. Palacios, J. Rodríguez Carbajal, J. M. Traveras (eds). Cysticercosis of the Nervous System. Charles C. Thomas, Springfield, Cap. 4:27-54.

Fleury A., Gomez T., Alvarez I., Meza D., Huerta M., Chavarria A., Carrillo Mezo R. A., Lloyd C., Dessein A., Preux P. M., Dumas M., Larralde C., Sciutto E. (2003). High prevalence of calcified silent neurocysticercosis in a rural village of Mexico. Neuroepidemiology. 22(2):139-145.}

Fleury A., Morales J., Bobes R.J., Dumas M., Yánez O., Piña J., Carrillo-Mezo R., Martínez J.J., Fragoso G., Dessein A., Larralde C., Sciutto E. (2006). An epidemiological study of familial neurocysticercosis in an endemic Mexican community. Trans R Soc Trop Med Hyg. 100(6):551-8.

Fleury A., Moreno Garcia J., Valdez Aguerrebere P., de Sayve Duran M., Becerril Rodriguez P., Larralde C., Sciutto E. (2010). Neurocysticercosis, a persisting health problem in Mexico. PLoS Negl Trop Dis. 4(8): e805

Flisser A., Gauci C. G., Zoli A., Martinez-Ocana J., Garza-Rodriguez A., Dominguez-Alpizar J. L., Maravilla P., Rodriguez-Canul R., Avila G., Aguilar-Vega L., Kyngdon C., Geerts S., Lightowlers M. W. (2004). Induction of protection against porcine cysticercosis by vaccination with recombinant oncosphere antigens. Infect Immun., 72: 5292-97.

Flisser A., Correa D. (2010). Neurocysticercosis May No Longer Be a Public Health Problem in Mexico. Plos Negl Trop Dis, 4(12):e8831 doi:10.1371/journal.pntd.0000831

Flores Pérez I., Aluja A. S. de y Martínez J. J. (2006). Efectos en el desarrollo del metacestodo de *Taenia solium* inducidos por dosis bajas de radiación Gamma. Rev. Vet. Méx. , Vol. 37:3

González AE, Gauci CG, Barber D, Gilman RH, Tsang VC, Garcia HH, Verastegui M, Lightowlers MW. (2005). Vaccination of pigs to control human neurocysticercosis. Am J Trop Med Hyg., 72(6):837-9.

Harrison L.J., Garate T., Bryce D. M., Gonzalez L. M., Foster-Cuevas M., Wamae L. W., Onyango-Abuje J. A., Parkhouse R. M. (2005). Ag-ELISA and PCR for monitoring the vaccination of cattle against *Taenia saginata* cysticercosis using an oncospheral adhesion protein (HP6) with surface and secreted localization. Trop Anim Health Prod. 37:103-20.

Herrera G. C., Aluja A. S. de y Méndez A. R. (2007). El uso de la ultrasonografía para el diagnóstico de la cisticercosis porcina. Rev. Vet. México 38;1:125-133.

Huerta M, Aluja A. S. de, Fragoso G, Toledo A, Villalobos N, Hernandez M, Gevorkian G, Acero G, Diaz A, Alvarez I, Avila R, Beltran C, Garcia G, Martinez JJ, Larralde C, Sciutto E. (2001). Synthetic peptide vaccine against *Taenia solium* pig cysticercosis: successful vaccination in a controlled field trial in rural Mexico. Vaccine. 20(1-2):262-6.

Instituto Nacional de Estadística Geografía e Informática, Censo de Población y Vivienda 2010. INEGI, México.

Johnson K.S., Harrison G.B., Lightowlers M.W., O'Hoy K.L., Cougle W.G., Dempster R.P., Lawrence S.B., Vinton J.G., Heath D.D., Rickard M.D. (1989). Vaccination against ovine cysticercosis using a defined recombinant antigen. Nature, 338: 585-587.

Keilbach N, Aluja A, Sarti E. (1989). A programme to control teniosis and cyticercosis (*Taenia solium*), experiences in a Mexican village. Acta Leiden. 57(2):181-189.

Larralde C., Padilla A., Hernández M., Govezensky T., Sciutto E., Gutiérrez G., Tapia-Conyer R., Salvatierra B., Sepúlveda J. (1992). Seroepidemiology of cysticercosis in Mexico. Salud Pública Mex. 34(2): 197-210.

Larralde C., y Aluja A. S. de (2006). Cisticercosis guía para profesionales de la salud. México: FCE, Secretaría de Salud, Instituto Nacional de Salud Pública, Fundación Mexicana para la Salud.

Manoutcharian K., Díaz-Orea A., Gevorkian G., Fragoso G., Acero G., González E., Aluja A. S. de, Villalobos N., Gómez-Conde E., Sciutto E. (2004). Recombinant bacteriophage-based multiepitope vaccine against *Taenia solium* pig cysticercosis. Vet Immunol Immunopathol. May; 99(1-2):11-24.

Manoutcharian K, Terrazas L.I., Gevorkian G., Acero G., Petrossian P., Rodriguez M., Govezensky T. (1999). Phage-displayed T-cell epitope grafted into immunoglobulin heavy-chain complementarity-determining regions: an effective vaccine design tested in murine cysticercosis. Infect Immun. 67(9):4764-70.

Manoutcharian K. Rosas, G. Hernández, M. Fragoso, G. Aluja, A. Villalobos, N. Rodarte, L. F. Sciutto, E. (1996). Cysticercosis: identification and cloning of protective recombinant antigens. J Parasitol. 82(2): 250-4.

Martínez, M. J., Aluja A. S. de y Gemmell M. (2000), Failure to incriminate domestic flies *(Diptera: Muscidae)* as mechanical vectors of *Taenia* eggs *(Cyclophillidea: Taeniidae)* in rural Mexico. *Journal of Medical Entomology* 37(4):489-491.

Martínez, M. J., A. S. de Aluja, A. N. M. Villalobos, A. C. Jaramillo y M. Gemmell. (1997). "Epidemiología de la cisticercosis en cerdos de una comunidad rural del estado de Guerrero, México", Veterinaria México 28(4):281-286.

Martínez, M. J., Aluja A. S. de, R. G. Ávila, V. L. Aguilar, C. A. Plancarte y A. C. Jaramillo (2003). Teniosis y detección de anticuerpos anticisticercos en personas de una comunidad rural del estado de Guerrero. *Salud Pública de México* 45(2):84-89.

Molinari J. L.; Meza R.; Suarez B.; Palacios S.; Tato P.; Retana A. (1983). *Taenia solium*: immunity in hogs to the Cysticercus. Exp Parasitol., 55, 340-57.

Morales J., Martínez J.J., Rosseti M. Fleury A., Maza V., Hernández M, Villalobos N, Fragoso G, de Aluja AS, Larralde C, Sciutto E. (2008). Spatial Distribution of Taenia solium Porcine Cysticercosis within a Rural Area of Mexico. PloS. NeGL. Trop. Dis., 2(9):e284. Sep 3.

Morales J. T. Velasco, V. Tovar, G. Fragoso, A Fleury, C. Beltran, N. Villalobos, A. Aluja, L.F. Rodarte, E. Sciutto. and C. Larralde. (2002). Castration and pregnancy of rural pigs significantly increase the prevalence of naturally acquired *Taenia solium* cysticercosis. Veterinary Parasitol., June, 108:41-48.

Morales J., Martínez J.J. García-Castella. J., Peña N., Maza V., Villalobos N., Aluja AS., Fleury A., Fragoso G., Sarralde C. Sciutto E. (2006). *Taenia solium*: the complex interactions, of biological, social, geographical and commercial factors, involved in the transmission dynamics of pig cysticercosis in highly endemic areas. Ann Trop Med Parasitol, 100(2):123-35.

Ortiz-Trejo J.M., Correa-Chacón A.J., Sctelo-Ham E.I., Torres-Valenzuela A., Alvarado-Esquivel C. (2006). Risk factors associated with neurocysticercosis in a public hospital in México. Gac Med Mex. May-Jun;142(3):175-9. Spanish.

Pawlowski Z. S., Allan J., Sarti E. (2005). Control of Taenia solium taeniasis/cysticercosis: from research towards implementation. Int J Parasitol. 35, 1221-32.

Plancarte A., Flisser A., Gauci C.G., Lightowlers M.W. (1999). Vaccination against Taenia solium cysticercosis in pigs using native and recombinant oncosphere antigens. Int J Parasitol, 9:643-7.

Quiroz R.H. (2002). Parasitologia y enfermedades parasitarias de animales domésticos. Grupo Noriega Editores, Editorial Limusa.

Rassy D., Bobes R. J., Rosas G., Anaya V. H., Brehm K., Hernandez B., Cervantes J., Pedraza S., Morales J., Villalobos N., de Aluja A. S., Laclette, J. P. Nunes, C. M. Biondi, G. F. Fragoso, G. Hernández, M. Sciutto, E. (2010). Characterization of S3Pvac anti-cysticercosis vaccine components: implications for the development of an anti-cestodiasis vaccine. PLoS-One. 5(6):e11287

Rodríguez L. G. y Del Moral B.L.E. (2010). Perspectivas del sector porcícola mexicano para 2010: recuperación de los efectos de la crisis económica y de la influenza (A)H1/N1. Revista Trimestral de Análisis de Coyuntura Económica, Vol. III, No. 2, Abril-Junio.

Rosas G., Cruz-Revilla C., Fragoso G., López-Casillas F., Pérez A., Bonilla M. A., Rosales R., Sciutto E. (1998). Taenia crassiceps cysticercosis: humoral immune response and protection elicited by DNA immunization. J Parasitol. 84(3): 516-23

Rosas G., Fragoso G., Garate T., Hernandez B., Ferrero P., Foster-Cuevas M., Parkhouse R. M., Harrison L. J., Briones S. L., Gonzalez L. M., Sciutto E. (2002). Protective immunity against Taenia crassiceps murine cysticercosis induced by DNA vaccination with a Taenia saginata tegument antigen. Microbes Infect., 4, 1417-26.

Sánchez,A. L., J. Lindback, P. M. Schantz, M. Sone, H. Sakai, M. T. Medina y I. Ljungstrom (1999), "A population-based, case-control study of Taenia solium taeniasis and cysticercosis", Annals of Tropical Medicine and Parasitology 93(3A):247-258.

Sarti E., Flisser A., Schantz P., Gleizer M., Loya M., Plancarte A., Ávila G., Allan J., Craig P., Bronfman M., Wijeyaratne P. (1997). "Development and evaluation of a health education intervention against Taenia solium in a rural community in Mexico". Am J Tropl Med Hyg. 56(2):127-132.

Sarti E., P. M. Schantz, R. Lara-Aguilera, H. Gómez y A. Flisser (1988), "Taenia solium taeniasis and cysticercosis in a Mexican village", Tropical Medicine and Parasitology 39(3):194-198.

Sarti E., P. Schantz, A. Plancarte, M. Wilson, I. Gutiérrez, A. López, J. Roberts y A. Flisser (1992). Prevalence and risk factors for Taenia solium taeniasis and cysticercosis in humans and pigs in a village in Morelos, México. American Journal of Tropical Medicine and Hygiene 46:677-685.

Sciutto E., Aluja A., Fragoso G., Rodarte L.F., Hernández M., Villalobos M.N., Padilla A., Keilbach N., Baca M., Govezensky T. (1995). Immunization of pigs against Taenia solium cysticercosis factors related to effective protection. Vet Parasitol, 60(1-2):53-67.

Sciutto E., Fragoso G., de Aluja A.S., Hernández M., Rosas G., Larralde C. (2008). Vaccine against cysticercosis. Curr Top Med Chem. 8(5):415-23.

Sciutto E., Morales J., Martínez J.J., Toledo A., Villalobos M.N., Cruz-Revilla C., Meneses G., Hernández M., Díaz A., Rodarte L.F., Acero G., Gevorkian G., Manoutcharian K., Paniagua J., Fragoso G., Fleury A., Larralde R., De Aluja A.S., Larralde C. (2007). Further evaluation of the synthetic peptide vaccine S3Pvac against *Taenia solium* cysticercosis in pigs in an endemic town of Mexico. Parasitology, 134:129-133.

Sciutto E., Rosas G., Hernández M., Morales J., Cruz-Revilla C., Toledo A., Manoutcharian K. Gevorkian G., Blancas A., Acero G., Hernádez B., Cervantes J., Bobes R.J., Goldbaum F.A., Huerta M., Diaz-Orea A., Fleury A., de Aluja A.S., Cabrera-Ponce J.L., Herrera-Estrella L., Fragoso G., Larralde C. (2007). Improvement of the synthetic tri-peptide vaccine (S3Pvac) against porcine *Taenia solium* cysticercosis in search of a more effective, inexpensive and manageable vaccine. Vaccine, 25(8):1368-78

Sciutto E., Morales J., Camacho C., Nájera M., Fleury A., Fragoso G., Aluja A. S. de, Hernández M., Martínez J.J., Villalobos N. (In press). Meaning of the presence of anti-cysticercal antibodies in pigs: usefulness in sensing cysticercososis transmission.

SIAP-SAGARPA. 2010. Estadísticas sobre la producción porcina para los años 2008 y 2009. (Abril 2010). http://siap.gob.mx

Sorvillo F., Wilkins P., Shafir S., Eberhard M. (2011). Public health implications of cysticercosis acquired in the United States. Emerg Infect Dis. Jan;17(1):1-6.

Sorvillo F.J., DeGiorgio C. & Watermant S.H. (2007). Deaths from cysticercosis, United States. Emerg Infect Dis. 13: 230-235.

Sosa J. (2010). Determinación de la frecuencia de cisticercosis por *T. solium* mediante la prueba de ELISA y su impacto en algunos indicadores productivos en cerdos del traspatio de Morelos 2008-2009. Tesis de licenciatura, Facultad de Ciencias Agropecuarias, Universidad Autónoma del Estado de Morelos. Sept. *System,* Charles C. Thomas, Springfield Illinois, pp. 27-54.

Toledo A., Fragoso G., Rosas G., Hernández M., Gevorkian G., Lopez-Casillas F., Hernández B., Acero G., Huerta M., Larralde C., Sciutto E. (2001). Two epitopes shared by *Taenia crassiceps* and *Taenia solium* confer protection against murine *T. crassiceps* cysticercosis along with a prominent T1 response. Infect Immun. 69, 1766-73.

Toledo A., Larralde C., Fragoso G., Gevorkian G., Manoutcharian K., Hernández M., Acero G., Rosas G., Lopez-Casillas F., Garfias C. K., Vazquez R., Terrazas I., Sciutto E. (1999). Towards a *Taenia solium* cysticercosis vaccine: an epitope shared by *Taenia crassiceps* and *Taenia solium* protects mice against experimental cysticercosis. Infect Immun., 67, 2522-30.

Villagrán J. Olvera J. E. (1988). Cisticercosis humana: Estudio clínico patológico de 481 casos de autopsia, Patología 26:149–156.

12

Control of Schistosomiasis and Soil-Transmitted Helminthiasis in Sub-Saharan Africa: Challenges and Prospects

Louis-Albert Tchuem Tchuenté
University of Yaoundé I, Laboratory of Parasitology and Ecology,
Centre for Schistosomiasis and Parasitology, Yaoundé
Cameroon

1. Introduction

Schistosomiasis and soil-transmitted helminthiasis (STH) are the most common types of parasitic infections in the world. These diseases have major health and socio-economic repercussions, and constitute an important public health problem in developing countries. Human schistosomiasis is caused by six species of schistosomes, i.e. *Schistosoma haematobium, Schistosoma mansoni, Schistosoma japonicum, Schistosoma mekongi, Schistosoma intercalatum* and *Schistosoma guineensis*; and is endemic in 78 countries, where 779 million people are at risk of infection. *S. haematobium* is responsible for urogenital schistosomiasis, and the other species cause intestinal schistosomiasis. It is estimated that 207 million people are infected (WHO, 2002; Steinmann et al. 2006). STH, also known as intestinal worm infection, is caused by four main species of worms commonly known as roundworms (*Ascaris lumbricoides*), whipworms (*Trichuris trichiura*) and hookworms (*Ancylostoma duodenale* and *Necator americanus*). It is estimated that STH affects more than 2 billion people worldwide, and the greatest numbers of infections occur in sub-Saharan Africa, the Americas, China and east Asia (WHO, 2006; Hotez et al., 2006; Brooker et al., 2006; Awasthi et al., 2003).

These diseases affect the poorest of the poor and infections are particularly abundant among people living in rural or deprived urban settings with low socio-economic status, lack of clean water and poor sanitation (Hotez et al., 2006). The morbidity caused by these worms is commonly associated with heavy infection intensities. Compared with any other age group, school-aged children and pre-school children are the most vulnerable group and they harbor the greatest numbers of intestinal worms. As a result, they experience growth stunting and diminished physical fitness as well as impaired memory and cognition (Crompton and Nesheim, 2002; Stephenson et al., 2000; Bethony et al., 2006). These adverse health consequences combine to impair childhood educational performance and reduce school attendance (Miguel & Kremer, 2004; Hotez et al., 2008). Studies have demonstrated that children may acquire helminth infections early in life (Sousa-Figueiredo et al., 2008; Stothard et al., 2008); which causes initial organ damage that can remain subclinical for years and manifest overtly only later, in adulthood (WHO, 2006; Odogwu et al., 2006).

Despite the existence of tools in the 1970s and 1980s, control was sustained for a prolonged period only in few countries and almost no progress was made in sub-Saharan African countries, the most affected part of the world. In the 1990s, interest in the control of these diseases in Africa waned. Therefore, as with other neglected tropical diseases (NTDs), schistosomiasis and STH control has been overshadowed by other health priorities. The highest priority of the international health community was given to the 'big three', i.e. HIV/AIDS, tuberculosis and malaria, with less attention to other infections related to poverty (Molyneux et al., 2005).

Recent years have witnessed an increased interest in the control of NTDs, and today there exists a global momentum for the control of these diseases. The control of NTDs has become a priority on the agenda of many governments, donors and international agencies. The World Health Organization (WHO) has played a major role in this prospect. Indeed, under the aegis of WHO, all member states of WHO (over 200 countries) have endorsed in May 2001 the World Health Assembly resolution WHA 54.19, with as a major objective the regular treatment of at least 75% of all school-aged children at risk of morbidity by 2010. The renewed impetus for schistosomiasis and STH control has generated a greater political commitment, as well as an unprecedented opportunity for cost-effective action (Molyneux et al., 2005). This momentum has encouraged many countries to establish national action plans and programmes to control schistosomiasis, STHs and other NTDs (Hotez et al., 2009; Tchuem Tchuenté & N'Goran, 2009). Within the past decade, significant progress has been made on large scale treatments through integrated control of schistosomiasis, STH and other NTDs, thanks to a number of international organizations, donor foundations, bilateral institutions and non-governmental organizations that responded to the 2001 WHO's call for action (Savioli et al., 2009). Today, treatment is cost-effective and the 'preventive chemotherapy' is currently the strategy of choice (WHO, 2006). With a support from the American (USAID) and British (DFID) governments, as well as the Bill and Melinda Gates Foundation, the pharmaceutical industry, and many not-for profit organizations, millions of children are regularly treated for schistosomiasis, STH and other NTDs. However, the control of these diseases is a long-term undertaking which involves several challenges. This paper highlights the progress made and also focuses on some main challenges that are reviewed and discussed.

2. Epidemiology and burden of schistosomiasis and STH

Schistosomiasis and STH transmission are intimately associated with poverty and poor sanitation. For schistosomiasis, infecion is caused by penetration of the skin by larvae in water; whereas for STH, infection is caused by the ingestion of parasite eggs from contaminated food or dirty hands – in the case of *A. lumbricoides* and *T. trichiura* – or by active penetration of the skin by larvae in the soil – in the case of hookworms. People who get infected carry parasite eggs in the feces or in the urine (in the case of urinary schistosomiasis), and in areas where there is no latrine systems the soil and water around the villages and communities are contaminated with feces or urine containing worm eggs. Although schistosomiasis and STH infections occur predominantly in rural areas, the social and environmental conditions in many unplanned slums and squatter settlements of developing countries are ideal for their persistence (Crompton & Savioli, 1993). In endemic populations, infections are aggregated: most infected individuals in a community will have infections of a light or moderate intensity, while a few will be heavily infected. Heavily infected individuals suffer most of the clinical consequences of the infections and are the major source of infection for the rest of the community (WHO, 2002).

The epidemiology of helminth infections is influenced by several key determinants, including environment, population heterogeneity, age, household clustering, genetics and polyparasitism (Hotez et al., 2008). In recent years, considerable progress has been made in the use of geographical information system (GIS) and remote sensing (RS) to better understand helminth ecology and epidemiology, and to develop low-cost ways to identify target populations for treatment. GIS and RS were used to describe the global distribution of schistosomiasis and STH infections and to estimate the number of infections in school-age children in sub-Saharan Africa.

There is considerable geographical variation in the occurrence of infections (Brooker et al., 2009). In general, changes with age in the average intensity of helminth infections tend to be convex, rising in childhood and declining in adulthood. For schistosomiasis, *A. lumbicoides* and *T. trichiura*, the heaviest and most frequent infections are in children aged 5–15 years, with a decline in intensity and frequency in adulthood (Gilles, 1996). In contrast, hookworm frequently exhibits a steady rise of intensity of infection with age, peaking in adulthood (Bethony et al., 2002). Household clustering of infected individuals has been demonstrated for STH (Forrester et al., 1988), and this can persist through time, as shown by familial predisposition to heavy infection with *A. lumbricoides* and *T. trichiura* (Forrester et al., 1990). Because morbidity is associated with worm burden rather than the absence or presence of infection, prevalence is commonly combined with worm burden (intensity of infection) to assess the epidemiological situation for schistosomiasis and STH infections. Worm burden is commonly measured by the number of eggs per gram (EPG) of feces or eggs per 10ml of urine (Anderson, 1982; Montresor et al., 1998). Prevalence and intensity of infections are used to classify communities into transmission categories, which enable to determine the appropriate type of mass treatment a community should receive (WHO, 2006). Both should be assessed in monitoring the impact of deworming campaigns.

3. Control of schistosomiasis and STH

3.1 Progress towards the 2010 global target
Progress in implementing schistosomiasis and STH control programmes has been slow but steady. Since 2006, there has been an overall increase in the number of people treated for schistosomiasis and STH. The increase in treatments has occurred entirely in the African Region, where the number of people treated more than doubled from 2006 to 2009 (WHO, 2011). This number increased by 93% in 2010. The increase in the number treated suggests that both governments and their donor partners are now investing in schistosomiasis control (WHO, 2012). In 2010, 18 over 42 schistosomiasis endemic countries in the African region and 34/46 STH endemic countries or territories reported their treatment data to WHO. Overall, 27,983,327 people were treated for schistosomiasis, and 91,025,863 children for STH (Table 1).

Characteristics	Schistosomiasis	STH
No. endemic countries	42	46
No. countries reporting MDA data	18	34
No. people requiring treatment	220 578 484	283 800 000
No. people treated	27 983 327	91 025 863
No. pre-school aged children treated	-	42 711 551
No. school aged children treated	-	48 314 312

Table 1. African Regional summary of children treated for schistosomiasis and STH, 2010

Figure 1 illustrates the progress in Africa ten years after the 2001 WHA resolution. Although significant progress has been made over the past years to significantly reduce schistosomiasis and STH infection prevalence below low risk, or to regularly implement mass drug administration (MDA) in several countries, the global achievement is still very far from the WHO's target of regular deworming of at least 75% of school-age children at risk. Indeed, from the data of epidemiological coverage of STHs, it was estimated that only 15% of school-aged children at risk of infection have been treated with preventive chemotherapy in 2008 (WHO, 2010). School-based deworming interventions still cover only a minority of children considered to be at risk despite the low cost of these interventions and their significant impact on health. More worrying, the number of people treated for schistosomiasis in Sub-Saharan Africa is estimated to be only 6.71% of the people infected (WHO, 2011). The major constraint to controlling schistosomiasis continues to be the limited access to praziquantel (Hotez et al., 2010). In the African Region, only few countries (18 in 2008) have achieved the 75% treatment target.

3.2 Taking advantage of integrated control of NTDs

In the developing world, polyparasitism is the norm rather than the exception (Molyneux et al., 2005; Fleming et al., 2006; Tchuem Tchuenté et al., 2003). In large parts of the world, particularly in Africa, most children are infected by more than one species of helminth. These NTDs frequently overlap geographically and they impose a great burden on poor populations, affecting the same individuals. Therefore, the current strategy for NTD control is to integrate interventions for multiple diseases (Molyneux et al., 2005). This integrated approach is the basis for cost-effectiveness and streamlined efficiency. Also, because many of the drugs used for mass treatment are provided free of charge by major multinational pharmaceutical companies, the MDA approach is the most cost-effective global public health control measure (Hotez et al., 2007). Schistosomiasis and STH infections are the most prevalent and widespread of the common NTDs, and they overlap in many parts with many of the other NTDs. Therefore, an integration of schistosomiasis and STH control with other helminth control programmes and a good coordinated use of (donated) drugs would be highly beneficial for their control. This would indeed allow to take advantage of drug donation and co-administration, and to optimize the preventive chemotherapy.

Within the past decade, significant progress has been made on large-scale treatment of schistosomiasis and STH through integrated control with other NTDs, thanks to a number of international organizations, donor foundations, bilateral institutions and non-governmental organizations that responded to the 2001 WHO's call for action (Savioli et al., 2009). With a support from the American (USAID) and British (DFID) governments, as well as the Bill and Melinda Gates Foundation, the pharmaceutical industry, and many not-for profit organizations, millions of children are regularly treated for schistosomiasis, STH and other NTDs. Today, an integrated control of NTD using the preventive chemotherapy is operating in more than 15 countries. Within the first three years (2006-2009) of implementation of the USAID NTD Control Program, the number of persons reached each year increased progressively, with a cumulative total of 98 million persons receiving 222 million treatments (Linehan et al., 2011). In West Africa, nearly 13.5 million doses of albendazole have been administered against STH between 2004 and 2006 in Burkina Faso, Mali and Niger, with coverage rates varying between 67.0% and 93.9% (Garba et al., 2009). Monitoring and evaluation activities after large-scale administration of praziquantel for schistosomiasis and albendazole for STH showed a significant decrease in the intensity of infections. Also, there was a significant increase in haemoglobin concentration after 1 and 2

(A)

(B)

 Countries likely to have achieved interruption of transmission or towards elimination

 Countries with on-going large-scale schistosomiasis control programme

 Countries with limited or no schistosomiasis control programme

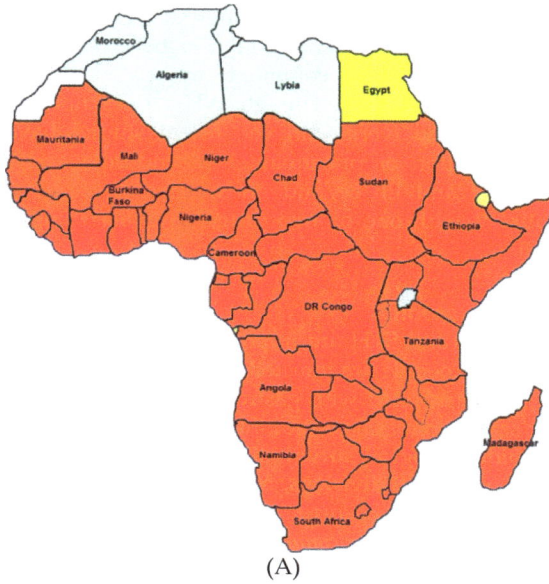

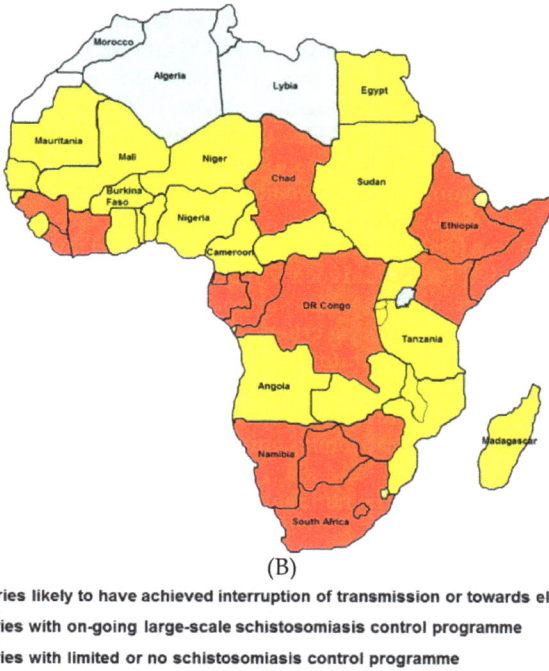

Fig. 1. Comparative status of schistosomiasis control in Africa at the end of the 20th century (A) and in 2010 (B).

years of treatment (Fenwick et al., 2009). Combination of ivermectin and albendazole, and co-administration of praziquantel and albendazole or mebendazole have been proven to be safe, with no side effects outside those commonly associated with each of these drugs (Horton et al., 2000; Olds et al., 1999). Though WHO does not formally recommends combination of praziquantel and ivermectin yet, recent studies have demonstrated the safety of triple co-administration of praziquantel, albendazole and ivermectin in areas where schistosomiasis, STH and LF or/and onchocerciasis are co-endemic and where several rounds of treatment with one or two drugs have been implemented in the past (Mohammed et al., 2008).

3.3 A country example: Cameroon
In Cameroon, schistosomiasis and STH are important parasitic diseases. Recent estimates indicate that at least 2 million people are infected with schistosomiasis, 5 million are at risk and more than 10 million are infected with gastrointestinal helminths (Minsante, 2005). In 1983, a pilot project for schistosomiasis control, funded by USAID, was set up. Within this framework a national epidemiological survey of schistosomiasis and STH was conducted between 1985 and 1987. Overall, 49 divisions, 504 schools and 23 850 schoolchildren were investigated. The results showed the occurrence of *S. haematobium, S. mansoni, S. guineensis, A. lumbricoides, T. trichiura* and *N. americanus* as the major helminth species. The highest transmission levels of schistosomiasis occured in the northern part, whereas STH were more prevalent in the southern part of the country (Ratard et al., 1990, 1991; Brooker et al., 2000). When considering all these helminthic diseases, no region of the country is spared. However, this pilot project stopped in 1989 when the USAID support ended.
Taking advantage of the renewed momentum for NTDs, the national programme for the control of schistosomiasis and STH was created in March 2003. There is a strong political commitment from the Ministries of Public Health and Basic Education. These two ministries work in close collaboration and this inter-sectorial engagement is consolidated by the fact that the national steering committee for the control is co-chaired by the Minister of Public Health and the Minister of Basic Education, as president and vice-president, respectively. The Cameroonian proposal for support to SCI was presented by the Minister of Public Health himself who attended the SCI advocacy meeting in London in July 2003. Therefore, the non-selection of Cameroon for SCI support came both as a surprise and a disappointment. Beyond the main ranking criteria, including the existence of a strategic plan for control, the strong political commitment and the quality of the proposal, the SCI selection was finally made on a regional combination of three East African countries and three West African countries, with emphasis on country-regional collaboration and consortium. In spite of this, the Cameroonian government made necessary efforts to ensure the success of the schistosomiasis and STH control, as it was among the priority programmes of the country. Hence, the national control programme was officially launched on 25 March 2004.
The action of the programme during the past few years was intense and multifaceted, with a number of key achievements. Based on the limited resources available, the priority activities were centred on three major activities: (1) the production of various strategic documents necessary for the implementation of the activities and advocacy; (2) the advocacy and the mobilisation of partners and funding; and (3) the implementation of activities in selected areas. A strong emphasis was put on advocacy, the results of which were encouraging for future activities and plans. The most important was the selection of Cameroon as the first

start-up country for mebendazole donation in Africa. Indeed, in 2005 Johnson & Johnson established a partnership with the Task Force for Child Survival and Development (currently The Task Force for Global Health) to develop a programme to donate mebendazole via a multi-disciplinary initiative designed to address intestinal worm infections in the most at-risk children of the world. Cameroon was selected as the start-up country for this drug donation programme because of its leadership and commitment to eliminating infections as a major public health problem (http://www.janssenpharmaceutica.be/download_Cameroen_N.asp). With regard to control, a pilot phase was completed in February 2006 in one health district, where approximately 20,000 school-aged children were treated with praziquantel and albendazole. Subsequently, the activities were extended to one entire region of the ten regions in Cameroon, i.e. the Adamawa region in the northern part of the country. This was implemented with support from partners, including the World Food Programme (WFP), the Canadian Co-operation, the United Nations International Children's Emergency Fund (UNICEF) and SCI/Medpharm (which donated the drugs praziquantel and albendazole). Deworming was conducted in all 500 primary schools in this region, and approximately 150,000 school-aged children were treated in May 2006. Overall, 700 head teachers, 500 representatives of parent teacher associations, and 2500 teachers were trained. In addition, parasitological surveys for schistosomiasis and STH were conducted in 40 selected schools where stool and urine samples were collected from a total of 1830 children.

The mebendazole donation enabled the national control programme to scale-up activities rapidly. As a result, deworming activities were increased to encompass all ten regions. In 2007, Cameroon launched a nationwide deworming campaign, and 4 million school-aged children were treated. The launching ceremony allowed the government and partners to further reaffirm their commitment and to galvanise communities, international development agencies, non-governmental organisations (NGOs) and other stakeholders to join in the effort to implement fundamental improvements in disease control and prevention. The country has in place school-based and community-directed channels and in the programme teachers and community drug distributors administer the drugs to children along with health and hygiene education. The major activities conducted are: (1) training of health and education personnel, (2) sensitization and education of communities about the disease, the risks of infection and measures for prevention, (3) promotion of hygiene, safe water and sanitation systems in communities, and (4) deworming of children. Since 2007, 4 million school-age children are treated annually with mebendazole, with the involvement of over 75,000 trained teachers and head teachers. Control of STH is primarily implemented through school-based distribution of mebendazole, co-administered with praziquantel where schistosomiasis is endemic. In addition, albendazole is co-administered with ivermectin during the community-directed treatment for LF. Furthermore, over 2.7 million children aged 1–5 years are dewormed during child health week campaigns implemented twice a year (Tchuem Tchuenté and N'Goran, 2009).

Moreover, parasitological surveys were conducted in selected schools in all 63 health districts of the Centre, East and West regions of Cameroon, in order to update the disease distribution map, to assess the impact of previous deworming campaigns, and to determine where treatment with PZQ should be extended. The results showed significant variation of schistosomiasis and STH prevalence between schools, villages, districts and regions. In comparison to previous mapping data collected 25 years ago, the results showed an increase of schistosomiasis transmission in several health districts, where PZQ MDA was not implemented so far. On the contrary, there was a significant decline of STH infection prevalence and intensities in all three regions, with an overall decline of prevalence from 90.06% (95% CI: 89.45-90.63%) to 24.11% (95% CI: 23.37-24.86%). Based on the prevalence data, the continuation of annual or bi-annual MDA for STH was recommended, as well as an extension of PZQ treatment in identified moderate and high risk communities for schistosomiasis (Tchuem Tchuenté et al., 2012). These results show the positive impact of annual deworming campaigns, and illustrate the progressive success of the national programme for the control of schistosomiasis and STH in Cameroon. This is illustrated in Figure 2. Parasitological surveys are in progress in the remaining regions of Cameroon for the update mapping.

4. Challenges

The control of schistosomiasis and STHs is a long-term undertaking, which involves several challenges. The first challenge is to mobilize the funds required for successful actions. Unlike some of the stigmatising NTDs with 'visible' morbidity such as onchocerciasis and LF which have successfully raised funding for the implementation of control activities, little funding are globally available for the implementation of schistosomiasis and STH control alone. Therefore, for their schistosomiasis and STH control programmes, endemic countries should take advantage of the opportunities resulting from the global growing financial resources generated by the new partnerships and impetus for NTD control. The recent changes in the international agenda and the increasing funding opportunities provide leverage for the control of schistosomiasis and STHs. The piggyback and integrated control approaches – based on a complementary co-administration of relevant drugs – are the basis for cost-effectiveness and streamlined efficiency. However, pigging back on other interventions or integration with other health programmes requires the setting up of clear efficient coordination mechanisms in order to optimize the use of resources mobilized from various partners. Among other challenges, the most important are the co-ordination at various levels, the country ownership and leadership, the scale up of control, the sustainability of control programmes, the strengthening of partnerships and institutional capacities, the implementation of operational research, monitoring and evaluation, and the development of new diagnostic tools.

4.1 Co-ordination
The NTD control programmes involve many partners and stakeholders, different diseases, several funding sources, and multiform resources. The main challenge is to set up clear efficient coordination mechanisms in order to optimize the resources mobilised from all partners. To ensure transparency in all processes, there is a need for a coordination mechanism for funding, drug supplies and integrated control of NTDs to enable all stakeholders to share information. The coordination mechanism should be at global, regional and country levels. The precise form of this co-ordination mechanism needs to be explored and agreed amongst stakeholders. At national level, the Ministry of Health should play the central role in this co-ordination.

4.2 Country ownership and leadership
In order to ensure the sustainability and the success of NTD control programmes, country leadership in the coordination of activities is essential. Each partner may have its own vision and own interest, and the ones who bring the money also sometimes decide what to do.

(A)

STH prevalence

○ 0%
○ 0.1 - 19.9%
● 20 - 49.9%
● ≥ 50%

(B)

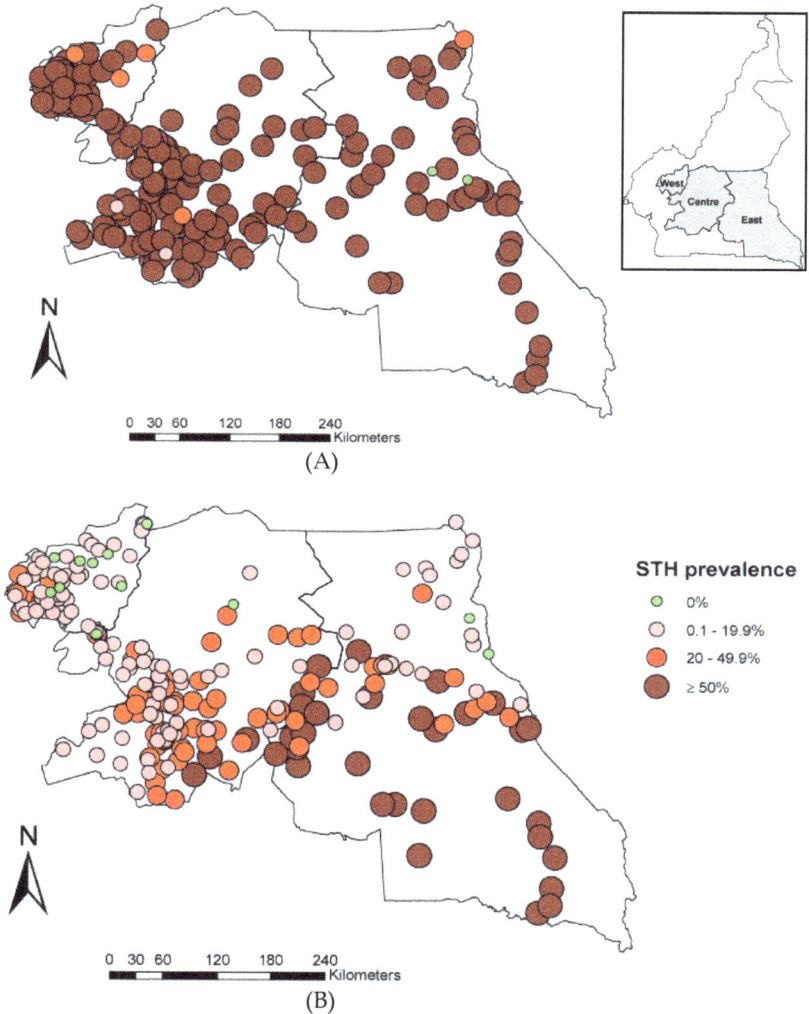

Fig. 2. Comparative maps of the overall soil-transmitted helminthiasis prevalence between the years 1985-1987 (A) and 2010 (B) in the Centre, East and West regions of Cameroon.

Sometimes, many people in a country are working for the same thing, but with different targets because there are different donors. Country ownership brings many gains, including development of local capacity and expertise. There should be a strong political commitment to tackle NTDs in endemic countries. Indeed, examples of success stories are from those countries (e.g. Japan, Morocco and China) that had clear ambitious goal, with high government and national commitment, funding mobilization and leadership. For example, in early 1963 STH occurred in Okinawa, Japan at high prevalence up to 40% in adult population. Through the development of an ambitious 'zero parasites' campaign a successful control was conducted and within a period less than 10 years STHs and other parasites were eradicated in Okinawa. In contrary, lack of ambitious control is remarkable in Sub-Saharan Africa where many countries have passive attitude, waiting for partners to decide and to tell them what to do. African governments should develop more positive and ambitious approach for the control of NTDs, and donors and agencies beyond disease endemic countries — the agents of aid to developing countries — will need to accept that countries must have ownership of their health systems and total control over decisions about the health of their people.

4.3 Scale up of control

In order reach the target set by WHA for the different NTDs, there is a need to accelerate the extent of treatment. The extension of regular deworming coverage as a public health intervention to reach all individuals at risk remains a challenge. There is also a challenge to tackle the big countries such as Nigeria, Democratic Republic of Congo, Ethiopia and Tanzania which count for 60% of at risk population not covered by preventive chemotherapy yet. In the context of multi-disease integrated control, the current tendency in sub-Saharan Africa is to integrate helminth control within the community-directed interventions, taking advantages of the long experience and gains of onchocerciasis and LF control programmes through the establishment of community-directed treatment with ivermectin (CDTI) in all countries supported by the African Programme for Onchocerciasis Control – APOC (Sékétéli et al., 2002; Amazigo et al., 2002). Yet, in the majority of countries, STHs are more widely distributed than both onchocerciasis and LF. Therefore, the challenge will be to extend MDA coverage in those areas where CDTI does not exist. Countries should thus act cautiously and anticipate to avoid to neglect STH and schistosomiasis control in those endemic areas. School-based deworming is probably the simple, cost-effective and best sustainable way to expand coverage of children. With more schools than clinics, and more teachers than health workers, the existing and extensive education infrastructure provides the most efficient way to reach the highest number of school-age children and to reach the WHO target of covering at least 75% of all school-aged children in need. The recent increases of donated anthelminthic medicines by Merck KGaA (praziquantel), Johnson & Johnson (mebendazole) and GlaxoSmithKline (albendazole) constitute a real boost towards the achievement of this goal.

4.4 Sustainability

To roll back the NTDs, it is necessary to continue and maintain the implementation of control activities during very long period. The programme should be long-term, and financial and implementation plans should be made accordingly. This would avoid one of the major errors of the past where most of the programmes were supported by short-term external funds and stopped immediately when funds ceased. To ensure sustainability, countries should, from the beginning, envisage strategies to: (1) keep the momentum, interest and enthusiasm for the control of the diseases; (2) organize and finance in a sustained way the distribution of drugs to those who need them; (3) mobilize funding for operational costs for drug distribution, health education materials, baseline data collection, monitoring and evaluation, etc.; (4) ensure the availability and affordability of the drugs at community level in endemic areas; (5) integrate programme activities within the existing health structures and networks; and (6) strengthen the health system and national capacity at all levels, especially in the peripheral and remote areas which manage the greater number of communities and infected persons. One of the key questions is how to guarantee the continuation of control after the decline or interruption of external funds.

4.5 Strengthening of partnership
An efficient control requires multisector collaboration and multilateral funding. No single organization can hope to achieve this goal alone. School-aged children are the target group for schistosomiasis and STH, so the collaboration between the Ministry of Health and the Ministry of Education should be reinforced. The target group for the different filarial infections is the entire population and the control strategy is based on community-directed interventions, which requires ownership by the communities and strong partnership with NGOs. Overall, partnership with other government departments and NGOs concerned with water supply, sanitation and development projects should be developed and reinforced.

4.6 Strengthening of institutional capacities
The integration of control activities within the health services is fundamental for the sustainability of the programme. However, most of the existing structures do not have the capacity to ensure the implementation of these activities, leading to programme failure. Therefore, the strengthening of the health system is a requirement for the long-term viability of the control programme. Furthermore, an efficient participation of schools and communities in the disease control requires a reinforcement of capacity of the school system and the community ownership.

4.7 Operational research
It is important to support operational research to fulfill gaps and improve the implementations of the control. For example, the understanding of some key issues, such as baseline epidemiology, morbidity assessment, drug efficacy testing and monitoring of drug resistance, is of vital importance.

4.8 Monitoring and evaluation
Regular monitoring and evaluation are necessary to ensure that programmes are efficiently implemented and that the beneficiaries gain the maximum benefit. This is particularly challenging given the diversity of tools and indicators. Substantial progress has been made towards the development of standardized tools for monitoring and evaluating NTD control programmes. WHO is currently developing guidelines based on the experience to date with integrated preventive chemotherapy interventions.

4.9 Better diagnostic tools
Because of its simplicity and relatively low-cost, the Kato–Katz technique (Katz et al., 1972) is widely used for epidemiological field surveys and is recommended by the WHO for surveillance and monitoring of schistosomiasis and STH control programmes (WHO, 1991; Montresor et al., 1998). Though the specificity is very high, the sensitivity of Kato–Katz in single stool sample examination is limited by day-to-day variation in egg excretion leading to measurement error in estimating the presence of infection. This is particularly accentuated in areas with high proportions of light intensity infections (Hall, 1981; Booth et al., 2003; Tarafder et al., 2009). In the current era of preventive chemotherapy, the intensification of large-scale interventions and repeated mass deworming will significantly reduce the prevalence and intensities of schistosomiasis and STH infections (Savioli et al., 2004; Kabatereine et al., 2007). As consequence of the increase of low-intensity infections, more light infections will be often missed if single stool samples are examined by Kato–Katz method, resulting in high underestimation rates. Therefore, there is a need to develop and

validate more sensitive diagnostic tools for accurate surveillance and monitoring of schistosomiasis and STH control programmes, and for monitoring of drug efficacy. Some studies recommended multiple stool samples in order to avoid underestimating the 'true' prevalence and transmission potential of schistosomiasis and STH infections. Indeed, it was demonstrated that Kato–Katz examination of 3 instead of 1 stool specimen increased the sensitivity of helminth diagnosis, most notably for hookworm (Steinmann et al., 2008; Knopp et al., 2008) and intestinal schistosomiasis (De Vlas and Gryseels, 1992; Lin et al., 2008). Recent studies suggested that urine circulating cathodic antigen (CCA) assays maybe an appropriate test for the diagnosis of S. mansoni in moderate transmission zones (Shane et al., 2011; Stothard et al., 2011; Tchuem Tchuenté et al., 2012). Several alternative stool examination techniques have been tested for the detection of STH infections. FLOTAC, a new technique mainly used in the veterinary field, was suggested as a suitable diagnostic tool particularly in situations of low parasite infection intensities (Cringoli, 2006). Recent studies found that a single FLOTAC examination was more sensitive than triplicate Kato–Katz thick smears for the diagnosis of low-intensity STH infections (Knopp et al., 2009). In particular, the FLOTAC technique improves the ability to diagnose human hookworm infections accurately (Utzinger et al., 2008), which is generally underestimated when using Kato–Katz thick smears due to a rapid disintegration of hookworm eggs and the constraint to read the slides very shortly (within 30 min) after preparation (Dacombe et al., 2007). FLOTAC was thus suggested as a suitable method for a rigorous surveillance of helminth control programmes, monitoring of STH transmission and verification of local elimination (Knopp et al., 2009). McMaster, another flotation technique commonly used in veterinary parasitology, is an alternative diagnostic tool. The results of a comparative study of four techniques, i.e. ether-based concentration, Parasep Solvent Free, McMaster and FLOTAC, showed that despite the fact that McMaster was less sensitive than FLOTAC, the former technique was the most feasible and easy to perform under field conditions. McMaster appeared as a promising technique of choice when using fecal egg counts for monitoring of drug efficacy against STHs (Levecke et al., 2009). Overall, several techniques are available for the detection of STH infections, with significant difference in the cost, sensitivity, simplicity and field applicability. Though a true 'gold standard' test with 100% accuracy does not exist, Kato–Katz thick smears is so far commonly and widely used as the basic and 'default' technique for helminth epidemiology, despite some limitations.

Further efforts should be made to validate other detection tools (Tchuem Tchuenté, 2011). The choice of a specific diagnostic assay should be governed by the objective of the activity, and according to the stage of helminth control (Berquist et al., 2009). As the accuracy of a given diagnostic technique may vary significantly according to helminth transmission level, tools should be adapted when moving from morbidity control to elimination of infection. Moving toward the surveillance and elimination phases requires more sensitive techniques such as antibody detection. However, sero-diagnostic tools for detection of helminth infections require blood sample collection (invasive), access to affordable, high-quality reagents; which are important limiting factors for their integration into large-scale national control programmes. These are probably some of the reasons why today only a few countries have adopted antibody detection as a key strategy in helminth diagnosis (Berquist et al., 2009).

4.10 New paradigm shift: Moving from control to elimination

In the past years, the costs of PZQ and the lack of resources were major constraints for the control of schistosomiasis. Today, there exists new impetus for the control, with increasing funding opportunity and donated PZQ by pharmaceutical companies. Therefore, there is an opportuny to take up the challenge, to be more ambitious and to move from control to elimination where feasible. To do this there is a need to adapt the current threshold for intervention (i.e. prevalence > 10%) and to carefully define the implementation unit for PZQ mass administration. Treatment algorithms should be re-defined based on current knowledge and experiences.

5. Conclusion

During the past several decades, many attempts have been made to control schistosomiasis, STH and other NTDs. Important advances have been made such as the development of praziquantel, albendazole and mebendazole, the current drugs of choice for these NTDs, which amplified treatment possibilities to the majority of people who need it. Although few control successes were achieved, the global objective is long way off and these diseases remain important public health problems in developing countries. Fulfilling the mandate of the World Health Assembly resolution 54.19 will require the regular treatment of hundreds of millions of children over decades. A successful control of schistosomiasis and STHs across the endemic regions calls for strengthening health system and interventions, ensuring access to anthelminthic drugs in all health services, co-implementation and the coordinated use of the different anthelminthic drugs, promotion of access to safe water, adequate sanitation and health education, and mobilization of resources to sustain control activities. The challenge also includes an improvement of drug efficacy for a much better rapid impact. Indeed, the low cure rate of the recommended drugs for STH, at the single dose as commonly used, highlights the need for an alternative strategy based either on a multiple-days treatment regimen, an alternating use of albendazole and mebendazole from one deworming round to another, or the use of an alternative drug. A multiple day treatment would obviously increase the costs, but the immediate and long-term benefits would be priceless. Today, there exist new impetus to global helminth control and a series of favourable factors for implementing successful control programmes. There are several and increasing funding opportunities, and we have a great opportunity to properly take up the challenge and relieve poor communities from disease burden that jeopardise their development. There is an urgent need for well co-ordinated and transparent use of multisource funds to increase efficiency and to avoid duplication of efforts. We should act cautiously and address the dilemma between costs and efficacy of interventions, and between control and elimination. Time is right to act more ambitiously and to set the agenda for schistosmiasis and STH elimination.

6. Acknowledgements

The author gratefully acknowledges all partners and stakeholders who contribute towards the successful control of schistosomiasis and STH in Cameroon.

7. References

Amazigo, U.V., Obono, O.M., Dadzie, K.Y., Remme, J., Jiya, J., Ndyomugyenyi, R., Roungou, J.B., Noma, M., Sékétéli, A. (2002). Monitoring community-directed treatment programmes for sustainability: lessons from the African Programme for Onchocerciasis Control (APOC). *Ann. Trop. Med. Parasitol.* 96 (Suppl. 1), S75–S92.

Anderson, R.M. (1982). Population Dynamics of Infectious Diseases: *Theory and Applications*. Chapman and Hall, London, United Kingdom, 377 pp.

Awasthi, S., Bundy, D.A., Savioli, L. (2003). Helminth infections. *British Medical Journal* 327, 431-433.

Berquist, R., Johansen, M.V., Utzinger, J. (2009). Diagnostic dilemmas in helminthology: what tools to use and when? *Trends Parasitol.* 25, 151-156.

Bethony, J., Brooker, S., Albonico, M., Geiger, S.M., Loukas, A., Diemert, D., Hotez, P.J. (2006). Soil-transmitted helminth infections: ascariasis, trichuriasis, and hookworm. *Lancet* 367, 1521-1532.

Bethony, J., Chen, J., Lin, S., Xiao, S., Zhan, B., Li, S., Xue, H., Xing, F., Humphries, D., Yan, W., Chen, G., Foster, V., Hawdon, J.M., Hotez, P.J. (2002). Emerging patterns of hookworm infection: influence of aging on the intensity of Necator infection in Hainan Province, People's Republic of China. *Clin. Infect. Dis.* 35, 1336-1344.

Booth, M., Vounatsou, P., N'Goran, E.K., Tanner, M., Utzinger, J. (2003). The influence of sampling effort and the performance of the Kato-Katz technique in diagnosing *Schistosoma mansoni* and hookworm co-infections in rural Côte d'Ivoire. *Parasitology* 127, 525-531.

Brooker, S., Clements, A.C.A., Bundy, D.A.P. (2006). Global epidemiology, ecology and control of soil-transmitted helminth infections. *Advance in Parasitology* 62, 221-261.

Brooker, S., Donnelly, C.A. and Guyatt, H.L. (2000). Estimating the number of helminthic infections in the Republic of Cameroon from data on infection prevalence in schoolchildren. *Bulletin of the World Health Organization* 78, 1456-1465.

Brooker, S., Kabatereine, N.B., Smith, J.L., Mupfasoni, D., Mwanje, M.T., Ndayishimiye, O., Lwambo, N.J.S., Mbotha, D., Karanja, P., Mwandawiro, C., Muchiri, E., Clements, A.C.A., Bundy, D.A.P., Snow, R.W. (2009). An updated of human helminth infections: the example of East Africa. *Int. J. Health Geogr.* 8, 42.

Cringoli, G. (2006). FLOTAC, a novel apparatus for a multivalent faecal egg count technique. *Parasitologia* 48, 381-384.

Crompton, D.W., Savioli, L. (1993). Intestinal Parasitic Infections and Urbanization. *Bull. World Health Organ.* 71, 1-7.

Crompton, D.W.T., Nesheim, M.C. (2002). Nutritional impact of intestinal helminthiasis during the human life cycle. *Ann. Rev. Nutr.* 22, 35-59.

Dacombe, R.J., Crampin, A.C., Floyd, S., Randall, A., Ndhlovu, R., Bickle, Q., Fine, P.E.M. (2007). Time delays between patient and laboratory selectively affect accuracy of helminth diagnosis. *Trans. R. Soc. Trop. Med. Hyg.* 101, 140-145.

De Vlas S.J., Gryseels B. (1992). Underestimation of *Schistosoma mansoni* prevalences. *Parasitology Today* 8: 274-277.

Fenwick, A., Webster, J.P., Bosque-Oliva, E., Blair, L., Fleming, F.M., Zhang, Y., Garba, A., Stothard, J.R., Gabrielli, A.F., Clements, A.C.A., Kabatereine, N.B., Toure, S., Denbele, R., Nyandindi, U., Mwansa, J., Koukounari, A. (2009). The Schistosomiasis Control Initiative (SCI): rationale, development and implementation from 2002-2008. *Parasitology* 136, 1719-1730.

Fleming, F.M., Brooker, S., Geiger, S.M., Caldas, I.R., Correa-Oliveira, R., Hotez, P.J., Bethony, J.M. (2006). Synergistic associations between hookworm and other helminth species in a rural community in Brazil. *Trop. Med. Int. Health* 11, 56-64.

Forrester, J.E., Scott, M.E., Bundy, D.A., Golden, M.H. (1988). Clustering of *Ascaris lumbricoides* and *Trichuris trichiura* infections within households. *Trans. R. Soc. Trop. Med. Hyg.* 82, 282–288.

Forrester, J.E., Scott, M.E., Bundy, D.A.P., Golden, M.H.N. (1990). Predisposition of individuals and families in Mexico to heavy infection with *Ascaris lumbricoides* and *Trichuris trichiura*. *Trans. R. Soc. Trop. Med. Hyg.* 84, 272–276.

Garba, A., Touré, S., Dembelé, R., Boisier, P., Tohon, Z., Bosqué-Oliva, E., Koukounari, A., Fenwick, A. (2009). Present and future schistosomiasis control activities with support from the Schistosomiasis Control Initiative in West Africa. *Parasitology* 136, 1731–1737.

Gilles, H. (1996). Soil-transmitted helminths (geohelminths). In: *Tropical Diseases*. Cook, G. (Ed.), Manson's. W.B. Saunders, London, United Kingdom, pp. 1369–1412.

Hall, A. (1981). Quantitative variability of nematode egg counts in faeces: a study among rural Kenyans. *Trans. R. Soc. Trop. Med. Hyg.* 75, 682–687.

Horton, J., Witt, C., Ottensen, E.A., Lazdins, J.K., Addiss, D.G., Awadzi, K., Beach, M.J., Belizario, V.Y., Dunyo, S.K., Espinel, M., Gyapong, J.O., Hossain, M., Ismail, M.M., Jayakody, R.L., Lammie, P.J., Makunde, W., Richard-Lenoble, D., Selve, B., Shenoy, R.K., Simonsen, P.E., Wamae, C.N., Weerasooriya, M.V. (2000). An analysis of the safety of single dose, two drug regimens used in programmes to eliminate lymphatic filariasis. *Parasitology* 121, S147–S160.

Hotez, P.J., Brindley, P.J., Bethony, J.M., King, C.H., Pearce, E.J., Jacobson, J. (2008). Helminth infections: the great neglected tropical diseases. *The Journal of Clinical Investigation* 118, 1311-1321.

Hotez, P.J., Bundy, D.A.P., Beegle, K., Brooker, S., de Silva, N., Montresor, A., Engels, D., Drake, L., Chitsulo, L., Michaud, C., Bethony, J.M., Oliveira, R., Xiao, S.H., Fenwick, A., Savioli, L. (2006). Helminth infections: soil-transmitted helminth infections and schistosomiasis. In: *Disease Control Pririoties in Developing Countries*, 2nd Edition. D. Jamison, M. Claeson, J. Breman and A. Meacham, eds. New York: Oxford University Press.

Hotez, P.J., Fenwick, A., Savioli, L., Molyneux, D.H. (2009). Rescuing the bottom billion through control of neglected tropical diseases. *Lancet* 373, 1570-1575.

Hotez, P.J., Molyneux, D.H., Fenwick, A., Kumaresan, J., Ehrlich Sachs, S., Sachs, J.D., Savioli, L. (2007). Control of neglected tropical diseases. *N. Engl. J. Med.* 357, 1018–1027.

Hotez, P.J., Engels, D., Fenwick, A., Savioli, L. (2010). Africa is desperate for praziquantel. *Lancet*, 376: 496–498.

Kabatereine, N.B., Brooker, S., Koukounari, A., Kazibwe, F., Tukahebwa, E.M., Fleming, F.M., Zhang, Y.B., Webster, J.P., Stothard, J.R., Fenwick, A. (2007). Impact of a national helminth control programme on infection and morbidity in Ugandan schoolchildren. *Bull. World Health Organ.* 85, 91–99.

Katz, N., Chaves, A., Pelligrino, J. (1972). A simple device for quantitative stool thicksmear technique in schistosomiasis mansoni. *Rev. Inst. Med. Trop. Sao Paulo* 14, 397–400.

Knopp, S., Mgeni, A.F., Khamis, I.S., Steinmann, P., Stothard, J.R., Rollinson, D., Marti, H., Utzinger, J. (2008). Diagnosis of soil-transmitted helminths in the era of preventive chemotherapy: effect of multiple stool sampling and use of different diagnostic techniques. *PLoS Negl. Trop. Dis.* 2, e331.

Knopp, S., Rinaldi, L., Khamis, I.S., Stothard, J.R., Rollinson, D., Maurelli, M.P., Steinmann, P., Marti, H., Cringoli, G., Utzinger, J. (2009). A single FLOTAC is more sensitive than triplicate Kato-Katz for the diagnosis of low-intensity soil-transmitted helminth infections. *Trans. R. Soc. Trop. Med. Hyg.* 103, 347–354.

Levecke, B., De Wilde, N., Vandenhoute, E., Vercruysse, J. (2009). Field validity and feasibility of four techniques for the detection of Trichuris in Simians: a model for monitoring drug efficacy in public health? *PLoS Negl. Trop. Dis.* 3, e366.

Lin D.D., Liu J.X., Liu Y.M., Hu F., Zhang Y.Y., et al. (2008). Routine Kato-Katz technique underestimates the prevalence of *Schistosoma japonicum*: a case study in an endemic area of the People's Republic of China. *Parasit. Int.* 57, 281-286.

Linehan, M., Hanson, C., Weaver, A., Baker, M., Kabore, A., Zoerhoff, K.L.; Sankara, D., Torres, S., Ottensen, E. (2011). Integrated implementation of programs targeting naglected tropical diseases through preventive chemotherapy: proving the feasibility at national scale. *American Journal of Tropical Medicine and Hygiene*, 84, 1: 5-14.

Miguel, E., Kremer, M. (2004). Worms: Identifying impacts on education and health in the presence of treatment externalities. *Econometrica* 72, 159–217.

Minsante (2005). Programme National de Lutte contre la Schistosomiase et les Helminthiases Intestinales: Plan stratégique 2005-2010. Ministère de la Santé Publique, Cameroun.

Mohammed, K.A., Haji, H.J., Gabrielli, A.F., Mubila, L., Biswas, G., Chitsulo, L., Bradley, M.H., Engels, D., Savioli, L., Molyneux, D.H. (2008). Triple co-administration of ivermectin, albendazole and praziquantel in Zanzibar: a safety study. *PLoS Negl. Trop. Dis.* 2 (1), e171.

Molyneux, D. H., Hotez, P., Fenwick, A. (2005). Rapid impact interventions: how a policy of integrated control for Africa's neglected tropical diseases could benefit the poor. *PLoS Medicine* 2, 1064–1070.

Molyneux, D.H., Hotez, P.J., Fenwick, A. (2005). Rapid impact interventions: how a policy of integrated control for Africa's neglected tropical diseases could benefit the poor. *PLoS Medecine* 2, 1064-1070.

Montresor, A., Crompton, D.W.T., Hall, A., Bundy, D.A.P., Savioli, L. (1998). Guidelines for the Evaluation of Soil-transmitted Helminthiasis and Schistosomiasis at Community Level: A Guide for Managers of Control Programmes. *World Health Organization*, Geneva.

Odogwu, S.E., Ramamurthy, N.K., Kabatereine, N.B., Kazibwe, F., Tukahebwa, E.,Webster, J.P., Fenwick, A., Stothard, J.R. (2006). Intestinal schistosomiasis in infants (3 years of age) along the Ugandan shoreline of Lake Victoria. *Ann. Trop. Med. Parasitol.* 100, 315–326.

Olds, G.R., King, C., Hewlett, J., Olveda, R., Wu, G., Ouma, J., Peters, P., McGarvey, S., Odhiambo, O., Koech, D., Liu, C.Y., Aligui, G., Gachihi, G., Kombe, Y., Parraga, I., Ramirez, B., Whalen, C., Horton, R.J., Reeve, P. (1999). Double blind, placebocontrolled study of concurrent administration of albendazole and praziquantel in schoolchildren with schistosomiasis and geohelminths. *J. Infect. Dis.* 179, 996–1003.

Ratard, R. C., Kouemeni, L. E., Ekani Bessala, M. M., Ndamkou, C. N., Greer, G. J., Spilsburg, J., Cline, B. L. (1990). Human schistosomiasis in Cameroon. I.

Distribution of schistosomiasis. *American Journal of Tropical Medicine and Hygiene* 42, 561–572.

Ratard, R. C., Kouemeni, L. E., Ekani Bessala, M. M., Ndamkou, C. N., Sama, M. T., Cline, B. L. (1991). Ascariasis and trichuriasis in Cameroon. *Transactions of the Royal Society of Tropical Medicine and Hygiene* 85, 84–88.

Savioli, L., Albonico, M., Engels, D., Montresor, A. (2004). Progress in the prevention and control of schistosomiasis and soil-transmitted helminthiasis. *Parasitol. Int.* 53, 103–113.

Savioli, L., Gabrielli, A.F., Montresor, A., Chitsulo, L., Engels, D. (2009). Schistosomiasis control in Africa: 8 years after World Health Assembly Resolution 54.19. *Parasitology* 136, 1677–1681.

Sékétéli, A., Adeoye, G., Eyamba, A., Nnoruka, E., Drameh, P., Amazigo, U.V., Noma, M., Agboton, F., Aholou, Y., Kale, O.O., Dadzie, K.Y. (2002). The achievements and challenges of the African Programme for Onchocerciasis Control (APOC). *Ann. Trop. Med. Parasitol.* 96 (Suppl. 1), S15–S28.

Shane H.L.L., Verani J.R., Abudho B., Montgomery S.P., Blackstock A.J., Mwinzi P.N.M., Butler S.E., Karanja D.M.S., Secor W.E. (2011). Evaluation of urine CCA assays for detection of *Schistosoma mansoni* infection in Western Kenya. *PLoS Negl. Trop. Dis.* 5(1): e951. doi:10.1371/journal.pntd.0000951.

Sousa-Figueiredo, J.C., Basanez, M.G., Mgeni, A.F., Khamis, I.S., Rollinson, D., Stothard, J.R. (2008). A parasitological survey, in rural Zanzibar, of pre-school children and their mothers for urinary schistosomiasis, soil-transmitted helminthiases and malaria, with observations on the prevalence of anaemia. *Ann. Trop. Med. Parasitol.* 102, 679–692.

Steinmann, P., Du, Z.W., Wang, L.B., Wang, X.Z., Jiang, J.Y., Li, L.H., Marti, H., Zhou, X.N., Utzinger, J. (2008). Extensive multiparasitism in a village of Yunnan Province, People's Republic of China, revealed by a suite of diagnostic methods. *Am. J. Trop. Med. Hyg.* 78, 760–769.

Steinmann, P., Keiser, J., Bos, R., Tanner, M., Utzinger, J. (2006). Schistosomiasis and water resources development: systematic review, meta-analysis, and estimates of people at risk. *Lancet Infectious Diseases* 6, 411-425.

Stephenson, L.S., Latham, M.C., Ottesen, E.A. (2000). Malnutrition and Parasitic Helminth Infections. *Parasitology* 121 (Suppl.), S23–28.

Stothard, J.R., Imison, E., French, M.D., Sousa-Figueiredo, J.C., Khamis, I.S., Rollinson, D. (2008). Soil-transmitted helminthiasis among mothers and their pre-school children on unguja island, zanzibar with emphasis upon ascariasis. *Parasitology* 135, 1447–1455.

Stothard J.R., Sousa-Figuereido J.C., Betson M., Adriko M., Arinaitwe M., et al. (2011). *Schistosoma mansoni* infections in young children: when are schistosome antigens in urine, eggs in stool and antibodies to eggs first detectable? *PLoS Negl. Trop. Dis.* 5(1): e938. doi:10.1371/journal.pntd.0000938

Tarafder, M.R., Carabin, H., Joseph, L., Balalong Jr., E., Olveda, R., McGarvey, S.T. (2009). Estimating the sensitivity and specificity of Kato–Katz stool examination technique for detection of hookworms, *Ascaris lumbricoides* and *Trichuris trichiura* infections in humans in the absence of a 'gold standard'. *Int. J. Parasitol.*, doi:10.1016/j.ijpara.2009.09.003.

Tchuem Tchuenté, L.A. (2011). Control of soil-transmitted helminths in sub-Saharan Africa: Diagnosis, drug efficacy concerns and challenges. *Acta Tropica* 120S, S4– S11.

Tchuem Tchuenté, L.A., N'Goran, E.K. (2009). Schistosomiasis and soil-transmitted helminthiasis control in Cameroon and Côte d'Ivoire: implementing control on a limited budget. *Parasitology* 136, 1736-1745.

Tchuem Tchuenté, L.A., Behnke, J.M., Gilbert, F., Southgate, V.R., Vercruysse, J. (2003). Polyparasitism with *Schistosoma haematobium* and soil-transmitted helminth infections among school children in Loum, Cameroon. *Tropical Medicine and International Health* 8, 975–986.

Tchuem Tchuenté, L.A., Kamwa Ngassam, R.I., Sumo, L., Ngassam, P., Dongmo Noumedem, C., Luogbou, D.G.O., Dankoni, E., Kenfack, C.M., Feussom Gipwe, N., Akame, J., Tarini, A., Zhang, Y., Angwafo III, F.F. (2012); Mapping of schistosomiasis and soil-transmitted helminthiasis in the regions of Centre, East and West Cameroon. *PLoS Negl. Trop. Dis.* (in press).

Tchuem Tchuenté L.A., Kueté Fouodo C.J., Kamwa Ngassam R.I., Sumo L., Dongmo Noumedem C., Kenfack C.M., Feussom Gipwe N., Dankoni Nana E., Stothard J.R., Rollinson D. (2012). Evaluation of circulating cathodic antigen (CCA) urine-tests for diagnosis of *Schistosoma mansoni* infection in Cameroon. *PLoS Negl. Trop. Dis.* (in press).

Utzinger, J., Rinaldi, L., Lohourignon, L.K., Rohner, F., Zimmermann, M.B., Tschannen, A.B., N'Goran, E.K., Cringoli, G. (2008). FLOTAC: a new sensitive technique for the diagnosis of hookworm infections in humans. *Trans. R. Soc. Trop. Med. Hyg.* 102, 84–90.

World Health Organization (2002). Prevention and control of schistosomiasis and soil-transmitted helminthiasis. Report of a WHO Expert Committee. WHO *Technical Report Series* No. 912. World Health Organization, Geneva.

World Health Organization (2006). Preventive chemotherapy in human helminthiasis: coordinated use of anthelminthic drugs in control interventions : a manual for health professionals and programme managers. World Health Organization Press, Geneva.

World Health Organization (2010). Soil-transmitted helminthiasis: number of children treated 2007-2008: update on the 2010 global target. *Weekly Epidemiological Record* 16, 85: 141-148.

World Health Organization (2011). Schistosomiasis: number of people treated, 2009. *Weekly Epidemiological Record* 9, 86: 73-80.

World Health Organization (2012). Schistosomiasis: population requiring preventive chemotherapy and number of people treated in 2010. *Weekly Epidemiological Record* 4, 87: 37–44.

World Health Organization (1991). Basic Laboratory Methods in Medical Parasitology. World Health Organization, Geneva.

13

Molecular Diagnosis and Monitoring of Benzimidazole Susceptibility of Human Filariids

Adisak Bhumiratana[1,2,3], Apiradee Intarapuk[3], Danai Sangthong[3],
Surachart Koyadun[4], Prapassorn Pechgit[1] and Jinrapa Pothikasikorn[5]
[1]*Department of Parasitology and Entomology, Faculty of Public Health,*
Mahidol University, Bangkok
[2]*Center for EcoHealth Disease Modeling and Intervention Development Research,*
Faculty of Public Health, Mahidol University, Bangkok
[3]*Environmental Pathogen Molecular Biology and Epidemiology Research Unit,*
Faculty of Veterinary Medicine, Mahanakorn University of Technology, Bangkok
[4]*Ministry of Public Health, Department of Disease Control, Office of*
Disease Prevention and Control 11 Nakhon Si Thammarat
[5]*Department of Microbiology, Faculty of Science, Mahidol University, Bangkok*
Thailand

1. Introduction

Lymphatic filarial nematode parasites, mainly *Wuchereria bancrofti* and *Brugia malayi,* are causing agents of lymphatic filariasis in humans, which can be effectively treated with antifilarial drugs including diethylcarbamazine (DEC) and ivermectin. Albendazole, an effective benzimidazole compound, acts as a board-spectrum anthelminthic drug, and when combined with either one of antifilarial drugs, it exerts synergistic effects on reduction of peripheral microfilaremia in lymphatic filariasis cases. However, the varying parasite infection levels in those treated with DEC or ivermectin alone or in combination with albendazole are due to differences in drug responses. The additional clearance of infection with albendazole relative to what is observed with DEC or ivermectin alone suggests that albendazole has different parasite target(s). The homologous *β-tubulin* gene of human and veterinary filariids that β-tubulin homologs have conserved domains structurally related to other orthologs among the nematodes, cestodes, trematodes and vertebrate hosts, is responsible for benzimidazole susceptibility. The genetic inheritance of resistance in nematode parasites can undergo under selection of benzimidazole compounds in a way that albendazole resistance mechanism involves one of two single amino acid substitutions from phenylalanine to tyrosine in parasite β-tubulin at position 167 or 200. This genetically-stable marker has shown promise for molecular diagnosis and monitoring of *W. bancrofti* infections that carry responsible genotypes associated with benzimidazole susceptibility or resistance. In particular, this approach can augment the surveillance and monitoring of mass treatment impacts on the parasite populations in target areas where long-running elimination programs for lymphatic filariasis are implemented at a large-scale by using a regionally-adopted combination therapy with antifilarial drugs, recommended by the World Health Organization.

2. Lymphatic filariasis towards elimination

2.1 Factors that favor elimination

Lymphatic filariasis (LF) is a mosquito-borne parasitic disease caused by three main species of thread-like filarial nematode parasites belonging to the superfamily Filarioidea, which are *Wuchereria bancrofti* and *Brugia malayi*, and lesser extent by *Brugia timori*. These endoparasitic nematode lifestyles have a highly conservative life-cycle development sequence in which they develop their metamorphosis in both human and mosquito (Fig. 1). The adult worms that cause clinical manifestations of the disease are dioecious. Male and female worms have separate reproductive system in their pseudocoelomatic body cavity and they live in the

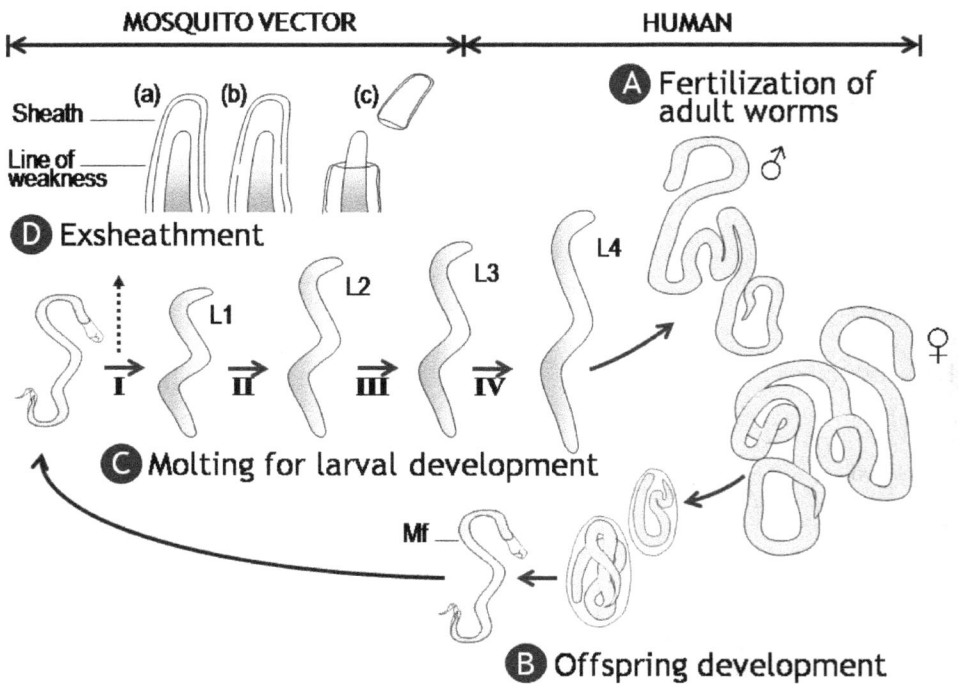

Fig. 1. A development sequence of filarial nematode parasite in human and mosquito (A-D). After the induction of L3 infection in susceptible human host, the mature filarial female worm (A) that possesses fecundicity and fertilization can produce microfilariae (Mf). These offsprings develop from fertilized eggs (B) in the uterus of female worm. They are ingested during the bite of mosquito vector, and consequently, a 5-stage molting progression (B) initially starts after exsheatment of the Mf in mosquito's midgut (C). In this regard, the probable mechanisms involve: (a) proposed anterior of line of weakness, (b) internal digestion of the sheath, and (c) exsheatment of anterior end. Third stage larvae (L3) possess post-infective stage development in mosquito thoracic muscle and then migrate to the proboscis. They are transmitted by infective mosquito during a blood meal, and that they become the L4 (or L5) and mature adult worms in the lymphatic system in human.

human lymphatic system, i.e., lymphatic vessels, with 5-15 years of life expectancy (Table 1). Only when its fecundic lifespan is capable of mating does the lymphatic-dwelling female worm produce advanced stage of sheathed larvae called "microfilariae". These short-living offsprings then penetrate the blood circulation. For a complete life cycle, the microfilariae are ingested by susceptible female mosquito during a blood meal in which they can develop further into larval stages L1-L2 to infective L3 stage. Transmission occurs when the infected mosquito transmits this L3 stage to susceptible persons during other blood meals. The naturally acquired transmission is associated with both intrinsic and extrinsic factors that can regulate the parasitic worm burdens in an endemic population (Fig. 2).

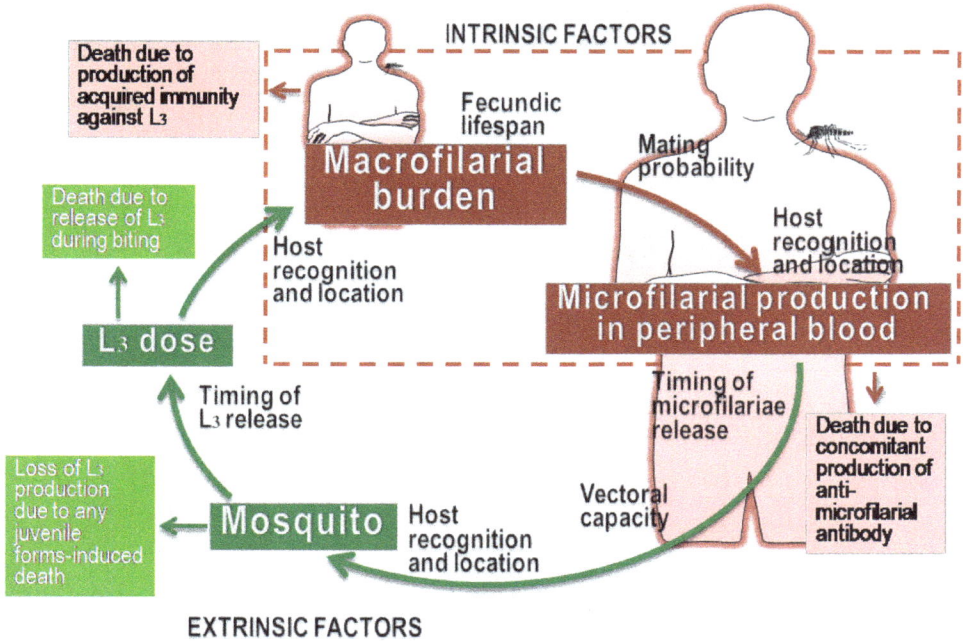

Fig. 2. An explanatory model of human-parasite-vector interactions and favorable factors that influence its adaptation in hosts. The lymphatic filarial infections in humans depend on extrinsic factors of incoming L3 inocula and host recognition and location, and a proportion of adult worms with fecundicity and mating probability. Transmission is influenced by host-vector combination (host location and recognition of mosquito feeding habits), microfilarial loads in blood with timing of microfilariae release, and vectoral capacity (longevity and low refractoriness). Long lifespan of the mosquito and timing of L3 release are favorable factors of transmission.

As such, understanding of how these filarial nematode parasites can be removed from the human hemisphere is to understand basically the biology of their life cycle. How do the parasite taxa succeed their complete life cycle in the certain conditions under which they evoke host exploitation strategies? The biology of the parasitic symbionts can disclosure the parasite diversity and fitness shaped by hosts and environmental constraints that the parasites can evolve the adaptation, i.e., the ability to control the physiology and behavior of their host for their own benefit. It has been known so far their distribution among hosts and strategies of host exploitation are restricted in number of host species. The *W. bancrofti*, which is highly host-specific parasite, is sessile to human while other zoonotic *Brugia* taxa exploit other non-human reservoir hosts. This host-specificity variation does not account for the origin of the parasitism as they succeed their parasitism and share common transmission pattern and complex life cycle in vertebrate hosts and arthropods. The geographical variation, on the other hand, can be restrained by selective pressures from the hosts, or the physio-chemical environments such as therapeutic agents and insecticides, or due to phylogenetic constraints. Such this selection can be explained by the experimental infections, mainly using *Brugia* species in rodents (e.g., jirds, hamsters, rats and mice), dogs, ferrets, cats and monkeys. All of which were proposed not just for understanding vertebrate immunology, pathology and chemotherapy, but also for exploring the interactions of the parasite and host. Among these host-parasite systems, *B. pahangi* that infects naturally cats in the Southeast Asia is experimentally appropriate for studies of infection and disease dynamics (Table 1).

Parameter	Cat	Human
Parasite	*Brugia pahangi*	*Wuchereria bancrofti* *B. malayi, B. timori*
Longevity (years)	7-8	5-15
Mature female worm length (cm)	3-7	5-10
Location of :		
Adult	Lymphatics	Lymphatics
Microfilariae	Blood	Blood
Vector	Mosquito	Mosquito
Typical infection/disease sequlae[a]	Infection – Loss of infection – Pathology	Infection – Loss of infection – Pathology

[a]For both host-parasite systems, infection patterns encapsulate a spectrum ranging from asymptomatic persistent microfilaremia to symptomatic amicrofilaremia or complete refractoriness to infection. Adapted from Grenfell et al (1991).

Table 1. Correlation between feline and human lymphatic filariasis

Because of their conservation of complex life-cycle development between feline and human lymphatic filarial parasites, it induces the infection and clinical sequelae in susceptible cats, and hence, resembles that of *Brugia* and *Wuchereria* in humans. However, the parasite does not always succeed their population diversity by increasing its fitness in the hosts (Fig. 2). Its population dynamic is primarily influenced by naturally acquired immunity (i.e., a type of concomitant immunity), which plays a significant role in host selection pressure to restrict a parasitic worm burden (Bundy et al, 1991; Grenfell et al, 1991; Mitchell, 1991; Grenfell and Micheal, 1992). This immunity against incoming L3 cannot remove them from the infection in humans but restrict a number of L3 by a production of concomitant immunity. Variability of adult worm burden results in a proportion of microfilaremic and amicrofilaremic persons in the population. The circulating microfilariae have short life cycle in human blood circulation; a proportion of the microfilariae can be removed by anti-microfilarial antibody

(Simonsen et al, 1996; 2008; Ravindran et al, 2003). They develop two molts (L1 and L2) and induce the infection in susceptible mosquito vectors while the infected mosquitoes can regulate melanization involved in innate immune defense and wound healing to the penetration of filarial nematodes (Zou et al, 2010; Castillo et al, 2011). In blood-engorged mosquitoes that harbor high microfilarial density, they can induce death due to the vector intolerance against development of juvenile forms, and consequently, this leads to loss of L3. Furthermore, release of the L3 does not always permit a passage at an equal number during other blood meal taken by the infective mosquito due to the vector tolerance. Thus, they are naturally killed by host immune, vector barrier, and physical environment; these contributing factors can favor the LF elimination in humans.

As was, LF becomes one of six potentially eradicable diseases of which the criteria for assessing their eradicability (CDC, 1993) are based not only on the scientific feasibility of understanding the biological information mentioned earlier and practical use of the public health interventions and other methods to be applied or used in existing national control program, but also on the political will or popular support of executing the implementation of LF control strategies. First, the scientific feasibility depends basically on the disease vulnerability. Unlike the *W. bancrofti* that exists only in humans, the *B. malayi* spends an enzoonotic life-cycle in which the parasite is transmitted by the potent mosquito and thrive in domestic cats as non-human reservoir, and a *per se* epizoonotic cycle in which the parasite is transmitted and thrive through which the mosquito vector takes blood meal from infected cats, and subsequently, transmit the infective stage to humans during other blood meal. Controversially, the humans carrying *B. malayi* infection can serve as a source for the infection to permit a passage to the animal reservoir through bites of the mosquito vector. Nonetheless, both diseases do not always ease their spread into the population as a result of the naturally-induced immunity and duration of microfilarial production in susceptible individuals or communities (Maizels and Lawrence, 1991; Ottesen, 1992) (Fig. 2). More important, the infections can be both easily diagnosed using advanced tools and effectively treated with the antifilarial drugs that are safe, inexpensive and easily deployed. The feasibility of elimination has been shown that the operation of the pragmatic diagnostic methods or interventions is demonstrable at a large scale in the target populations. Last, the political will/popular support is pivotal for the program manager to capture information required to analyze situations of the perceived burden of LF that is figured out by a large number of suffering and disabled persons worldwide (WHO, 2002; 2008; 2010): the details are available at the websites of the Global Program to Eliminate Lymphatic Filariasis (GPELF) (http://www.who.int/lymphatic_filariasis/disease/en/) and Global Alliance to Eliminate Lymphatic Filariasis (http://www.filariasis.org). Also, the National Program to Eliminate Lymphatic Filariasis (PELF) by which the resource mobilization and funding structure are administered must be allied, by adopting the GPELF's strategies, to practical considerations of interventions, methods, logistic supplies (medical and field-work), delivery processes, expenditures (unit costs and cost-effectiveness), integration of control activities into existing health systems services (or other health development programs), socio-economic impacts on gaining health benefits, community awareness and acceptance, and ecological disturbances to target disease, non-target disease and the environment. For the resource-limited countries as allied nations, a national budget plan that notifies outsources and fund raising needs the subsidy of the internationally collaborative program.

2.2 Mass chemotherapy as elimination strategy

Ideally, the success of controlling the disease depends definitely on the objectives and ultimate goals of disease control spectrum (CDC, 1993); with this regard, the rational management of LF elimination differs with control (Table 2). As recommended by the World Health Organization (WHO), two pillars of global elimination strategies emphasize interruption of transmission and elimination of the infection in humans, and the other large-scale morbidity control to prevent disease and disability (WHO, 1999a; 2002; 2008; 2010). Principle outcomes of the GPELF reduce numbers of microfilaremic persons and disease cases as preventing new infection introduced among the population at risk of, or affected with, the infection. To meet this criteria, the GPELF proposes a mainstay of elimination strategy effectively available for mass drug administration (MDA) in target population; a combined treatment with diethylcarbamzine citrate (DEC) 6 mg/kg plus 400 mg albendazole (in *W. bancrofti* transmssion areas where *Onchocerca volvulus* is not coendemic), or with 200 µg ivermectin plus 400 mg albendazole (in *W. bancrofti* transmssion areas where *O. volvulus* is coendemic) (Ottesen et al, 1997; 1999; Ottesen, 2000; WHO, 1999a; 2000; 2001; 2002). An annual MDA with coverage of 60-80% for 4-5 years is considered to be effective enough to interrupt transmission in control areas in the absence of vector control (Gyapong et al, 2005). Also, new options for mass treatment of at risk population are effectively available: DEC-fortified salt for 1 year; and a combination of single annual dose of albendazole plus DEC, followed by DEC-fortified salt (Weaver et al, 2011). The ample supply and distribution of DEC-fortified salt can be administered in some countries.

2.3 Surveillance and monitoring systems

As for presenting dynamics of the infection and disease in nature (Grenfell et al, 1991; Srividya et al, 1991; Ottesen, 1992; Meyrowitsch et al, 1995), the parasites cause a wide spectrum of clinical manifestations in the affected population that are characterized by asymptomatic microfilaremia, acute lymphatic inflammation and chronic lymphatic pathology (WHO, 1992a; 1992b; 1994). Susceptible persons develop clinically LF as a result of prolonged exposure to multiple infective bites of potent mosquitoes from several months to years. On the other hand, the people living for at least 6 months are at the greatest risk for the infection. The chronic filariasis cases represent a tip of the iceberg, as microfilaremic carriers are the reservoir of the infection to others. The prevalence and intensity of the infection in humans depends mainly upon a number of microfilaremic persons and a geometric mean of microfilarial loads in the affected population. These proximate measures are indicative of the degrees of endemicity. The prevalence and geographical distribution of the disease are important not just for determination of its potential transmission in mosquito, but also for diagnosis and surveillance in different endemic settings. Therefore, the recognition of what is the filarial origin of the disease and where the affected individuals or communities are is fundamental for public health importance to identify the solution and control rationale. Diagnostic approaches that emphasize the detection and specific identification of microfilaremic infection in the individual by using most standard microscopic methods are important component of LF control program, which is aimed to reduce number of microfilaremic persons. The suitable blood collection and microscopic diagnosis in health settings can be effectively available to identify anyone infected, and subsequently, treated with antifilarial drug regimens. However, this specific objective of control is less important as the elimination is desired not just to interrupt transmission and clear human infection on a large-scale, but also to reduce the morbidity attributed to the disease and hence improve both personal-focused hygiene and health care to all beneficiaries in target population at risk (Table 2).

	Control	Elimination
1. Definition	- Reduction of microfilaremia prevalence	- Reduction of microfilaremia prevalence as arbitrarily qualitative or quantitative level of control as no longer a public health problem
2. Outcome indicators as options for monitoring tools	- Annual infection prevalence; microfilaremia rate (a microfilaremic number surveyed in endemic population) - Disease rate (a number of disease cases surveyed in endemic population) - Annual transmission potential (ATP) (i.e., a number of infective bite per annum which acquire the infection) as mosquito infection rate is not useful indicator	- Degrees to which transmission is interrupted; microfilaremia rate mosquito infection rate and antigenemia rate - Disease rate is not useful indicator
2.1 Objective	- **To assess whether the control program achieves its goals or desired outcomes** (e.g., reduction in microfilaremia and/or disease prevalence)	- **To assess whether the elimination program achieves its goals or desired outcomes**[†] (e.g., reduction in microfilaremia prevalence, antigenemia prevalence)
3. Process indicators as options for monitoring and evaluation tools	- Coverage of selective treatment and follow-up, as mosquito net utilization, insecticide spraying and reservoir control can be useful indicators	- Mass treatment coverage, drug compliance coverage (e.g., adverse drug reactions prevalence and severe adverse event reports), KAP survey
3.1 Objective	- **To assess how well the various components of the control program are functioning** (e.g., the number of newly and follow-up microfilaremic persons treated with antifilarial drugs)	- **To assess how well the various components of the elimination program are functioning**[‡] (e.g., the number of new infections, the number of drug tablets distributed)

Adapted from the GPELF (http://www.who.int/lymphatic_filariasis/disease/en/).
†,‡Outcome indicators can be optionally used for monitoring systems; longitudinal surveillance of populations in sentinel sites, cross-sectional "spot checks" in other sites, and auxiliary "background" surveillance.
KAP - Knowledge, attitudes and practices.

Table 2. Rational approaches to lymphatic filariasis control and elimination

Tools	Advantages for the applications	Chief obstacles when applied or used in demonstrated areas	References
ICT Filariasis	• Simple-to-use rapid diagnostic test kit commercially available for use in qualitative detection of *W. bancrofti* adult worm circulating antigens present in whole blood/serum/plasma samples; stronger positive test line equivalent to higher antigen levels; • Sensitive and specific for anytime-of-day determination of active infection (antigenemic) whether microfilaremia is present, or the treatment is given; • Highly reproducible and practical when lots of large-scale blood samples (100 μl each) are analyzed either under the field conditions by not-well-trained field workers or in laboratory settings (with 100 μl each of serum/plasma samples freshly prepared or frozen) by laboratory personnel in order to assess the human infection rates in areas known as endemic for *W. bancrofti* or respective areas of emergence/reemergence; • Suitable for rapid assessment survey to detect the early infection in endemic carriers including migrants, refugees, any persons who work in endemic areas (mine in rainforest and border) for years, or visitors to the areas; • Suitable to monitor and evaluate the infection in humans inhabiting in risk areas in initial surveillance before MDA; drug responses during MDA; and the new infection in post-MDA areas whether they are certified as eliminated areas	• Costly; • Indicate, but not quantify, the level of the circulating antigens; somehow, provides false-negative identifications with the infections harboring very low antigen titers; • Cannot differentiate the status between infection and disease, occurrence and recurrence, or sensitivity and resistance • Primarily requires standardization and quality control of lots of samples (finger-prick blood) that are collected and analyzed	Weil & Liftis, 1987 Weil et al, 1987; 1996; 1997 Freedman et al, 1997 Ramzy et al, 1999 Bhumiratana et al, 1999; 2002; 2004; 2005 Nguyen et al, 1999 Phantana et al, 1999 Simonsen et al, 1999 Omar et al, 2000 Pani et al, 2000; 2004 Sunish et al, 2002; 2003 Braga et al, 2003 Engelbrecht et al, 2003 Koyadun et al, 2003 Nuchprayoon et al, 2003 Siriaut et al, 2005 Ruberanziza et al, 2009 Foo et al, 2011

Tools	Advantages for the applications	Chief obstacles when applied or used in demonstrated areas	References
Og4C3 ELISA	• Commercially available diagnostic test kit, and principally the same when use in qualitative and quantitative detection of active *W. bancrofti* infection, but more sensitive and specific than the ICT Filariasis; • Highly reproducible when lots of large-scale serum/plasma samples (100 μl each of freshly prepared or frozen samples) are analyzed in the public health reference laboratory or research institutes in order to assess the human infection rates, and to monitor and evaluate the infection or drug responses in individuals or in the target population under the circumstances described above;	• Costly, labor-intensive and intrusive • Cannot differentiate the status between infection and disease, occurrence and recurrence, or sensitivity and resistance • Primarily requires standardization and quality control of lots of venous blood samples (subsequently prepared for sera or plasma) that are collected, transported, stored and analyzed; • Also requires well-trained field workers and laboratory personnel	More & Copeman, 1990 Turner et al, 1993 Chanteau et al, 1994a; 1994b Lammie et al, 1994 McCarthy et al, 1995 Rocha et al, 1996 Nicolas, 1997 Ismail et al, 1998 Eberhard, 1997 Simonsen and Dunyo, 1999 Nuchprayoon et al, 2003 Bhumiratana et al, 2004; 2005
Polymerase chain reaction (PCR)	• Very highly sensitive and specific for the microfilaremic infections with *W. bancrofti* and *B. malayi* in humans and mosquitoes distinguishable from other filarial nematode parasites such as *O. volvulus, D. immitis, D. repens* and *B. pahangi*; • Highly reproducible and practical when lots of samples as low as 20 μl human blood, individual mosquito (dissected or whole body), or mosquito pool, are analyzed in the public health reference laboratory or research institutes in order to assess the human and	• Too costly, labor-intensive, intrusive, in-house developed tool • Primarily requires standardization and quality control of lots of samples (finger-prick or venous blood, or pooled wild-caught mosquitoes) that are collected, transported, stored and analyzed; • Also requires well-trained field workers or	Chanteau et al, 1994c Lizotte et al, 1994 McCarthy et al, 1996 Siridewa et al, 1996 Williams et al, 1996 Zhong et al, 1996 Ramzy et al, 1997 Nicolas et al, 1999 Cox-singh et al, 2000 Thanomsub et al, 2000 Pradeep Kumar et al, 2002

Tools	Advantages for the applications	Chief obstacles when applied or used in demonstrated areas	References
	mosquito infection rates, and to monitor and evaluate the infections or drug responses in individuals or in the target population under the circumstances described above; • Can differentiate the status between infection (microfilaremia) and disease, occurrence (new infection) and recurrence, or sensitivity and resistance; • Detection limit of as low as one Mf per blood volume tested (up to 1 ml), or one juvenile larva (L1, L2 or L3) per pooled mosquitoes (up to 100)	laboratory personnel and accessory equipments for DNA preparation and analysis of PCR products; • Cannot differentiate larval stages (L1, L2 or L3) in infected mosquitoes	Fischer et al, 2003 Kanjanavas et al, 2005 Nuchprayoon et al, 2005; 2007 Rao et al, 2006 Mishra et al, 2007 WHO, 2009 Bhumiratana et al, 2010 Pechgit et al, 2011 Takagi et al, 2011

Table 3. Direct determination tools for use as part of the Global Program to Eliminate Lymphatic Filariasis

To meet this objective, a large-scale transmission control requires a current magnitude and geographical distribution of the disease in the at-risk population. To understand the extent to which the target population needs to be designed for MDA and monitored whether the MDA implementation is effective, such surveillance and monitoring systems are required. To identify the communities with, or at risk of, the infection, for instance, the direct assessment techniques (Table 3) are required for practical use both in initial surveillance for filarial infection and in monitoring and evaluating the effectiveness of mass treatment, as part of the GPELF (WHO, 1999a; 1999b; Ottesen, 2000). In this regard, the mass treatment with more effective antifilarial drug regimens as well as the availability of other existing and alleviating control measures has been deliberately implemented to meet such these highly achievable objectives of the elimination. Nonetheless, in addition to what is recommended by WHO, the GPELF requires for ground-breaking development of systems, protocols and tools that will be able to be convincingly applied to or routinely used in the PELF to fix undesirable events of mass treatment impacts in different complex epidemiological settings (Kyelem et al, 2008; Ottesen et al, 2008; WHO, 2008; 2010).

3. Parasite infection and drug responsiveness

3.1 Microfilaremia and drug-responsive microfilaremia

In an endemic population that represents the infection and disease dynamics in nature, the asymptomatic microfilaremia is a stage of the active infection with filarial adult worms (Srividya et al, 1991; Meyrowitsch et al, 1995), which regulate host immune responses (hypoimmune responsiveness) in infected individuals (Bundy et al, 1991; Grenfell et al, 1991; Maizels and Lawrence, 1991; Mitchell, 1991; Grenfell and Micheal, 1992; Ottesen, 1992;

Simonsen et al, 1996; 2008; Ravindran et al, 2003). This phenomenon results in immunotolerance, i.e., a prolonged induction of the balance of immune defense to the parasites stimulated by the adult worms, in most asymptomatic microfilaremic persons. The female adult worm involves in regulation of the host microfilaremia. The fecundicity (a period of pregnancy) allows its fertilization to produce a diverse number of the offspring microfilariae. Although the proportion of microfilariae can be removed from the blood circulation in patients, there are the plenty of microfilariae, which circulate in the peripheral blood and show the appearance both nocturnally and diurnally. This microfilarial periodicity or circadian cycle of the parasite in humans is clinically unimportant for treatment but very important for its epidemiologic implication, which plays a significant role in diagnosis, surveillance and epidemiology. The parasite infection is the foundation for the processes that not only determine the infection prevalence but also monitor and evaluate the effectiveness of the treatment with the antifilarial drugs in infected individuals. In this regard, the amount of microfilaremia seems to be a function of naturally-acquired infection loads, which refers to as the most viable microfilariae, and drug-responsive microfilaremia refers to as the affected parasite population that harbors a diverse range of viable and non-viable microfilariae (Pechgit et al, 2011). These outcome indicators are useful for monitoring and evaluating the benzimidazole susceptibility of the filarial nematode parasites in the population in areas of the PELF implementing the MDA 2-drug regimen either albendazole plus DEC or albendazole plus ivermectin.

However, the MDA 2-drug regimen is not the only factor that shapes the parasite population under complex epidemiological settings. Of note, the *W. bancrofti* populations have ability to provoke the genetic variability that shows the important implications in the endemic populations targeted by the MDA (Pradeep Kumar, 2000). The existence of genetic diversity of *W. bancrofti* populations that has greater heterogeneity under DEC therapy and vector control gives rise to questioning about the development of drug resistance in LF, which possibly occurs in the target populations. The selection pressure is an intensity of selection affecting the frequency of genes in a parasite population. The selection that increases or decreases the susceptibility of the parasite population depends on the frequency of the alleles involved. The genetic polymorphism occurring in the *W. bancrofti* population under the selection pressure(s) may evoke gradually under specified conditions to yield the fitness, which can be determined by a genotype in the parasite population. The increase in the parasite fitness can be estimated by the equilibrium frequencies of the alleles (genotypes) at heterozygote advantage in a hypothethical population. That is, rapid establishment of advantageous alleles in the *W. bancrofti* population, called "selection sweep", may evoke with advantageous drug-resistant genotypes epidemiologically linked to other factors shaped by the host and environment (Schwab et al, 2006: 2007; Churcher et al, 2008). Eventually, it may reduce the genetic variation in the population.

3.2 Benzimidazole-susceptibility of the parasite

This chapter emphasizes microfilaremia responsiveness in the population under the suppression of the PELF implementing MDA 2-drug regimen, 6 mg/kg DEC plus 400 mg albendazole. The microfilaremia responses against the DEC are the foundations of understanding how the albendazole exerts the effects on the parasite population in addition to what is observed by DEC alone. The DEC is known as the oldest of the antifilarial drugs used in the LF control. The single-dose drug acts as microfilaricide as does the effective ivermectin (de Silva et al, 1997; Ottesen, 2000; Molynuex et al, 2003; Ottesen et al, 2008) while its macrofilaricidal activity is not definitely effective against adult worms (Eberhard et al, 1991; Norões et al, 1997; Dreyer et al, 1998; Rajendran et al, 2002; 2004; Oliveira-Menezes et al, 2007). The adult worm loads that are age-dependent (Lammie et al, 1994; Rajendran et al, 2002) are susceptible to treatment with the DEC alone or even combination with albendazole (Norões et al, 1997; Rajendran et al, 2002). It was seen that DEC alone disturbs the microfilarial sheath of some filarial species while it has effects on the oogenesis and fertilization of female adult worms. Nonetheless, little is known about the filarial nematode parasites whether they evoke resistance mechanism against DEC due to the lack of deepening its mechanism of action, particularly the availability in parasite tissues and the selectivity on parasite targets. Oliveira-Menezes et al (2007) demonstrated that DEC has minor effects on alterations of the cuticle or surface of both male and female adult worms; these responsible parasites were collected from the *W. bancrofti*-infected patients treated with DEC, as compared to those isolated from the untreated patients. Additionally, such alterations are seen in adult worms recovered from the patients treated with DEC plus albendazole. The possible explanation is that the potential adulticidal effect of albendazole relative to what is observed by the DEC alone. The subtle alterations imply the distinct morphologic characteristics of the parasite itself or the complex host-parasite interactions, and if implemented and continuously prolonged, the annual mass treatment with DEC plus albendazole has not yet become an apparent issue, particularly the impacts on the parasite population adaptation. Of note, the *O. volvulus* parasite develops the mechanism involved in resistance to ivermectin (Awadzi et al, 2004). Do the filarial nematode parasites have mimicry in the resistance mechanisms to ivermectin and albendazole? However, detailed study of the parasite resistance to albendazole has not been established.

Focus is on the MDA 2-drug that acts as effective microfilaricide while its aberrant activity that influences microfilaremia response to its efficacy in microfilaricidal activity. Provided this phenomenon occurs, the expected outcomes of such drug failure will impact on solving the solutions and paving the implications of how they will adapt under the certain circumstances and how we will also mitigate their adaptation. Most studies enlightened the understanding of this effective deworming MDA 2-drug, which plays the significance of reduction of the infection prevalence. A single-dose combined treatment with DEC plus albendazole has short- and long-term effects on *W. bancrofti* microfilaremics in the endemic populations (Ismail et al, 1998; Ottesen et al, 1999; El Setouhy et al, 2004; Rajendran et al, 2004). Compared to those receiving DEC alone, an additional benefit of the combined drugs results in decline in annual cyclic infection prevalence due to progressive reduction in density of *W. bancrofti* microfilaremia. Although its macrofilaricidal effect on clearance of *W. bancrofti* antigenemia has been reported (McCarthy et al, 1995; Eberhard, 1997; Rajendran et al, 2002; 2004; Koyadun et al, 2003; Bhumiratana et al, 2004; Siriaut et al, 2005; Bhumiratana et al, 2005; Yongyuth et al, 2006), the DEC alone or co-administered with the albendazole does not clear rapidly the antigenemia. The MDA with the DEC alone will recover an increase in the antigenemia prevalence of *W. bancrofti* unless there is yearly-round MDA in the population (Rajendran et al, 2002). A 400 mg single oral-dose albendazole regimen is broad-spectrum effective against helminthiases (Albonico, 1994; de Silva et al, 1997; Beach et al, 1999; Ottesen et al, 1999; Horton, 2000) and, as co-administered orally with DEC, a synergistic and long-term effect on geohelminths has been proven useful for 'beyond-lymphatic filariasis' elimination program (Ottesen et al, 1997; 1999; Ismail et al, 1998; Horton et al, 2000; Ottesen, 2000; Mani et al, 2002; 2004; Molynuex et al, 2003; Yongyuth et al, 2006).

Few reports established the evidence that the human filarial nematode parasites provoke molecular mechanism involved in benzimidazole sensitivity/resistance until recently findings of the genetically-induced resistance against benzimidazole compounds have been well documented in veterinary nematode parasites (Beech et al, 1994; Kwa et al, 1995; Humbert et al, 2001; Bennett et al, 2002; Drogemuller et al, 2004; Robinson et al, 2004; Cole et al, 2006; Ghisi et al, 2007). Resistance to albendazole in veterinary nematodes is known to be caused by either one of two single amino acid substitutions from phenylalanine to tyrosine in parasite β-tubulin at position 167 or 200. The genetically stable *W. bancrofti* β-tubulin gene responsible for a molecular mechanism of drug resistance has been proposed as that of the veterinary helminth parasites is performed under selection of albendazole and ivermectin. The *W. bancrofti* population isolated from the patients treated with a combination of albendazole and ivermectin had significantly higher genotypic frequencies associated with resistance at position 200 (Schwab et al, 2005). A resistance mutation was not detected at position 167. Hoti et al (2003, 2009) reported that the polymorphism in the codon of this residue in *W. bancrofti* populations representing geographically distant areas of India, through sequencing exon 5 region of *β-tubulin* isotype 1 gene. The nucleotide sequence data showed that *W. bancrofti* isolates from wide geographic areas of India had codon for Phe (TTC) at position 200, suggesting that the parasite might be genetically sensitive to benzimidazole. Similarly, Bhumiratana et al (2010) and Petchgit et al (2011) demonstrated that the *W. bancrofti* population recovered from the dynamic cross-border migrant population from areas that have been targeted by the MDA 2-drug regimen (300 mg DEC plus 400 mg albendazole) elicits the genetic background of benzimidazole susceptibility; a resistance mutation has not been observed at position 167 or 200. However, the albendazole, anthelmintic benzimidazole, is being co-administered with an antifilarial drug such as DEC, part of the PELF implementing in many endemic countries. But this drug is known to result in the faster development of drug resistance in the veterinary nematode parasites and hence it is necessary to monitor drug sensitivity among the responsible *W. bancrofti* populations.

4. Molecular diagnosis and monitoring of benzimidazole susceptibility

4.1 Parasite beta-tubulin encoding gene as molecular marker

Molecular mechanisms of benzimidazole resistance in nematode parasites are hypothesized. However, detailed study of benzimidazole resistance in trichostrongylids found that the β-tubulin encoding gene involved in benzimidazole susceptibility is responsible for the genetic inheritance of resistance in the veterinary nematode parasites under selection with benzimidazole that involves one of two single amino acid substitutions from phenylalanine (Phe) to tyrosine (Tyr) in parasite β-tubulin at position 167 or 200 (Beech et al, 1994; Kwa et al, 1993; 1994; 1995; Roos et al, 1990; Elard et al, 1996; Elard and Humbert, 1999; Humbert et al, 2001; von Samson-Himmelstjerna et al, 2002; Winterrowd et al, 2003; Drogemuller et al, 2004; Cole et al, 2006; Ghisi et al, 2007). The potential point mutation occurs at the DNA level by nucleotide substitution for the codon for amino acid position 200 of the *β-tubulin* gene, a substitution of TTC (Phe) with TAC (Tyr). This irreversible change brings about distinguishment of the responsible parasite population between benzimidazole-sensitive and -resistant nematodes. This principal mechanism for benzimidazole resistance is postulate to involve changes in the selectivity of the benzimidazoles on the primary structure of β-tubulin molecules, a building block of the microtubule in the parasites (Lacey, 1988; Lacey and Gill, 1994; Robinson et al, 2004).

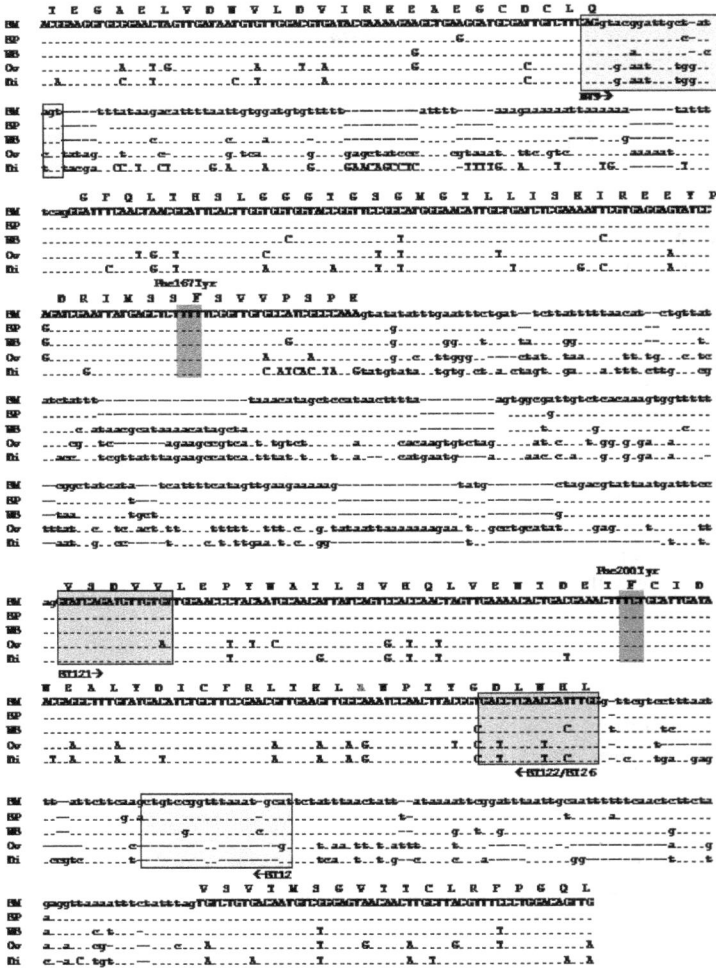

Fig. 3. ClustalW alignment of the filarial β-tubulin gene. The partial nucleotide sequence representatives (accession no. and positions): *Brugia malayi* (BRQD553TR, 3-789), *Brugia pahangi* (M36380, 2267-3054), *Wuchereria bancrofti* (AY705383, 109-916), *Onchocerca volvulus* (AF019886, 1582-2400) and *Dirofilaria immitis* (HM596854, 1462-2244) are shown as coding (upper case) and non-coding (lower case) sequences. The deduced amino acid sequences for the conserved domains are shown for all taxa aligned; *D. immitis* and *O. volvulus* have one amino acid substituted at position Ala218Thr. The gap is performed on the maximum homology (insertion/deletion), which represents conserved (•) and degenerate nucleotide residues and the regions designed to amplify specifically the target sequences based on the W*btubb* primer sets (light-gray boxes), both forward (→) and reverse (←). Hypothetically, two amino acid substitutions at positions Phe167Tyr and Phe200Tyr (dark-gray boxes) retained in DNA fragments (141 and 174 bp) could be identified using the PCR detection system described by Bhumiratana et al (2010) and Pechgit et al (2011).

Intriguingly, such mimicry in molecular mechanism for benzimidazole resistance in the filarial nematode parasites has been increasingly investigated, based basically on the molecular characterization of the homologous β-*tubulin* gene retained in their genome and the advantageous fitness of benzimidazole-resistant genotypes in the population (Roos et al, 1995; Elard et al, 1998; Elard et al, 1999; Silvestre et al, 2001; Silvestre and Humbert, 2002). The nematode parasites possess the single-copy homologous *β-tubulin* (*tubb*) gene that encodes a β-tubulin polypeptide, 448 amino acids (Met1 to Glu448). Hypothetically similar to that of trichostrongylids, the binding of benzimidazoles to conserved domains (of the exons 4 to 6) leads to blocking an assembly of tubulin (TUBB), and thus disrupting structural formation of microtubule (cytoskeleton protein) in the nematode parasites. The nucleotide sequences of the homologous *β-tubulin* gene as molecular marker and other related TUBB gene family of the nematode parasites can be retrieved from the genome databases: the GenBank at the National Center for Biotechnology Information (NCBI), http://www.ncbi.nlm.nih.gov/genbank/, the European Molecular Biology Laboratory (EMBL) http://www.ebi.ac.uk/, and the DNA DataBank of Japan (DDBJ) http://www.ddbj.nig.ac.jp/. The website of nematode and neglected genomics (http://www.nematodes.org/fgn/index.html) establishes genome database, especially for the filarial genome project (FGP), which includes published complete *B. malayi* genome. Meanwhile, the homologous sequences of *B. malayi β-tubulin* gene can be obtained from the TIGR genome database (http://www.tigr.org/tdb/e2k1/bma1).
The structural organization of homologous *tubb* genes of two filarial nematode parasites, *B. pahangi* (Guenette et al, 1991) and *D. immitis* (Bourguinat et al, 2011), has been shown for the establishment of complete coding sequences that span 9 discrete exons: exon 1 (Met1 to Lys19), exon 2 (Phe20 to Asp55), exon 3 (Gly56 to Gln131), exon 4 (Gly132 to Lys174), exon 5 (Val175 to Leu228), exon 6 (Val229 to Gln292), exon 7 (Met293 to Arg324), exon 8 (Glu325 to Thr386) and exon 9 (Ala387 to Glu448). The homology is 78% at DNA level due to bias of codon usage and insertion/deletion of intron sequences (Fig. 3). Among these, the exons 4 and 5 confer hypothetical point mutation at amino acid positions Phe167Tyr (or TTT/TAT) and Phe200Tyr (or TTC/TAC), based only on the second nucleotide base changed in the codons. In the homologous segment of its closely related taxa, *W. bancrofti β-tubulin* (W*btubb*) gene that possesses two distinct exons, 4 (Gly132 to Lys174) and 5 (Val175 to Leu228), with flanking intron sequences (Fig. 3) shares the homology at DNA level with *B. malayi* and *B. pahangi* (93% similarity), compared to *O. volvulus* and *D. immitis* (76% similarity) (Bhumiratana et al, 2010; Pechgit et al, 2011). This target DNA has been proved useful for designing W*btubb* locus-specific primers to discriminate between W*btubb* and other homologs of human and animal filariids. Based on its usefulness in molecular diagnosis and monitoring of the infection carrying the benzimidazole-sensitive or resistant phenotypes, the PCR applications of this molecular marker for *W. bancrofti* have been well documented (Hoti et al, 2003; 2009; Schwab et al, 2005; Bhumiratana et al, 2010; Pechgit et al, 2011).

4.2 Polymerase chain reaction-based approaches

In contrary to the antigen detection methods such as ICT Filariasis and Og4C3 ELISA that provide the proof of *W. bancrofti* antigenemic infection in human blood, the microfilarial DNA detection by PCR provides the evidence of *W. bancrofti* microfilaremic infection in human blood and mosquito (Table 3). As a result of the existence of genetically stable

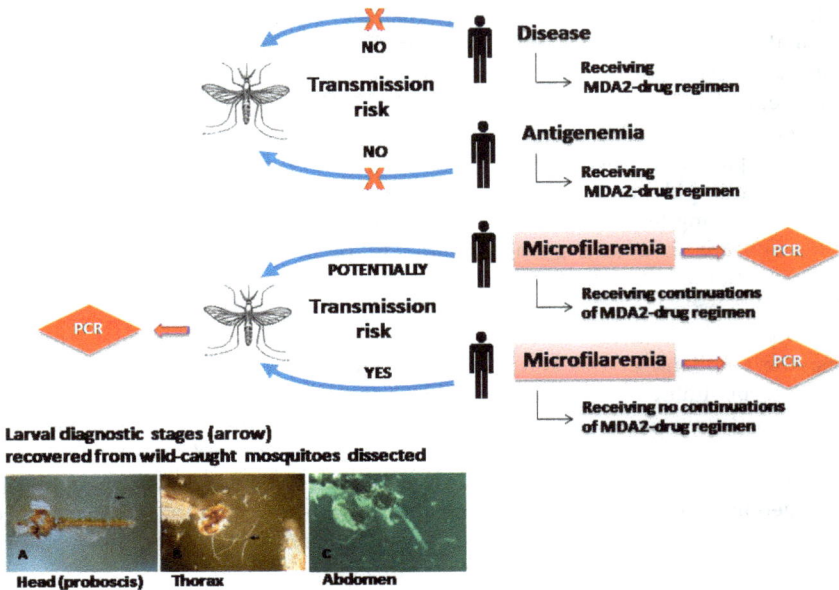

Fig. 4. A purposed scheme for PCR detection of *W. bancrofti* benzimidazole-susceptible isolates in human blood and mosquito.

Primer Name	Sequence (5′ to 3′)	Direction	Length (bases)	Expected amplicon size (bp)	Hypothetical nucleotide positions	Susceptible(S)/ resistant(R) genotypes investigated	Reference
BT9	CAGGTACAGATT GCTACAGT	Forward	20	607[c]	(TTT)167(TAT)	S/Phe167	Bhumiratana
BT12	GCGATTTAAACC CGACAGC	Reverse	19		(TTC)200(TAC)	S/Phe200	et al (2010)
BT121[a]	GGATCCGTATCA GATGTTGTG	Forward	21	174[d]			Bhumiratana
BT122[b]	GAATTCCAAGTG GTTGAGGTCG	Reverse	22		(TTC)200(TAC)	S/Phe200	et al (2010)
Wt2F	GTATCAGATGTT GTGTTG	Forward	18	475[e]			Hoti et al
Wt2R	ACGACTTGAATG AGTTGTC	Reverse	19		(TTC)200(TAC)	S/Phe200	(2003)
Wbbt2 F	TATCAGATGTTG TGTTGG	Forward	18	475[f]			Hoti et al
Wbbt2 R	CTGTTGAG AAGTTCAGCA	Reverse	19		(TTC)200(TAC)	S/Phe200	(2009)

5′modifications with additional recognition sequences: [a]*Bam*H I (GGATCC) and [b]*Eco*R I (GAATTC).
[c][d]Retrieved *Wuchereria bancrofti* genome accession nos.: AY705383 and GU190718–24.
[e]Retrieved *Brugia pahangi* genome accession nos.: M36380.
[f]Retrieved *Wuchereria bancrofti* genome accession nos.: EF190199-190209, EF492870-492878.

Table 4. The *β-tubulin* isotype 1 gene-specific primers used in the PCR amplification of *W. bancrofti* benzimidazole-susceptible isolates

W. bancrofti β–tubulin gene, the nested PCR amplification can work well with the microfilaremic infection that responds to treatment with MDA 2-drug regimen (DEC plus albendaozle) (Pechgit et al, 2011). This newly developed PCR assay in addition to promising advanced tool (Hoti et al, 2003; 2009; Bhumiratana et al, 2010) has the potential benefits in the molecular diagnosis and monitoring of the infection, as compared to the other PCR amplification methods previously described elsewhere (Table 3). The concepts for PCR assays based on the Wb*tubb* locus-specific primers (Table 4) have been proposed in two applicable formats: the locus-specific nested PCR and allele-specific nested PCR. These applications have established the advantages on how to circumvent some common counterintuitive problems of conventional PCR with regards to both parasite genome analysis and low-copy gene detection; such detailed study has been well established by Pechgit et al (2011). The *W. bancrofti* microfilarial DNA detection methods depends much on the purity and quantity of the microfilariae recovered from different blood sample preparations. The purified aggregate parasite number in the absence of human host white blood cells, for example, are ideal for the quality of DNA extract, which serves as target sequences in the PCR reactions. In general, most PCR methods for the detection of *W. bancrofti* distinguishable from other filarial nematode parasites in human and mosquito is based on the repetitive *Ssp* I sequences, which are highly copy number per haploid genome. However, PCR amplification based on this *Ssp* I locus provides the positive identifications of the parasite infection existed in specimens of choice. The assay does not determine the infection that responds to benzimidazole sensitivity/resistance; such responsible *W. bancrofti* parasite population is amplified based on the β–tubulin gene which is single copy in haploid genome. Therefore, the amplification is performed using the Wb*tubb* locus-specific nested PCR and allele-specific nested PCR that provides the proof of the *W. bancrofti* infection carrying benzimidazole-sensitive/resistant phenotypes; methodologically, the technical requirements for their applications have been described by Pechgit et al (2011) and Hoti et al (2009). More specific, based on our experience, the Wb*tubb* locus-specific nested PCR with thermocycling modifications using touchdown and touchup cycles has been applied or used in detection and characterization of *W. bancrofti* infection both in human blood from patients untreated or treated with DEC plus albendazole and in wild-caught mosquito, provided such infections carrying benzimidazole-sensitive/resistant strains are the same source of the parasite population (Fig. 4). Hypothesis is that whether the parasite infection is genetically predisposed to the MDA 2–drug regimen (DEC plus albendazole) in areas under suppression of PELF, it will have frequencies of benzimidazole-susceptible homozygous allele (*SS*) greater than benzimidazole-susceptible heterozygous allele (*Sr*) and homozygous resistant allele (*rr*), which are associated with albendazole resistance, unless the parasite fitness is increased. This also permit the monitoring and evaluation of the parasite fitness to better understand theoretically and hypothetically evolutionary biology and ecology of the parasite, by which the human hosts play a key as a major source of selective pressures on the adaptation of parasite population constrained by environmental conditions.

5. Future perspectives

The GPELF has been deployed into the endemic countries implementing MDA 2-drug regimes (i.e., single annual doses of albendazole in combination with DEC or ivermectin) to reduce microfilaremia prevalence to levels low enough (principally lower than transmission threshold) to interrupt transmission of the disease in the absence of vector control. Based on scientific information on drug resistance to anthelmintics, the issue of albendazole resistance in the *W. bancrofti* parasite has assumed increasing importance since the GPELF is implemented on a large-scale in at-risk populations in different complex epidemiological settings, and predictably, the implementation phrase of the program will increase. Many studies have shown some vulnerability in how the parasite has the ability to evoke molecular mechanisms for resistance to anthelminthics as the nematodes of veterinary importance have developed resistance against both albendazole and ivermectin. Furthermore, there have been lines of evidence that the vulnerability of helminthiasis control programs that employ the MDA with these drugs is associated with several factors that facilitate the promotion of drug-resistant strains. At the same time, the factors are considered concerning the new options of drug combinations with different parasite targets or modes of actions to keep active shelf-life of DEC because the filarial nematode parasites have long life-span and complex life-cycle development. Likewise, to better understand what is relative to achieve MDA's goal to confront growing trend of drug resistance, it is essential for the development of molecularly diagnosing and monitoring the benzimidazole sensitivity/resistance in areas of long-running PELF program implementation using albendazole plus DEC or albendazole plus ivermectin. More applicable tools which will be validated in effective manner are also required to explore the genetic basis for resistance to anthelminthics.

6. References

Albonico, M. (1994). A randomized controlled trial comparing mebendazole and albendazole against *Ascaris*, *Trichuris* and hookworm infections. *Trans R Soc Trop Med Hyg* 88, 585–589.

Awadzi, K., Boakye, D.A., Edwards, G., Opoku, N.O., Attah, S.K., Osei-Atweneboana, M.Y. et al. (2004). An investigation of persistent microfilaridermias despite multiple treatments with ivermectin, in two onchocerciasis-endemic foci in Ghana. *Ann Trop Med Parasitol* 98, 231–249.

Beach, M.J., Streit, T.G., Addiss, D.G., Prospere, R., Roberts, J.M., Lammie, P.J. (1999). Assessment of combined ivermectin and albendazole for treatment of intestinal helminth and *Wuchereria bancrofti* infections in Haitian schoolchildren. *Am J Trop Med Hyg* 60, 479–486.

Beech, R.N., Prichard, R.K., Scott, M.E. (1994). Genetic variability of the beta-tubulin genes in benzimidazole-susceptible and resistant strains of *Haemonchus contortus*. *Genetics* 138, 103–110.

Bennett, A.B., Anderson, T.J., Barker, G.C., Michael, E., Bundy, D.A. (2002). Sequence variation in the *Trichuris trichiura* beta-tubulin locus: implications for the development of benzimidazole resistance. *Int J Parasitol* 32, 1519–1528.

Bhumiratana, A., Koyadun, S., Suvannadabba, S., Karnjanopas, K., Rojanapremsuk, J., Buddhirakkul, P., et al. (1999). Field trial of the ICT Filariasis for diagnosis of *Wuchereria bancrofti* infections in an endemic population of Thailand. *Southeast Asian J Trop Med Public Health* 30, 562–568.

Bhumiratana, A., Wattanakull, B., Koyadun, S., Suvannadabba, S., Rojanapremsuk, S., Tantiwattanasup, W. (2002). Relationship between male hydrocele and infection prevalences in clustered communities with uncertain transmission of *Wuchereria bancrofti* on the Thailand-Myanmar border. *Southeast Asian J Trop Med Public Health* 33, 7–17.

Bhumiratana, A., Siriaut, C., Koyadun, S., Satitvipawee, P. (2004). Evaluation of a single oral dose of diethylcarbamazine 300 mg as provocative test and simultaneous treatment in Myanmar migrant workers with *Wuchereria bancrofti* infection in Thailand. *Southeast Asian J Trop Med Public Health* 35, 591–598.

Bhumiratana, A., Koyadun, S., Srisuphanunt, M., Satitvipawee, P., Limpairojn, N., Gaewchaiyo, G. (2005). Border and imported bancroftian filariases: baseline seroprevalence in sentinel populations exposed to infections with *Wuchereria bancrofti* and concomitant HIV at the start of diethylcarbamazine mass treatment in Thailand. *Southeast Asian J Trop Med Public Health* 36, 390–407.

Bhumiratana, A., Pechgit, P., Koyadun, S., Siriaut, C., Yongyuth, P. (2010). Imported bancroftian filariasis: Diethylcarbamazine response and benzimidazole susceptibility of *Wuchereria bancrofti* in dynamic cross-border migrant population targeted by the National Program to Eliminate Lymphatic Filariasis in South Thailand. *Acta Trop* 113, 121–128.

Bourguinat, C., Keller, K., Prichard, R.K., Geary, T.G. (2011). Genetic polymorphism in *Dirofilaria immitis*. *Vet Parasitol* 176, 368–373.

Braga, C., Dourado, M. I., Ximenes, R. A. D. A., Alves, L., Brayner, F., Rocha, A., et al. (2003). Field evaluation of the whole blood immunochromatographic test for rapid bancroftian filariasis diagnosis in the northeast of Brazil. *Rev Inst Med Trop Sao Paulo*, 45, 125–129.

Bundy, D.A.P., Grenfell, B.T., Rajagopwlan, P.K. (1991). Immunoepidemiology of Lymphatic filariasis: the relationship between infection and disease. *Immunol Today* 12, A71–75.

Castillo, J.C., Reynolds, S.E., Eleftherianos, I. (2011). Insect immune responses to nematode parasites. *Trends Parasitol* (in press), doi:10.1016/j.pt.2011.09.001.

CDC. (1993). Recommendations of the International Task Force for Disease Eradication. *Morb Mortal Wkly Rep* 42(RR16), 1–38. [http://www.cdc.gov/mmwr/preview/mmwrhtml/00025967.htm]

Chanteau, S., Moulia-Pelat, J.P., Glaziou, P., Nguyen, N.L., Luquiaud, P., Plichart, C., et al. (1994a). Og4C3 circulating antigen: a marker of infection and adult worm burden in *Wuchereria bancrofti* filariasis. *J Infect Dis* 170, 247–250.

Chanteau, S., Glaziou, P., Luquiaud, P., Plichart, C., Moulia-Pelat, J.P., Cartel, J.L. (1994b). Og4C3 circulating antigen, anti-*Brugia malayi* IgG and IgG4 titers in *Wuchereria bancrofti* infected patients, according to their parasitological status. *Trop Med Parasitol* 45, 255–257.

Chanteau, S., Luquiaud, P., Failloux, A.B., Williams, S.A. (1994c). Detection of *Wuchereria bancrofti* larvae in pools of mosquitoes by the polymerase chain reaction. *Trans R Soc Trop Med Hyg* 88, 665–666.

Churcher, T.S., Schwab, A.E., Prichard, R.K., Basáñez, M.G. (2008). An analysis of genetic diversity and inbreeding in *Wuchereria bancrofti*: implications for the spread and detection of drug resistance. *PLoS Negl Trop Dis* 2, e211.

Cole, G.C., Jackson, F., Pomroy, W.E., Prichard, R.K., von Samson-Himmeltjerna, G., Silvestre, A., et al. (2006). The detection of anthelminthic resistance in nematodes of veterinary importance. *Vet Parasitol* 136, 167–185.

Cox-Singh, J., Pomrehnb, A.S., Wolfec, N.D., Rahmand, H.A., Lua, H., Singha, B. (2000). Sensitivity of the nested-polymerase chain reaction (PCR) assay or *Brugia malayi* and significance of 'free' DNA in PCR-based assays. *Int J Parasitol* 30, 1177–1179.

de Silva, N., Cuyatt, H., Bundy, D.A. (1997). Anthelminthics: a comprehensive review of their clinical pharmacology. *Drugs* 53, 769–788.

Dreyer, G., Addiss, D., Santos, A., Figueredo-Silva, J., Norões, J. (1998). Direct assessment in vivo of the efficacy of combined single-dose ivermectin and diethylcarbamazine against adult *Wuchereria bancrofti*. *Trans R Soc Trop Med Hyg* 92, 219–222.

Drogemuller, M., Schieder, T., von Samson-Himmelstjerna, G. (2004). Beta-tubulin complementary DNA sequence variations observed between cyathostomins from benzimidazole-susceptible and -resistant populations. *J Parasitol* 90, 868–870.

Eberhard, M.L. (1997). Clearance of *Wuchereria bancrofti* antigen after treatment with diethylcarbamazine or ivermectin. *Am J Trop Med Hyg* 57, 483–486.

Eberhard, M.L., Lammie, P.J., Dickinson, C.M., Roberts, J.M. (1991). Evidence of nonsusceptibility to diethylcarbamazine in *Wuchereria bancrofti*. *J Infect Dis* 163, 1157–1160.

Elard, L., Cabaret, J., Humbert, J.F. (1999). PCR diagnosis of benzimidazole-susceptibility or -resistance in natural populations of the small ruminant parasite, *Teladorsagia circumcincta*. *Vet Parasitol* 80, 231–237.

Elard, L., Comes, A.M., Humbert, J.F. (1996). Sequences of beta-tubulin cDNA from benzimidazole-susceptible and -resistant strains of *Teladorsagia circumcincta*, a nematode parasite of small ruminants. *Mol Biochem Parasitol* 79, 249–253.

Elard, L., Humbert, J.F. (1999). Importance of the mutation of amino acid 200 of the isotype 1 β-tubulin gene in the benzimidazole resistance of the small-ruminant parasite *Teladorsagia circumcincta*. *Parasitol Res* 85, 452–456.

Elard, L., Sauve, C., Humbert, J.F. (1998). Fitness of benzimidazole-resistant and -susceptible worms of *Teladorsagia circumcincta*, a nematode parasite of small ruminants. *Parasitology* 117, 571–578.

El Setouhy, M., Ramzy, R.M.R., Ahmed, E.S., Kandil, A.M., Hussain, O., Farid. H.A., et al. (2004). A randomized clinical trial comparing single- and multi-dose combination therapy with diethylcarbamazine and albendazole for treatment of bancroftian filariasis. *Am J Trop Med Hyg* 70, 191–196.

Engelbrecht, F., Oettl, T., Herter, U., Link, C., Philipp, D., Edeghere, H., et al. (2003). Analysis of *Wuchereria bancrofti* infections in a village community in northern Nigeria: Increased prevalence in individuals infected with *Onchocerca volvulus*. *Parasitol Int* 52, 13–20.

Fischer, P., Boakye, D., Hamburger, J. (2003). Polymerase chain reaction-based detection of lymphatic filariasis. *Med Microbiol Immunol* 192, 3–7.

Foo, P.K., Tarozzic, A., Mahajan, A., Yoong, J., Krishnan, L., Kopf, D., et al. (2011). High prevalence of *Wuchereria bancrofti* infection as detected by immunochromatographic card testing in five districts of Orissa, India, previously considered to be non-endemic. *Trans R Soc Trop Med Hyg* 105, 109–114.

Freedman, D.O., de Almeida, A., Miranda, J., Plier, D.A., Braga, C. (1997). Field trial of a rapid card test for *Wuchereria bancrofti*. *Lancet* 350, 1681.

Ghisi, M., Kaminsky, R., Maser, P. (2007). Phenotyping and genotyping of *Haemonchus contortus* isolates reveals a new putative candidate mutation for benzimidazole resistance in nematodes. *Vet Parasitol* 144, 313–320.

Grenfell, B.T., Micheal, E., Denham, D.A. (1991). A model for the dynamics of human lymphatic filariasis. *Parasitol Today* 7, 318–323.

Grenfell, B.T., Micheal, E. (1992). Infection and disease in lymphatic filariasis: an epidemiological approach. *Parasitology* 104(suppl), S81–90.

Guenette, S., Prichard, R.K, Klein, R.D., Matlashewski, G. (1991). Characterization of a beta-tubulin gene and a beta-tubulin gene products of *Brugia pahangi*. *Mol Biochem Parasitol* 44, 153–164.

Gyapong, J.O., Kumaraswami, V., Biswas, G., Ottesen, E.A. (2005). Treatment strategies underpinning the global programme to eliminate lymphatic filariasis. *Expert Opin Pharmacother* 6, 179–200.

Horton, J. (2000). Albendazole: a review of anthelminthic efficacy and safety in humans. *Parasitology* 121(suppl), S113–132.

Horton, J., Witt, C., Ottesen, E.A., Lazdins, J.K., Addiss, D.G., Awadzi, K., et al. (2000). An analysis of the safety of the single dose, two drug regimens used in programmes to eliminate lymphatic filariasis. *Parasitology* 121, S147–160.

Hoti, S.L., Subramaniyan, K., Das, P.K. (2003). Detection of codon of amino acid 200 in isotype 1 beta-tubulin gene of *Wuchereria bancrofti* isolates, implicated in resistance to benzimidazole in other nematodes. *Acta Trop* 88, 77–81.

Hoti, S.L., Dhamodharan, R., Subramaniyan, K., Das, P.K. (2009). An allele specific PCR assay for screening for drug resistance among *Wuchereria bancrofti* populations in India. *Indian J Med Res* 130, 193–199.

Humbert, J.F., Cabaret, J., Elard, L., Leignel, V., Silvestre, A. (2001). Molecular approaches to studying benzimidazole resistance in trichostrongylid nematode parasites of small ruminants. *Vet Parasitol* 101, 405–414.

Ismail, M.M., Jayakody, R.L., Weil, G.J., Nirmalan, N., Jayasinghe, K.S.A., Abeyewickrema, W., et al. (1998). Efficacy of single dose combinations of albendazole, ivermectin and diethylcarbamazine for the treatment of bancroftian filariasis. *Trans R Soc Trop Med Hyg* 92, 94–97.

Kanjanavas, P., Tan-ariya, P., Khawsak, P., Pakpitcharoena, A., Phantana, S., Chansiri, K. (2005). Detection of lymphatic *Wuchereria bancrofti* in carriers and long-term storage blood samples using semi-nested PCR. *Mol Cell Probes* 19, 169–172.

Koyadun, S., Bhumiratana, A., Prikchu, P. (2003). *Wuchereria bancrofti* antigenemia clearance among Myanmar migrants after biannual mass treatments with diethylcarbamazine, 300 mg oral-dose FILADEC tablet, in Southern Thailand. *Southeast Asian J Trop Med Public Health* 34, 758–767.

Kwa, M.S.G., Veenstra, J.G., Van Dijk, M., Roos, M.H. (1995). *β-Tubulin* genes from the parasitic nematode *Haemonchus contortus* modulate drug resistance in *Caenorhabditis elegans*. *J Mol Biol* 246, 500–510.

Kwa, M.S.G., Veenstra, J.G., Roos, M.H. (1993). Molecular characterisation of beta-tubulin genes present in benzimidazole-resistant populations of *Haemonchus contortus*. *Mol Biochem Parasitol* 60, 133–143.

Kwa, M.S.G., Veenstra, J.G, Roos, M.H. (1994). Benzimidazole resistance in *Haemonchus contortus* is correlated with a conserved mutation at amino acid 200 in beta-tubulin isotype 1. *Mol Biochem Parasitol* 63, 299–303.

Kwa, M.S.G., Veenstra, J.G., Van Dijk, M., Roos, M.H. (1995). *β-Tubulin* genes from the parasitic nematode *Haemonchus contortus* modulate drug resistance in *Caenorhabditis elegans*. *J Mol Biol* 246, 500–510.

Kyelem, D., Biswas, G., Bockarie, M.J., Bradley, M.H., El-Setouhy, M., Fischer, P.U., et al. (2008). Determinants of success in national programs to eliminate lymphatic filariasis: a perspective identifying essential elements and research needs. *Am J Trop Med Hyg* 79, 480–484.

Lacey, E. (1988). The role of the cytoskeletal protein, tubulin, in the mode of action and mechanism of drug resistance to benzimidazoles. *Int J Parasitol* 18, 885–936.

Lacey, E., Gill, J.H. (1994). Biochemistry of benzimidazole resistance. *Acta Trop* 56, 245–262.

Lammie, P.J., Hightower, A.W., Eberhard, M.L. (1994). Age specific prevalence of antigenemia in a *Wuchereria bancrofti*-exposed population. *Am J Trop Med Hyg* 51, 348–355.

Lizotte, M., Supali, T., Partono, F., Williams, S.A. (1994). A polymerase chain reaction assay for the detection of *Brugia malayi* in blood. *Am J Trop Med Hyg* 51, 314–321.

Maizels, R.M., Lawrence, R.A. (1991). Immunological tolerance: the key feature in human filariasis? *Parasitol Today* 7, 271–276.

Mani, T.R., Rajendran, R., Munirathinam, A., Sunish, I.P., Abdullah, S.M., Augustin, D.J. et al. (2002). Efficacy of co-administration of albendazole and diethylcarbamazine against geohelminthiases: a study from South India. *Trop Med Int Health* 7, 541–548.

Mani, T.R., Rajendran, R., Sunish, I.P., Munirathinam, A., Arunachalam, N., Satyanarayana, K. et al. (2004). Effectiveness of two annual, single-dose mass drug administrations of diethylcarbamazine alone or in combination with albendazole on soil-transmitted helminthiasis in filariasis elimination programme. *Trop Med Int Health* 9, 1030–1035.

McCarthy, J.S., Guinea, A., Weil, G.J., Ottesen, E.A. (1995). Clearance of circulating filarial antigen as a measure of the macrofilaricidal activity of diethylcarbamazine in *Wuchereria bancrofti* infection. *J Infect Dis* 172, 521–526.

McCarthy, J.S., Zhong, M., Gopinath, R., Ottesen, E.A., Williams, S.A., Nutman, T.B. (1996). Evaluation of a polymerase chain reaction-based assay for diagnosis of *Wuchereria bancrofti* infection. *J Infect Dis* 173, 1510–1504.

Meyrowitsch, D.W., Simonsen, P.E., Makunde, W.H. (1995). Bancroftian filariasis: analysis of infection and disease in five communities of north-eastern Tanzania. *Ann Trop Med Parasitol* 89, 653–663.

Mishra, K., Raj, D.K., Hazra, R.K., Dash, A.P., Supakar, P.C. (2007). The development and evaluation of a single step multiplex PCR method for simultaneous detection of *Brugia malayi* and *Wuchereria bancrofti. Mol Cell Probes* 21, 355–362.

Mitchell, G.F. (1991). Co-evolution of paarsites and adaptive immune responses. *Immunol Today* 12, A2–5.

Molynuex, D.H., Bradley, M., Hoeraul, A., Kyelem, D., Taylor, M.J. (2003). Mass drug treatment for lymphatic filariasis and onchocerciasis. *Trends Parasitol* 19, 516–522.

More, S.J., Copeman, D.B. (1990). A highly specific and sensitive monoclonal antibody-based ELISA for the detection of circulating antigen in bancroftian filariasis. *Trop Med Parasitol* 41, 403–406.

Nguyen, N.L., Plichart, C., Esterre, P. (1999). Assessment of immunochromatographic test for rapid lymphatic filariasis diagnosis. *Parasite* 6, 355–358.

Nicolas, L. (1997). New tools for diagnosis and monitoring of bancroftian filariasis parasitism: the Polynesian experience. *Parasitol Today* 13, 370–375.

Nicolas, L., Luquiaud, P., Lardeux, F., Mercer, D.R. (1999). A polymerase chain reaction assay to determine infection of *Aedes polynesiensis* by *Wuchereria bancrofti. Trans R Soc Trop Med Hyg* 90, 136–139.

Norões, J, Dreyer, G, Santos, A, Mendes, VG, Mendeiros, Z, Addiss, D. (1997). Assessment of the efficacy diethylcarbamazine on adult *Wuchereria bancrofti in vivo. Trans R Soc Trop Med Hyg* 91, 78-81.

Nuchprayoon, S., Porksakorn, C., Junpee, A., Sanprasert, V., Poovorawan, Y. (2003). Comparative assessment of an Og4C3 ELISA and an ICT filariasis test: A study of Myanmar migrants in Thailand. *Asian Pac J Allerg Immunol* 21, 253–257.

Nuchprayoon, S., Junpee, A., Poovorawan, Y., Scott, A.L. (2005). Detection and differentiation of filarial parasites by universal primers and polymerase chain reaction-restriction fragment length polymorphism analysis. *Am J Trop Med Hyg* 73, 895–900.

Nuchprayoon, S., Junpee, A., Poovorawan, Y. (2007). Random amplified polymorphic DNA (RAPD) for differentiation between Thai and Myanmar strains of *Wuchereria bancrofti. Filaria J* 6:6, doi:10.1186/1475–2883–6–6.

Oliveira-Menezes, A., Lins, R., Norões, J., Dreyer, G. (2007). Comparative analysis of a chemotherapy effect on the cuticular surface of *Wuchereria bnacrofti* adult worms in vivo. *Parasitol Res* 101, 1311–1317.

Omar, M.S., Sheikha, A.K., Al-Amari, O.M., Abdalla, S.E., Musa, R.A. (2000). Field evaluation of two diagnostic antigen tests for *Wuchereria bancrofti* infection among Indian expatriates in Saudi Arabia. *Southeast Asian J Trop Med Public Health* 31, 415–418.

Ottesen, E.A. (1992). Infection and disease in lymphatic filariasis: an immunological perspective. *Parasitology* 104(suppl), S71–79.

Ottesen, E.A. (2000). The global programme to eliminate lymphatic filariasis. *Trop Med Int Health* 5, 591–594.

Ottesen, E.A., Duke, B.O.L., Karam, M., Behbehani, K. (1997). Strategies and tools for the control/elimination of lymphatic filariasis. *Bull World Health Org* 75, 491–503.

Ottesen, E.A., Ismail, M.M., Horton, J. (1999). The role of albendazole in programmes to eliminate lymphatic filariasis. *Parasitol Today* 15, 382–386.

Ottesen, E.A., Hooper, P.J., Bradley, M., Biswas, G. (2008). The global programme to eliminate lymphatic filariasis: health impact after 8 years. *PLoS Negl Trop Dis* 2, e317. doi:10.1371/journal.pntd.0000317.

Pani, S.P., Hoti, S.L., Elango, A., Yuvaraj, J., Lall, R., Ramaiah, K.D. (2000). Evaluation of the ICT whole blood antigen card test to detect infection due to nocturnally periodic *Wuchereria bancrofti* in South India. *Trop Med Int Health* 5, 359–363.

Pani, S.P., Hoti, S.L., Vanamail, P., Das, L.K. (2004). Comparison of an immunochromatographic card test with night blood smear examination for detection of *Wuchereria bancrofti* microfilaria carriers. *Natl Med J India*, 17, 304–306.

Pradeep Kumar, N., Patra, K.P., Hoti, S.L., Das, P.K. (2002). Genetic variability of the human filarial parasite, *Wuchereria bancrofti* in South India. *Acta Trop* 82, 67–76.

Pechgit, P., Intarapuk, A., Pinyoowong, D., Bhumiratana, A. (2011). Touchdown-touchup nested PCR for low-copy gene detection of benzimidazole-susceptible *Wuchereria bancrofti* with a *Wolbachia* endosymbiont imported by migrant carriers. *Exp Parasitol* 127, 559–568.

Phantana, S., Sensathein, S., Songtrus, J., Klagrathoke, S., Phongnin, K. (1999). ICT filariasis test: a new screening test for Bancroftian filariasis. *Southeast Asian J Trop Med Public Health* 30, 47–51.

Rajendran, R., Sunish, I.P., Mani, T.R., Munirathinam, A., Abdullah, S.M., Arunachalarm, N. et al. (2002). The influence of the mass administration of diethylcarbamazine, alone or with albendazole, on the prevalence of filarial antigenaemia. *Ann Trop Med Parasitol* 96, 595–602.

Rajendran, R., Sunish, I.P., Mani, T.R., Munirathinam, A., Abdullah, S.M., Arunachalarm, N. et al. (2004). Impact of two annual single-dose mass drug administrations with diethylcarbamazine alone or in combination with albendazole on *Wuchereria bancrofti* microfilaraemia and antigenaemia in South India. *Trans R Soc Trop Med Hyg* 98, 174–181.

Ramzy, R.M.R., Farid, H.A., Kamal, I.H., Ibrahim, G.H., Morsy, Z.S., Faris, R., et al. (1997). A polymerase chain reaction-based assay for detection of *Wuchereria bancrofti* in human blood and *Culex pipiens*. *Trans R Soc Trop Med Hyg* 91, 156–160.

Ramzy, R.M.R., Helmy, H., El-Lethy, A.S.T., Kandil, A.M., Ahmed, E.S., Weil, G.J., et al. (1999). Field evaluation of a rapid format kit for the diagnosis of bancroftian filariasis in Egypt. *East Mediterr Health J* 5, 880–887.

Rao, R.U., Atkinson, L.J., Ramzy, R.M.R., Helmy, H., Farid, H.A., Bockarie, M.J., et al. (2006). A real-time PCR-based assay for detection of *Wuchereria bancrofti* DNA in blood and mosquitoes. *Am J Trop Med Hyg* 74, 826–832.

Ravindran, B., Satapathy, A.K., Sahoo, P.K., Mohanty, M.C. (2003). Protective immunity in human lymphatic filariasis: problems and prospects. *Med Microbiol Immunol* 192, 41–46.

Robinson, M.W., Mcferran, N., Trudgett, A., Hoey, L., Fairweather, I. (2004). A possible model of benzimidazole binding to beta-tubulin disclosed by invoking an inter-domain movement. *J Mol Graph Model* 23, 275–284.

Rocha, A., Addiss, D., Ribeiro, M.E., Norões, J., Baliza, M., Medeiros, Z., et al. (1996). Evaluation of the Og4C3 ELISA in *Wuchereria bancrofti* infection: infected persons with undetectable or ultra-low microfilarial densities. *Trop Med Int Health* 1, 859–864.

Roos, M.H., Boersema, J.H., Borgsteede, F.H.M., Cornelissen, J., Taylor, M., Ruitenberg, E.J. (1990). Molecular analysis of selection for benzimidazole resistance in the sheep parasite *Hemonchus contortus*. *Mol Biochem Parasitol* 43, 77–88.

Roos, M.H., Kwa, M.S.G., Grant, W.N. (1995). New genetic and practical implications of selection for anthelmintic resistance in parasitic nematodes. *Parasitol Today* 11, 148–150.

Ruberanziza, E., Mupfasoni, D., Karibushi, B., Rujeni, N., Kabanda, G., Kabera, M., et al. (2009). Mapping of lymphatic filariasis in Rwanda. *J Lymphoedema* 4, 20–23.

Schwab, A.E., Boakye, D.A., Kyelem, D., Prichard, R.K. (2005). Detection of benzimidazole resistance-associated mutations in the filarial nematode *Wuchereria bancrofti* and evidence for selection by albendazole and ivermectin combination treatment. *Am J Trop Med Hyg* 73, 234–238.

Schwab, A.E., Churcher, T.S., Schwab, A.J., Basáñez, M.G., Prichard, R.K. (2007). An analysis of the population genetics of potential multi-drug resistance in *Wuchereria bnacrofti* due to combination chemotherapy. *Parasitology* 134(Pt 7), 1025–1040.

Schwab, A.E., Churcher, T.S., Schwab, A.J., Basáñez, M.G., Prichard, R.K. (2006). Population genetics of concurrent selection with albendazole and ivermectin or diethylcarbamazine on the possible spread of albendazole resistance in *Wuchereria bancrofti*. *Parasitology* 133(Pt 5), 589–601.

Silvestre, A., Cabaret, J., Humbert, J.F. (2001). Effect of benzimidazole under-dosing on the resistant allele frequency in *Teladorsagia circumcincta* (Nematoda). *Parasitology* 123, 103–111.

Silvestre, A., Humbert, J.F. (2002). Diversity of benzimidazole-resistance alleles in populations of small ruminant parasites. *Int J Parasitol* 32, 921–928.

Simonsen, P.E., Dunyo, S.K. (1999). Comparative evaluation of three new tools for diagnosis of bancroftian filariasis based on detection of specific circulating antigens. *Trans R Soc Trop Med Hyg* 93, 278–282.

Simonsen, P.E., Lemnge, M.M., Msangeni, H.A., Jakobsen, P.H., Bygbjerg, I.C. (1996). Bancroftian filariasis: The patterns of filarial-specific immunoglobulin G1 (IgG1), IgG4, and circulating antigens in an endemic community of northeastern Tanzania. *Am J Trop Med Hyg* 55, 69–75.

Simonsen, P.E., Meyrowitsch, D.W., Jaoko, W.G., Malecela, M.N., Michael, E. (2008). Immunoepidemiology of *Wuchereria bancrofti* infection in two East African communities: Antibodies to the microfilarial sheath and their role in regulating host microfilaremia. *Acta Trop* 106, 200–206.

Siriaut, C., Bhumiratana, A., Koyadun, S., Anurat, K., Satitvipawee, P. (2005). Short-term effects of a treatment with 300 mg oral-dose diethylcarbamazine on nocturnally periodic *Wuchereria bancrofti* microfilaremia and antigenemia. *Southeast Asian J Trop Med Public Health* 36, 832–840.

Siridewa, K., Karunanayake, E.H., Chandrasekharan, N.V. (1996). Polymerase chain reaction based technique for the detection of *Wuchereria bancrofti* in human blood samples, hydrocele fluid, and mosquito vectors. *Am J Trop Med Hyg* 54, 72–76.

Srividya, A., Pani, S.P., Rajagopalan, P.K., Bundy, D.A.P., Grenfell, B.T. (1991). The dynamics of infection and disease in Bancroftian filariasis. *Trans R Soc Trop Med Hyg* 85, 255–259.

Sunish, I.P., Rajendran, R., Mani, T.R., Gajanana, A., Reuben, R., Satyanarayana, K. (2003). Long-term population migration: an important aspect to be considered during mass drug administration for elimination of lymphatic filariasis. *Trop Med Int Health* 8, 316–321.

Sunish, I.P., Rajendran, R., Mani, T.R., Munirathinam, A., Tewari, S.C., Hiriyan, J., et al. (2002). Resurgence in filarial transmission after withdrawal of mass drug administration and the relationship between antigenaemia and microfilaraemia - A longitudinal study. *Trop Med Int Health* 7, 59–69.

Takagi, H., Itoh, M., Kasai, S., Yahathugoda, T.C., Weerasooriya, M.V., Kimura, E. (2011). Development of loop-mediated isothermal amplification method for detecting *Wuchereria bancrofti* DNA in human blood and vector mosquitoes. *Parasitol Int* (in press), doi:10.1016/j.parint.2011.08.018.

Thanomsub, B.W., Chansiri, K., Sarataphan, N., Phantana, S. (2000). Differential diagnosis of human lymphatic filariasis using PCR-RFLP. *Mol Cell Probes* 14, 41–46.

Turner, P., Copeman, D.B., Gerisi, D., Speare, R. (1993). A comparison of the Og4C3 antigen capture ELISA, the knott test, an IgG4 assay and clinical sign, in the diagnosis of bancroftian filariasis. *Trop Med Parasitol* 44, 45–48.

von Samson-Himmelstjerna, G., Pape, M., von Witzendorff, C., Schnieder, T. (2002). Allele-specific PCR for the beta-tubulin codon 200 TTC/TAC polymorphism using single adult and larval small strongyle (Cyathostominae) stages. *J Parasitol* 88, 254–257.

Weaver, A., Brown, P., Huey, S., Magallon, M., Bollman, E. B., Mares, D., et al. (2011). A low-tech analytical method for diethylcarbamazine citrate in medicated salt. *PLoS Negl Trop Dis* 5, e1005, doi: 10.1371/journal.pntd.0001005.

Weil, G.J., Liftis, F. (1987). Identification and partial characterization of a parasite antigen in sera from humans infected with *Wuchereria bancrofti*. *J Immunol* 138, 3035–3041.

Weil, G.J., Jain, D.C., Santhanam, S., Malhotra, A., Kumar, H., Sethumadhavan, K.V.P. et al. (1987). A monoclonal antibody-based enzyme immunoassay for detecting parasite antigenemia in bancroftian filariasis. *J Infect Dis* 156, 350–355.

Weil, G.J., Ramzy, R.M.R., Chandrashekar, R., Gad, A.M., Lowrie Jr., R.C., Faris, R. (1996). Parasite antigenemia without microfilaremia in bancroftian filariasis. *Am J Trop Med Hyg* 55, 333–337.

Weil, G.J., Lammie, P.J., Weiss, N. (1997). The ICT Filariasis Test: a rapid-format antigen test for diagnosis of bancroftian filariasis. *Parasitol Today* 13, 401–404.

Who. (1992a). Lymphatic filariasis: disease and its control. Fifth Report of the WHO Expert Committee on Filariasis. Geneva: World Health Oragnization. *WHO Tech Rep Ser* 821, p. 1–71.

Who. (1992b). Informal consultation on evaluation of morbidity in lymphatic filariasis, Tuberculosis Research Centre, Madras 10-11 February 1992. Geneva: World Health Organization. Mimeographed document WHO/TDR/FIL/92.3.

Who. (1994). Lymphatic filariasis infection and disease: control strategies. Report of a consultative meeting held at the University Sains Malaysia, Penang, Malaysia, August 1994. Geneva: World Health Organization. Mimeographed document WHO/TDR/CTD/FIL/PENANG/94.1.

Who. (1999a). Informal consultation on epidemiologic approaches to lymphatic filariasis elimination: initial assessment, monitoring, and certification, Atlanta, Georgia, USA 2-4 September 1998. Geneva: World Health Organization. Mimeographed documented WHO/FIL/99.195.

Who. (1999b). Guidelines for certifying lymphatic filariasis elimination (including discussion of critical issues and rationale), following from Informal consultation on epidemiologic approaches to lymphatic filariasis elimination: initial assessment, monitoring, and certification, Atlanta, Georgia, USA 2-4 September 1998. Geneva: World Health Organization. Mimeographed documented WHO/FIL/99/197.

Who. (2000). Elimination of lymphatic filariasis. Report of informal consultative meeting on lymphatic filaraisis in SEA region, Bhubaneswar, Orissa, India, 23-25 February 2000.

Who. (2001). Regional strategic plan for elimination of lymphatic filariasis (2000-2004). South-East Asia Regional Office, New Delhi: World Health Organization. Mimeographed documented SEA/FIL/28.corr.1.

Who. (2002). Global programme to eliminate lymphatic filariasis: Annual report on lymphatic filariasis 2001. Geneva: World Health Organization. Mimeographed document WHO/CDS/CPE/CEE/2002.28.

Who. (2008). Global programme to eliminate lymphatic filariasis. *Wkly Epidemiol Rec* 83, 333–341.

Who. (2009). Report: The role of polymerase chain reaction technique for assessing lymphatic filariasis transmission. Geneva: World Health Organization, p.1–55. Mimeographed document WHO/HTM/NTD/PCT/2009.1.

Who. (2010). Progress report 2000–2009 and strategic plan 2010–2020 of the global programme to eliminate lymphatic filariasis: halfway towards eliminating lymphatic filariasis. Geneva: World Health Organization, p.1–93. Mimeographed document WHO/HTM/NTD/PCT/2010.6

Williams, S.A., Nicolas, L., Lizotte-Waniewski, M., Plichart, C., Luquiaud, P., Nguyen, L.N., et al. (1996). A polymerase chain reaction assay for the detection of *Wuchereria bancrofti* in blood samples from French Polynesia. *Trans R Soc Trop Med Hyg* 90, 384–387.

Winterrowd, C.A., Pomroy, W.E., Sangster, N.C., Johnson, S.S., Geary, T.G. (2003). Benzimidazole-resistant β-tubulin alleles in a population of parasitic nematodes (*Cooperia oncophora*) of cattle. *Vet Parasitol* 117, 161–172.

Yongyuth, P., Koyadun, S., Jaturabundit, N., Sampuch, A., Bhumiratana, A. (2006). Efficacy of a single-dose treatment with 300 mg diethylcarbamazine and a combination of 400 mg albendazole in reduction of *Wuchereria bancrofti* antigenemia and concomitant geohelminths in Myanmar migrants in Southern Thailand. *J Med Assoc Thai* 89, 1237–1248.

Zhong, M., McCarthy, J.S., Bierwert, L., Lizotte-Waniewski, M., Chanteau, S., Nutman, T.B., et al. (1996). A polymerase chain reaction assay for detection of the parasite *Wuchereria bancrofti* in human blood samples. *Am J Trop Med Hyg* 54, 357–363.

Zou, Z., Shin, S.W., Alvarez, K.S., Kokoza, V., Raikhel, A.S. (2010). Distinct melanization pathways in the mosquito *Aedes aegypti*. *Immunity* 32, 41–53.

14

Hyperinfection Syndrome in Strongyloidiasis

Cristiane Tefé-Silva[1], Eleuza R. Machado[2],
Lúcia H. Faccioli[2] and Simone G. Ramos[1]
[1]*Department of Pathology, Faculty of Medicine of Ribeirão Preto*
[2]*Department of Clinical Analyses, Toxicology and Bromatology Faculty of*
Pharmaceutics Sciences of Ribeirão Preto, University of São Paulo
Brazil

1. Introduction

Strongyloidiasis is an intestinal parasitosis found in tropical and subtropical areas, where the warm climates are suitable for parasite survival (Barr, 1978). It is a common cause of morbidity and mortality, particularly in developing countries, and infects over one-quarter of the world's population (Genta, 1989). Approximately 52 species are known to infect mammals, birds, reptiles and amphibians (Speare, 1989). The most common globally distributed human pathogen of clinical importance is *Strongyloides stercoralis* (Schad, 1989). Another species, *Strongyloides fuelleborni,* is a zoonotic parasite that infects primates and is found sporadically in humans in Africa (Pampiglione & Ricciardi, 1972). *S. stercoralis* is a ubiquitous soil-transmitted intestinal nematode that was first reported in 1876 in French soldiers working in Vietnam. It is unique among helminths in that it completes its life cycle inside a single human host. A unique feature of strongyloidiasis is the ability of the parasite to autoinfect the host, which makes *S. stercoralis* a significant public health problem (Grove, 1989).

2. Epidemiology

The epidemiology of *Strongyloides* infection is poorly understood because it is difficult to detect and can be underestimated (Albonico et al., 1999; Viney & Lok, 2007). However, it is estimated that from 30 a 100 million people are infected worldwide with *Strongyloides,* and can range from asymptomic to multiorgan failure (Genta, 1989). *Strongyloides* is found in tropical and subtropical areas and requires specific soil and climate conditions for its development. In North America, Latin America, Africa and Southeast Asia, the infection is endemic (Roxby et al., 2009). The risk of acquiring strongyloidiasis is higher in rural areas, among people who work with soil, and among lower socioeconomic groups (Vadlamudi et al., 2006; Viney & Lok, 2007). Walking barefoot in areas where human faeces containing the parasite are deposited increases the probability of acquiring the infection (Grove, 1994).

3. Parasite

S. stercoralis has free-living and parasitic life cycles, and the morphology of each differs. Parasitic worms are female adults that reproduce by parthenogenesis and measure approximately 1 - 10 mm in length by 27 -95 μm in width. Free-living adults are approximately 1 mm, live in the soil, and reproduce sexually; females are slightly larger than males (Speare, 1989). Embryonated eggs are thin-shelled and measure approximately 55 - 60 µm in length and 28 - 32 µm in width. Rhabditiform larvae are the first-stage larvae (210 µm) and develop into free-living larvae or third-stage infective larvae that measure approximately 490-630 µm and are capable of infecting the host (Schad, 1989).

4. Life cycle

The life cycle of *S. stercoralis* includes a parasitic cycle (within human hosts) and an environmental cycle (free-living larvae). The parasitic cycle occurs when the infective filariform larvae penetrate the skin and secrete metalloproteases that facilitate penetration. The main larval route is via the bloodstream to the lungs, where they break into the alveolar spaces within hours after infection, promote haemorrhage, ascend the respiratory tree, are swallowed, and migrate to the intestine. Alternatively, the larvae may migrate directly through connective tissues (Grove, 1994, 1996).

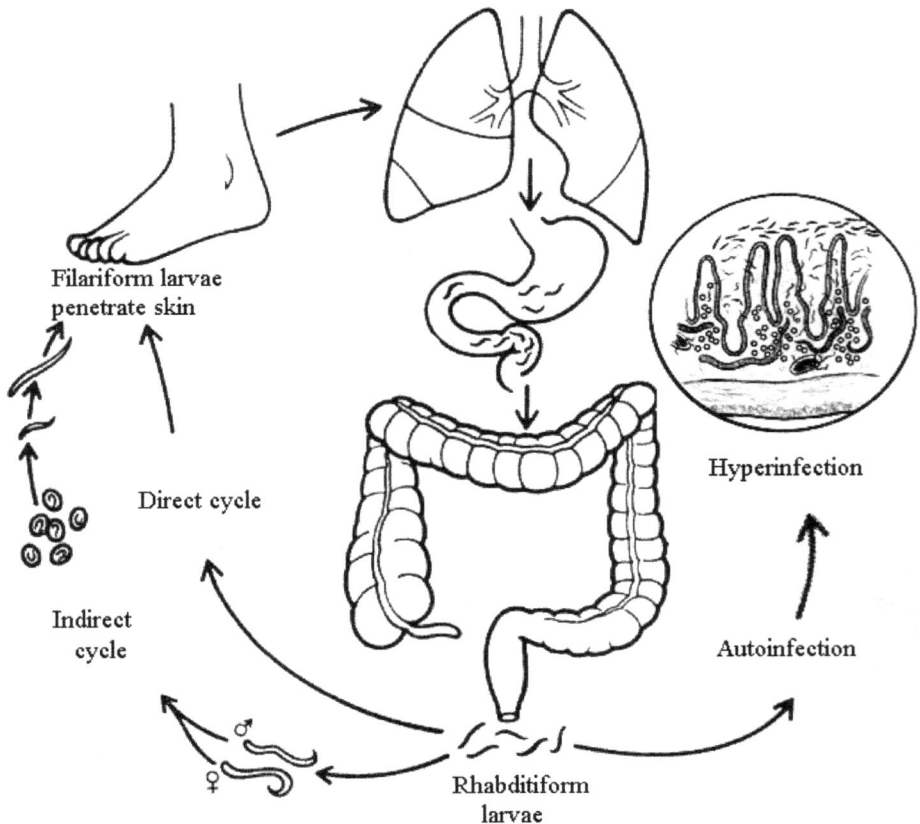

Fig. 1. Life cycle of *Strongyloides stercoralis* (modified from Carvalho & Da Fonseca Porto, 2004, and http://emedicine.medscape.com/article/229312-overview#a0104).

The infective larvae reach the small intestine, where they moult twice to become female adult worms. These females reproduce in the absence of males by parthenogenesis. The females are embedded in the intestinal mucosa and produce eggs in the duodenum. The rhabditiform larvae emerge from the hatching eggs and migrate into the intestinal lumen, then pass into the external environment with the faeces. Depending on temperature and humidity, the rhabditiform larvae may have two different life cycles in the environment: an indirect (heterogonic) life cycle, in which the rhabditiform larvae differentiate into free-living adults and release eggs that hatch and transform into infective larvae, or a direct (homogonic) life cycle, in which the rhabditiform larvae may moult directly into filariform larvae and repenetrate the host skin, restarting the cycle (Schad, 1989).

One characteristic that differentiates *S. stercoralis* from almost all other worms is its capacity to replicate within the host. Rhabditiform larvae in the bowel lumen transform into filariform larvae before excretion and invade the intestinal wall or the perianal skin, permitting ongoing cycles of autoinfection, an important feature of strongyloidiasis (Concha et al., 2005).

5. Clinical manifestation

The clinical presentation of strongyloidiasis varies with the status of the host´s immune system, and the infection is classified as acute, chronic or severe. Acute infections of strongyloidiasis manifest as a wide spectrum of clinical features ranging from asymptomatic disease to cutaneous (larva currens and urticaria), pulmonary (cough and tracheal irritation), and gastrointestinal symptoms (diarrhoea and constipation), although the majority of *S. stercoralis* infections are resolved (Mahmoud, 1996).

The ability of *S. stercoralis* to establish a cycle of autoinfection within the host results in chronic infections that can persist in an individual for decades. Chronic infections are often asymptomatic, but when symptoms occur they are usually mild, episodic and prolonged, including nausea, vomiting, diarrhoea, constipation, weight loss or cutaneous reactions (Grove, 1989).

Uncontrolled autoinfection of *S. stercoralis* is more likely to occur in immunosuppressed patients, leading to hyperinfection syndrome. The pulmonary phase of hyperinfection due to migrating larvae resembles Löffler syndrome with coughing and wheezing, asthma-like symptoms, haemorrhaging and pneumonia. In the intestine, symptoms include diarrhoea, nausea, vomiting, abdominal pain, and weight loss (Concha et al., 2005; Viney & Lok, 2007). Bacteremia is a common complication of hyperinfection syndrome and is caused by filariform larvae that may lead bacteria from the bowel to the bloodstream with subsequent secretion into the host circulation (Bamias et al., 2010). Pathogens such as *Streptococcus bovis*, *Escherichia coli*, *Klebsiella pneumonia* or *Enterobacter cloacae* are found during fatal complications of strongyloidiasis (Link & Orenstein, 1999). The mortality rate of dissemination associated with bacterial infections can reach approximately 90% (Igra-Siegman et al., 1981).

Dissemination occurs upon larval migration to organs beyond the range of the pulmonary phase, such as the liver, heart, lymph nodes, gallbladder, kidneys, pancreas, and brain (Keiser & Nutman, 2004). Petechiae and purpura have also been reported in disseminated cases as a result of larval migration through vessel walls, which promotes haemorrhage (Basile et al., 2010). Others complications of disseminated strongyloidiasis can occur and include syndromes such as cholecystitis, pancreatitis, paralytic ileus, intestinal perforation or infarction, peritonitis, and sepsis (Krishnan et al., 2006). Although unusual, brain involvement can occur in disseminated infections, with symptoms including headache, focal seizures, altered mental state, secondary bacterial meningitis and coma (Dutcher et al., 1990).

6. Hyperinfection syndrome

Since 1966, studies have reported that autoinfection may result in the dissemination of worms; denoted hyperinfection syndrome, the number of worms increases significantly, and worms are detectable in extraintestinal regions, with a mortality rate above 80% (Siddiqui & Berk, 2001). High-risk factors for hyperinfection and dissemination include corticosteroid therapy, malignancies, transplantation, malnutrition, hypogammaglobulinemia, and viral infections such as HIV (Human Immunodeficiency Virus) and HTLV-1 (Human T-Lymphotropic Virus Type 1) (Concha et al., 2005).

6.1 Corticosteroids
In recent decades, hyperinfection syndrome has increased significantly with the use of immunosuppressive drug therapy. Corticosteroids are widely prescribed drugs with potent immunosuppressive effects and are a major risk factor for the transformation of chronic strongyloidiasis into hyperinfection, which has a higher index of mortality (Armignacco et al., 1989; Al Maslamani et al., 2009). Corticosteroids are involved in the treatment of several diseases that are considered immunological abnormalities, such as lymphoma, rheumatoid arthritis, leprosy, chronic obstructive pulmonary disease (COPD), and polymyositis, leading to fatal hyperinfection in many cases (Keiser & Nutman, 2004).
However, the role of corticosteroids in susceptibility to severe *S. stercoralis* infection is poorly understood. One hypothesis is that both endogenous and exogenous corticosteroids promote immunosuppression by decreasing the number of inflammatory cells, such as eosinophils and mast cells, and suppressing the transcription of several cytokines. In addition, corticosteroids increase the apoptosis of Th2 lymphocytes (Genta, 1989). Corticosteroids may also have a direct effect on female worms by increasing the production of ecdysteroid-like molecules, hormones that control moulting in insects and possibly helminths (Genta, 1992). An increase in these molecules increases the moulting rate and transforms rhabditiform larvae into filariform larvae, increasing the worm burden and promoting hyperinfection and dissemination (Genta, 1992; Siddiqui et al., 2000).

6.2 Hematologic and others malignancies
Patients with hematologic malignancies have a high prevalence of *S. stercoralis* infection when compared with the global index. The reported cases of hematologic malignancies and *S. stercoralis* hyperinfection syndrome are associated with glucocorticoid treatment. The malignancy usually associated with *S. stercoralis* is lymphoma that is being treated with chemotherapy. Moreover, lung cancer has been associated with hyperinfection during the administration of immunosuppressive chemotherapy (Keiser & Nutman, 2004).

6.3 Transplantation
Hyperinfection syndrome is associated with transplants, and the progression of chronic intestinal infection before transplantation appears to be the most common mechanism.

Hyperinfection cases following organ transplant principally occur during the initial months after transplantation, but the infection was acquired before transplantation in the majority of cases (Roxby et al., 2009). Higher mortality rates occur from extraintestinal strongyloidiasis, which in most of these cases are related to corticosteroid therapy to treat rejection (Keiser & Nutman, 2004).

Renal transplants are most commonly associated with hyperinfection, which is related to immunosuppressive treatments (Devault et al., 1990; Rajapurkar et al., 2007; Valar et al., 2007). Cases of hyperinfection have been described in transplant recipients of other organs, such as the liver (Vilela et al., 2008; Rodrigues-Hernandez et al., 2009), heart (Schaeffer et al., 2004), pancreas (Ben-Yousseff et al., 2005), lung (Balagopal et al., 2009), and intestine (Patel et al., 2008). Hyperinfection in hematopoietic stem cell transplant patients may be due to immunosuppressive therapies (Dulley et al., 2008; Wirk & Wingard, 2008).

6.4 Malnutrition

An important cause of immunodeficiency that is related to hyperinfection is malnutrition, particularly in developing countries. Malnutrition promotes disruption of the intestinal mucosa, impairing the host's ability to expel the parasite from the gut (Olsen et al., 2009).

6.5 Hypogammaglobulinemia

Patients with immunodeficient conditions, such as hypogammaglobulinemia, may develop fatal hyperinfection. Case reports show that hypogammaglobulinemia is refractory to prolonged anthelmintic therapy (Brandt de Oliveira et al., 1981; Seet et al., 2005).

6.6 HIV

Although HIV infection predisposes a patient to hyperinfection due to immunosuppression, few cases of S. stercoralis and AIDS have been described (Marcos et al., 2008). The association between S. stercoralis and HIV principally occurs in endemic areas (Siddiqui & Berk, 2001). The hyperinfection syndrome can occur in patient with HIV with immune reconstruction syndromes increased after starting of highly active antiretroviral therapy (Brown et al., 2006). On the other hand, the infection with Strongyloides may contribute to serious nutritional deficiencies in HIV-infected individuals, such as anorexia and malabsorption (Lindo et al., 1998). However, the immunobiological and immunoregulatory mechanisms involving HIV and strongyloidiasis remain unclear.

6.7 HTLV-1

HTLV-1 is a virus that infects T cells and induces lymphocyte proliferation with the production of a Th1-type immune response in humans. The genome of the HTLV-1virus is diploid and, following interaction with the immune system, HTLV-1 enables the transcription of the viral DNA by integrating into the host genome effectively evading immune surveillance without killing the host (Iriemenan et al., 2010). Strongyloidiasis is strongly associated with HTLV-1, which predisposes patients to severe infections by depressing cell-mediated immunity or IgE responses (Grove, 1996; Carvalho & Da Fonseca Porto, 2004). Strongyloides and HTLV-1 may promote the Th1-type response in patients, increasing interferon levels and decreasing Th2-type responses, such as interleukin 4 (IL-4), IL-5, IL-13, and IgE, important host defences against helminths, and a decrease in this response allows not only an increasing in autoinfection but also decreased parasite killing.

In addition, this association reduces the efficacy of anthelmintic drugs, increasing the prevalence of infection (Montes et al., 2009; Iriemenam et al., 2010). Stool examinations should be performed with special attention to detect *S. stercoralis* larvae in all patients infected by HTLV-1 (Carvalho & Da Fonseca Porto, 2004).

7. Host-parasite interaction

The relationship between *S. stercoralis* and its host is complex, and little is known about the immunomodulatory mechanisms that regulate this interaction. Different factors are involved, including the capacity of the parasite to replicate, the adequacy of the host immune response, and the ability of the parasite to evade those responses (Grove, 1994; Trajman et al., 1997).

7.1 Cellular immune response

During helminthic infection, Th2-type cell-dependent host defences that involve CD4 cells are developed (Maizels & Yazdanbakhsh, 2003; Anthony et al., 2007). In human hosts and animal models, the cellular immune response to *Strongyloides* infection is characterised by intraepithelial and tissue eosinophils, neutrophils and mast cells with Th2-type production of cytokines such as IL-4, IL-5 and IL-13. Conversely, Th1-type responses are down-regulated during nematode infection (El-Malky et al., 2003; Paterson et al., 2008; Iriemenam et al., 2010).

7.1.1 Eosinophils

Eosinophils are essential against nonphagocytosable parasites, such as *Strongyloides*, that cannot be ingested because of their large size. Eosinophils defend the host by attacking the parasite via the FcεRI receptor, capturing antigens from the worms and presenting the antigens to T cells to initiate an antigen-specific immune response (Galioto et al., 2006; Padigel et al., 2006; Iriemenam et al., 2010). Others mechanisms may be involved, including antibody-dependent cellular cytotoxicity (ADCC) mediated by eosinophils on the parasite surface, which releases toxic molecules in an attempt to eliminate the parasite (Ligas et al., 2003; Klion & Nutman, 2004).

7.1.2 Mast cells

Mast cells have an important role in the defence against *S. stercoralis* by inhibiting the invasion of the adult worm into the intestinal epithelium, promoting the stimulation of gut motility, mucus release and expulsion of the parasites. In addition, mast cells induce the attraction and modulation of eosinophils (Kobayashi et al., 1998; Concha et al., 2005).

7.2 Cytokines

Strongyloidiasis promotes the robust Th2-type immune response with the production of cytokines, such as IL-3, IL-4, IL-5, IL-6, IL-9, IL-10 and IL-13. Contrarily, Th1-type responses are reduced during nematode infection (Wilkes et al., 2007; Patel et al., 2009).

IL-3 is important during *Strongyloides* infection stimulates the synthesis of potent mast cells and basophils enhancing the function of these cells (Abe et al., 1993). In addition, IL-3 can enhance the levels of intra-cellular IL-4 upon activating basophils, with anti-IgE and IL-3 contributing to an increase in eosinophils (Kimura et al., 2006; Lantz et al., 2008).

IL-4 has multiple immunoregulatory functions, including T-cell growth factor activity, B-cell regulation, serum IgE level enhancement, and stimulation of the growth and/or differentiation of macrophages, hematopoietic cells, and mast cells (Urban et al., 1991; Negrão-Correa et al., 2006; Wilkes et al., 2007). IL-4 decreases the fecundity and survival of adult worms and increases intestinal smooth muscle contraction, facilitating the expulsion of the parasite (Concha et al., 2005).

IL-5 regulates the production of eosinophil myelocyte precursors in bone marrow, the development of mature eosinophils after helminth infection and, in most instances, the production of a number of other cytokines, including IL-4 and IL-13, and chemokines such as RANTES and eotaxin (Herbert et al., 2000; Klion & Nutman, 2004; Mir et al., 2006).

IL-13 also participates in the defence mechanisms against helminths, promoting an increase in the intestinal fluid content and increased smooth muscle contractility, a phenomenon that may contribute to worm expulsion (Porto et al., 2001; Shea-Donohue & Urban, 2004; Patel et al., 2009).

7.3 Humoral immune response

The humoral immune response complements defence mechanisms against strongyloidiasis with the production of immunoglobulins by plasma cells. Several immunoglobulins, such as IgE, IgG and IgM, are essential for the elimination of the parasite (Ligas et al., 2003; Machado et al., 2005).

IgE antibodies can mediate the activation of accessory cells and the recognition of parasite antigens, promoting goblet cell mucus secretion and the degranulation of mast cells that release mediators affecting parasite survival (Machado et al., 2009). IgG and IgM can transfer immunity against the human parasite in the presence of the complement system and neutrophils (Abraham et al., 1995; Vadlamudi et al., 2006)

Laboratory models have suggested that both T and B cells mediate the immune response through an increase in immunoglobulins, eosinophils and mast cells and hyperplasia of goblet cells, which require interleukins and chemokines for their development and activation. In strongyloidiasis, dexamethasone seems to primarily suppress cytokines such as IL-1β, IL-4, VEGF, TNF-α, IFN-γ, IL-3, IL-4, IL-5, IL-10 and IL-12 and decreases the production of IgG and IgE antibodies during *S. venezuelensis* infection (Machado et al., 2011; Tefé-Silva et al., 2012).

7.4 Other responses

The complement system activates both classical and alternative pathways with chemoattraction and binding of granulocytes in association with effector cells, which are essential against *S. stercoralis* (Vadlamudi et al., 2006). Studies have reported that complement component C3 is required during *S. stercoralis* infection and facilitates eosinophil degranulation and larval death during the innate immune response (Kerepesi et al., 2006).

Strongyloides infection induces the production of leukotrienes, which are required to invoke the protective expulsion of parasites. Leukotrienes play an important role in controlling parasite burdens, as well as in altering the parasite reproductive cycle and eliminating the *S. venezuelensis* parasite (Machado et al., 2005).

8. Pathology

The pathology of strongyloidiasis differs in different stages of infection.

8.1 Acute infection

The obligate pulmonary phase of the parasite's life cycle typically occurs within hours after infection. During larval passage through the lungs, the parasite induces haemorrhage in the alveolar spaces, inflammatory infiltrate, and, occasionally, granuloma (Kinjo et al., 1998).

Histopathological analyses of human intestines have shown that *S. stercoralis* eggs and adult females colonise the duodenum and upper jejunum. Studies have also demonstrated the presence of oedema, duodenal villous atrophy, and crypt hyperplasia with disrupted epithelium due to the inhibition of cell proliferation and apoptosis (Coutinho et al., 2006; Werneck-Silva et al., 2006). Surface damage, ulceration, an increase in mucus secretion and functional changes in the intestine have also been reported. In many cases, the eosinophil infiltrates are associated with the intensity of the infection (Rivasi et al., 2006; Kishimoto et al., 2008).

8.2 Hyperinfection syndrome

The histology of lungs affected by hyperinfection syndrome revealed alveolar haemorrhage with large numbers of larvae in the alveoli, septa, pleurae and blood vessels. Many larvae were present throughout the walls of the tracheobronchial tree, with an increase in number toward the upper respiratory tract. Larvae in the lungs provoked inflammatory infiltrate

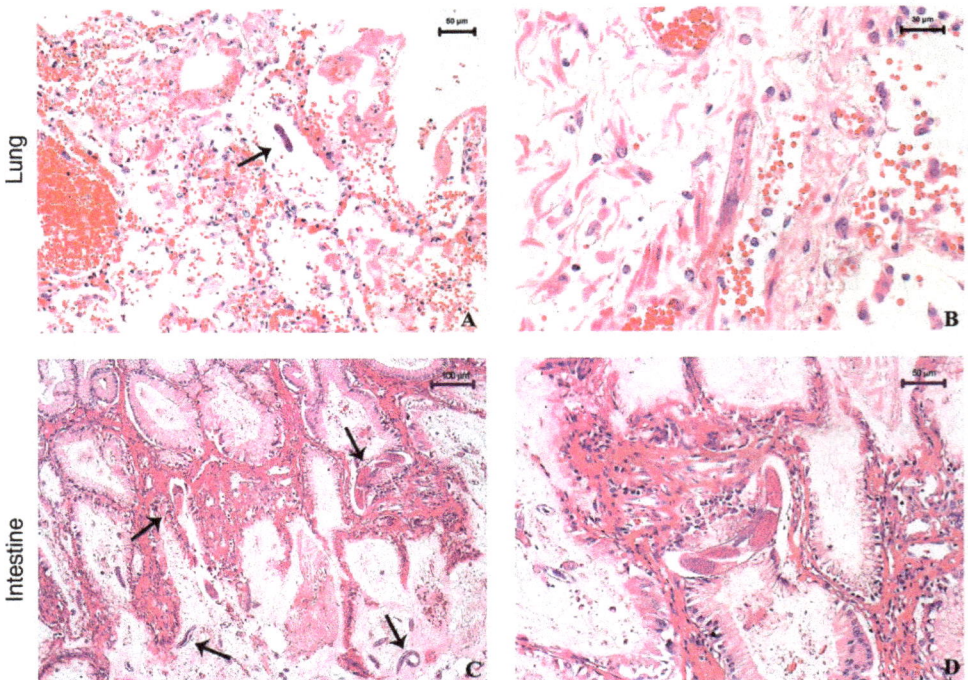

Fig. 2. Histopathology of *Strongyloides stercoralis* in the lungs and intestine of a 48-year-old woman with a gastric carcinoid tumor treated with chemotherapy. A and B: Pulmonary parenchyma. Note the presence of larvae in alveolar space (arrow). C and D: Female worms in the duodena (arrows). HE stain.

and were occasionally walled off by granulomas. Bronchopneumonia is probably a consequence of tissue damage inflicted by the invading larvae (Zumla & James, 2002).

In the human intestine, hyperinfection results in mucosal oedema, acute inflammation, mucosal haemorrhage, and focal ulceration with numerous *S. stercoralis* larvae, adult worms and ova embedded within the small bowel villi (Sathe &Madiwale, 2006; Al Maslamani et al., 2009).

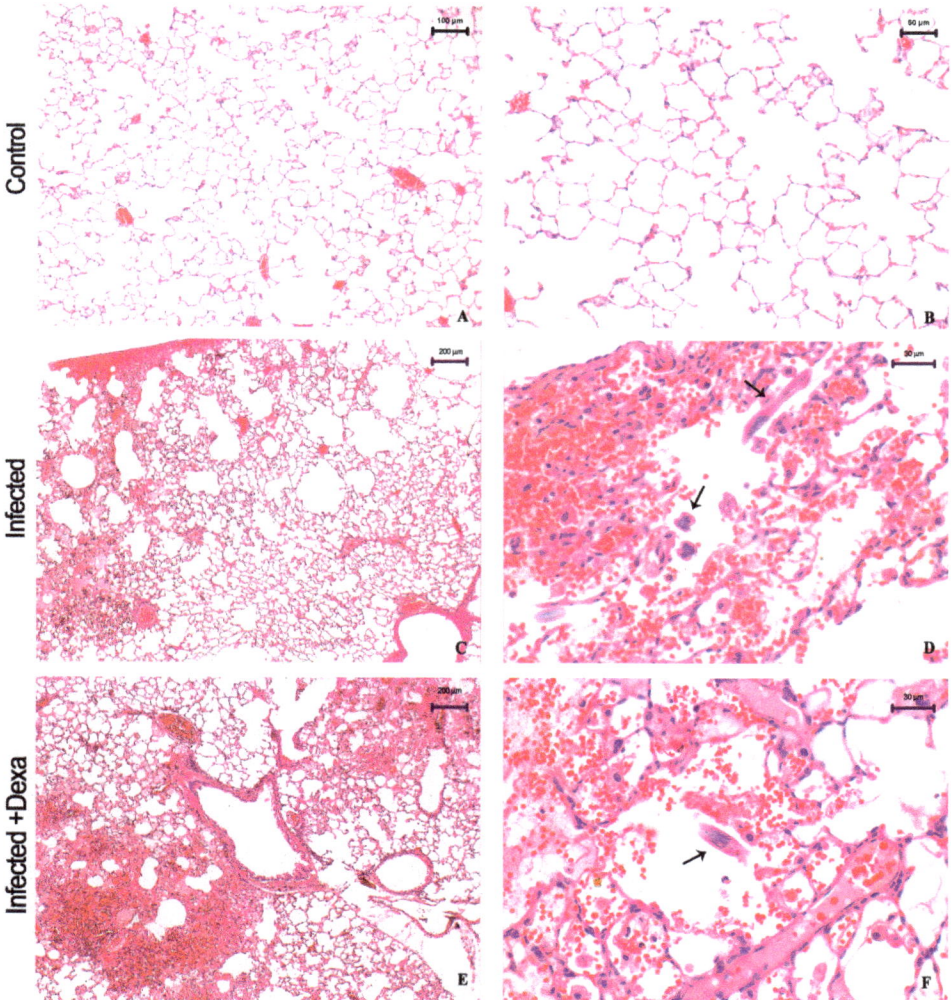

Fig. 3. Histopathology of the lungs of rats in an experimental model of strongyloidiasis on day 3 post-infection: A and B: Controls; C and D: Infected with *S. venezuelensis*. Note the scarce hemorrhagic foci with larvae in the alveolar spaces (arrows); E and F: Infected with *S. venezuelensis* and treated with dexamethasone. Note the prominent hemorrhagic foci showing larvae in the alveolar spaces (arrow). HE stain.

8.3 Hyperinfection syndrome in experimental models

Animal models are important for understanding the mechanism of hyperinfection. Studies in experimental models of *S. venezuelensis* infection have reported that filariform larvae were surrounded by inflammation mediated by eosinophils and mast cells in the lungs. The infection also promoted an important granulomatous response, sometimes entrapping the larvae, which is probably an attempt by the host to contain the parasite. In addition, airway

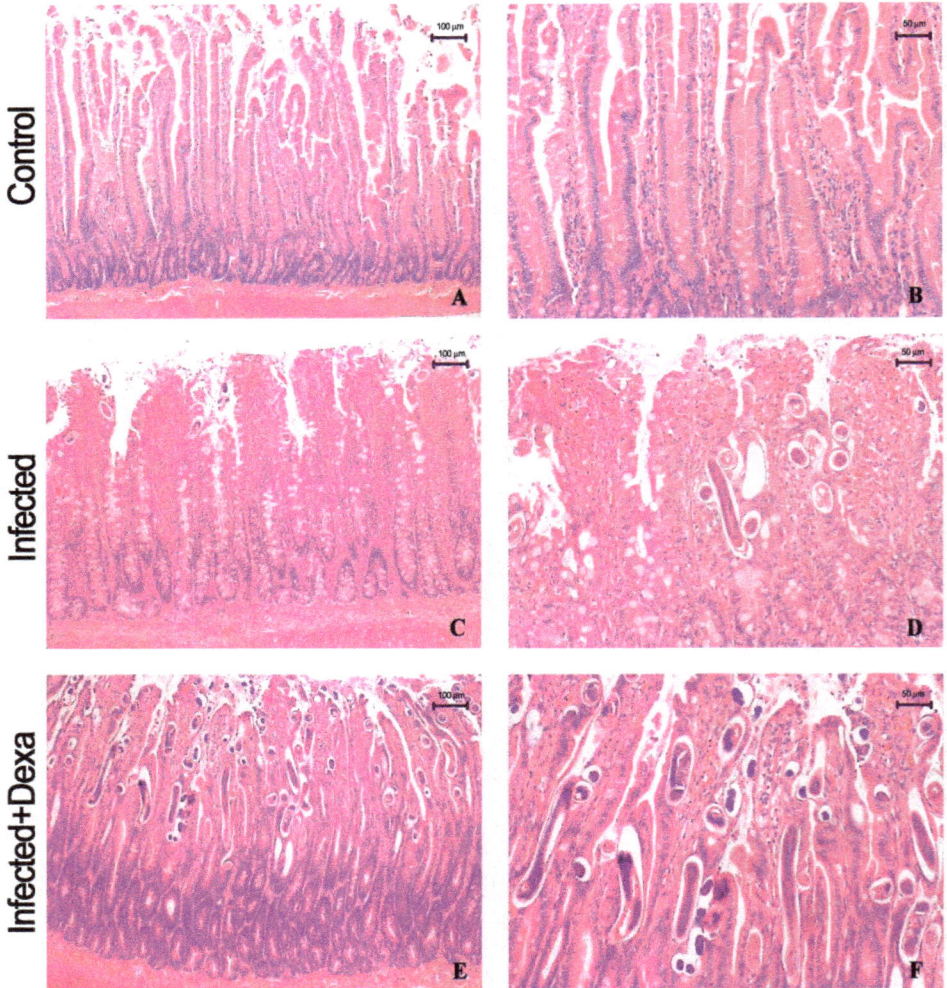

Fig. 4. Histopathology of the duodena of rats in an experimental model of strongyloidiasis on day 14 post-infection: A and B: Controls; C and D: Infected with *S. venezuelensis*. E and F: Infected with *S. venezuelensis* and treated with dexamethasone on day 14 post-infection. Note the massive mucosal invasion of fertile eggs and adult parasites, accompanied by erosion of the intestinal epithelial layer. HE stain.

remodelling similar to asthma, characterised by hyperplasia of goblet cells and increased bronchiolar wall thickness caused by oedema, hypertrophy of smooth muscle cells, neovascularisation and collagen deposition, was reported. In contrast, immunosuppression with dexamethasone interferes with the pulmonary cycle of *Strongyloides venezuelensis* infection and promotes greater haemorrhage, which is provoked by the substantial quantities of larvae that pass into the alveolar spaces, accompanied by a decrease in eosinophil and mast cell migration and impaired formation of granulomas (Tefé-Silva et al., 2008). In addition, dexamethasone treatment inhibited airway remodelling, contributing to the dissemination of the parasite (Tefé-Silva et al., 2012).

In the small intestine of rodents infected with *S. venezuelensis*, females and fertile eggs were observed in the wall of the gastrointestinal tract and invading the intestinal mucosa, with increased inflammatory exudate and eosinophils (Machado et al., 2005). Dexamethasone treatment promoted increased mucus production, which progressed to a massive mucosal invasion of fertile eggs and adult parasites that was accompanied by the erosion of the intestinal epithelial layer. Interestingly, the inflammatory response was relatively inconspicuous. Proliferative activity increased in the crypts and the villous fusion, resulting in an apparent reduction in the number of intestinal epithelial cells. In addition, dexamethasone enhanced parasite fertility and proliferation, with dissemination of the larvae to other visceral organs, such as the spleen, kidneys, heart, liver and brain (Machado et al., 2011).

Mice infected with *S. venezuelensis* and treated with dexamethasone showed increased blood neutrophil numbers and a reduction in eosinophil and mononuclear cell numbers in the blood, bronchoalveolar cells, and peritoneum when compared to *S. venezuelensis* infection in the absence of dexamethasone. In addition, dexamethasone impaired the host immune response, decreasing the production of cytokines such as tumour necrosis factor (TNF), interferon (IFN), interleukin-3 (IL-3), IL-4, IL-5, IL-10, and IL-12 in the lungs and circulating antibodies such as IgG, and IgE but increasing the overall parasite burden in the intestines and faeces (Machado et al., 2011).

9. Diagnosis

Strongyloidiasis is diagnosed on the basis of suspicion in patients with clinical signs and symptoms of the disease; however, in approximately 50% of cases, the infection is asymptomatic, complicating diagnosis. In some cases, diagnosis is difficult despite a low intestinal worm load and larval excretion in the faeces (Rajapurkar et al., 2007).

The classic triad of urticaria, abdominal pain and diarrhoea is suggestive of a diagnosis of strongyloidiasis. Parasites are usually found in the faeces; they are sometimes also seen in other body fluids or in tissue samples (Basile et al., 2010). The parasitological diagnosis is usually made after an examination of the faeces, and several diagnostic methods can be used to detect *S. stercoralis*, including stool examination, a modified Baermann technique, and stool culture on a blood agar plate. Enzyme-linked immunosorbent assays (ELISA) are used for serological diagnosis and have proven valuable in detecting both symptomatic and asymptomatic strongyloidiasis infection, with a high specificity for detecting IgG antibodies to *S. stercoralis* (Basile et al., 2010).

In patients with a disseminated infection, the diagnosis is relatively straightforward, given the high numbers of larvae that exist in the stool and, usually, in the sputum. White blood cell numbers may be elevated. Although an increase in eosinophils frequently occurs during infection, studies have shown that an absence of eosinophilia does not exclude a diagnosis of strongyloidiasis (Krishnan et al., 2006). Diagnosis through imaging is usually possible. Chest radiographs of some patients have shown infiltrate consistent with Loeffler's syndrome. Methods such as bronchoalveolar lavage and sputum culture are used to diagnose disseminated strongyloidiasis (Williams et al., 1988, Yassin et al., 2010). Duodenal fluid aspiration and intestine biopsy or the use of Enterotest ® may be required to detect the *Strongyloides* parasite (Yassin et al., 2010).

10. Treatment

Early identification of the disease and anthelminthic treatment results in a better prognosis for strongyloidiasis and, in many cases, prevents a fatal infection (Basile et al., 2010). *S. stercoralis* is resistant to anthelmintic drugs, and the parasite has the capacity to replicate and increase the worm burden again (Grove, 1996).

Thiabendazole, albendazole, and mebendazole are effective drugs against *S. stercoralis*. Thiabendazole was the drug of choice for treatment of strongyloidiasis, with a cure rate of up to 80%. Albendazole has variable therapeutic efficacy but has been used in hyperinfection syndrome and remains a viable treatment alternative to ivermectin. Mebendazole can be used to treat strongyloidiasis but is not recommended because of an association with liver dysfunction (Rajapurkar et al., 2007). Recently, there has been a change in the treatment of strongyloidiasis, as more studies support the choice of the drug ivermectin, which is effective at killing worms in the intestine. In patients with hyperinfection syndrome, ivermectin is considered the first-line therapy, and longer courses of treatment are indicated (Roxby et al., 2009).

Efficient treatment of strongyloidiasis depends on several factors that can decrease the efficacy of the drugs used for treatment, such as immunodeficiency, corticosteroid use, or co-infection with HTLV-1 (Vadlamudi et al., 2006). Prolonged or repeated treatment may be required in patients receiving immunosuppressive drugs.

Other measures, including decreasing the dosage of corticosteroids, discontinuing immunosuppressive therapies and treating bacterial infections, are essential elements in the treatment of these patients. In all cases, patients with strongyloidiasis, regardless of the severity of symptoms, must be treated to prevent long-term complications (Montes et al., 2010).

11. Control

Like other soil-transmitted nematode infections, strongyloidiasis can be controlled by improving sanitary conditions and properly disposing of faeces. Infected patients should be treated, even if they are asymptomatic, to preclude the possible onset of autoinfection. Immunosuppressants are contraindicated in these patients. Personal hygienic measures like proper protection of the skin to prevent contact with infected soil, community education about protective and hygienic measures, and prompt treatment of diagnosed cases would help prevent the disease (Vadlamudi et al., 2006).

12. Conclusion

Strongyloidiasis is an infection with a tendency to become chronic with an indolent course. However, in immunocompromised patients, especially those treated with corticosteroids, hyperinfection syndrome can compromise the prognosis of the patient. The mortality rates of hyperinfection are high, making *Strongyloides* infection an important global health problem. It is important to understand the biology and immunology of infection with *S. stercoralis* and the altered courses of infection that may occur when immune regulation is compromised. Clinicians who are aware of the possibility of hyperinfection are better equipped to diagnose, treat, or altogether prevent the fatal consequences of this lethal nematode.

13. Acknowledgments

We wish to thank Elaine Medeiros Floriano for excellent technical assistance and Mara R. Celes and Marcela S. Oliveira for photography assistance.

Financial support: This study was supported by the FAPESP (Fundação de Amparo à Pesquisa do Estado de São Paulo) and CNPq (Conselho Nacional de Desenvolvimento Científico e Tecnológico). Cristiane Tefé-Silva is supported by a scholarship through CNPq. Simone G. Ramos and Lúcia H. Faccioli are investigators at CNPq.

14. References

Abe, T., Sugaya, H., &Yoshimura, K. (1998). Analysis of T cell populations and IL-3 mRNA expression in mesenteric lymph node cells and intestinal intraepithelial lymphocytes in *Strongyloides ratti*-infected mice. *Journal of Helminthology,* Vol.72, No.1, (March), pp. 1-8, ISSN 0022-149X

Abraham, D., Rotman, H.L., Haberstroh, H.F., Yutanawiboonchai, W., Brigandi, R.A., Leon, O., Nolan, T.J., & Schad, G.A. (1995). *Strongyloides stercoralis*: protective immunity to third-stage larvae inBALB/cByJ mice. *Experimental Parasitology,* Vol.80, No.2, (March), pp. 297-307, ISSN 1090-2449

Al Maslamani, M.A., Al Soub, H.A., Al Khal, A.L., Al Bozom, I.A., Abu Khattab, M.J.,& Chacko, K.C. (2009). *Strongyloides stercoralis* hyperinfection after corticosteroid therapy: a report of two cases. *Annals of Saudi of Medicine,* Vol.29, No.5, (September-October), pp. 397-401, ISSN 0975-4466

Albonico, M., Crompton, D.W.T., & Savioli, L. (1999). Control strategies for human intestinal nematode infections. *Advances in Parasitology,* Vol.42, pp. 277–341, ISSN 0065-308X

Anthony, R.M., Rutitzky, L.I., Urban, J.F. Jr., Stadecker, M.J., & Gause, W.C. (2007). Protective immune mechanisms in helminth infection. *Nature Reviews Immunology,* Vol.7, pp. 975-987, ISSN 1474-1733

Armignacco, O., Capecchi, A., De Mori, P., & Grillo, L.R. (1989). *Strongyloides stercoralis* hyperinfection and the acquired immunodeficiency syndrome. *American Journal of Medicine,* Vol.86, No.2, (February), pp. 258, ISSN 0002-9343

Balagopal, A., Mills, L., Shah, A., & Subramanian, A. (2009). Detection and treatment of *Strongyloides* hyperinfection syndrome following lung transplantation. *Transplant Infectious Disease,* Vol.11, No.2, (April), pp. 149-154, ISSN 1399-3062

Bamias, G., Toskas, A., Psychogiou, M., Delladetsima, I., Siakavellas, S.I., Dimarogona, K., & Daikos, G.L. (2010). *Strongyloides* hyperinfection syndrome presenting as enterococcal meningitis in a low-endemicity area. *Virulence*, Vol.1, No.5, (September-October), pp. 468-470, ISSN 2150-5608

Barr, J.R. (1978). *Strongyloides stercoralis*. *Canadian Medical Association Journal*, Vol.118, No.8, (April), pp. 933-935, ISSN 1488-2329

Basile, A., Simzar, S., Bentow, J., Antelo, F., Shitabata, P., Peng, S.K., & Craft, N. (2010). Disseminated *Strongyloides stercoralis*: hyperinfection during medical immunosuppression. *Journal of the American Academy of Dermatology*, Vol.63, No.5, (November), pp. 896-902, ISSN 0190-9622

Ben-Youssef, R., Baron, P., Edson, F., Raghavan, R., & Okechukwu, O. (2005). *Strongyloides stercoralis* infection from pancreas allograft: case report. *Transplantation*, Vol.80, No.7, (October), pp. 997-998, ISSN 1534-0608

Brandt de Oliveira, R., Voltarelli, J.C., & Meneghelli, U.G. (1981). Severe strongyloidiasis associated with hypogammaglobulinaemia. *Parasite Immunology*, Vol.3, No.2, (Summer), pp. 165-169, ISSN 1365-3024

Brown, M., Cartledge, J.D., & Miller, R.F. (2006). Dissemination of Strongyloides stercoralis as an immune restoration phenomenon in an HIV-1-infected man on antiretroviral therapy. *International Journal of STD & AIDS*, Vol.15, No.8, (August), pp.560-661, ISSN 0956-4624

Carvalho, E.M. & Da Fonseca Porto, A. (2004). Epidemiological and clinical interaction between HTLV-1 and *Strongyloides stercoralis*. *Parasite Immunology*, Vol.26, No.11-12, (November-December), pp. 487-497, ISSN 1365-302

Concha, R., Harrington, W.Jr., & Rogers, A.I. (2005). Intestinal strongyloidiasis: recognition, management, and determinants of outcome. *Journal of Clinical Gastroenterology*, Vol.39, No.3, (March), pp. 203-211, ISSN 1539-2031

Coutinho, HB., Robalinho, T.I., Coutinho, V.B., Almeida, J.R., Filho, J.T., King, G., Jenkins, D., Mahida, Y., Sewell, H.F., & Wakelin, D. (1996). Immunocytochemistry of mucosal changes in patients infected with the intestinal nematode *Strongyloides stercoralis*. *Journal of Clinical Pathology*, Vol.49, No.10, (October), pp. 717-720, ISSN 1472-4146

DeVault, G.A.Jr., King, J.W., Rohr, M.S., Landreneau, M.D., Brown, S.T.III., & McDonald, J.C. (1990). Opportunistic infections with *Strongyloides stercoralis* in renal transplantation. *Reviews of Infectious Diseases*, Vol.12, No.4, (July-August), pp. 653-671, ISSN 0162-0886

Dulley, F.L., Costa, S., Cosentino, R., Gamba, C., & Saboya, R. (2009). *Strongyloides stercoralis* hyperinfection after allogeneic stem cell transplantation. *Bone Marrow Transplantation*, Vol.43, No.9, (May), pp. 741-742, ISSN 1476-5365

Dutcher, J.P., Marcus, S.L., Tanowitz, H.B., Wittner, M., Fuks, J.Z., & Wiernik, P.H. (1990). Disseminated strongyloidiasis with central nervous system involvement diagnosed antemortem in a patient with acquired immunodeficiency syndrome and Burkitts lymphoma. *Cancer*, Vol.66, No.11, (December), pp. 2417-2420, ISSN 1097-0142

El-Malky, M., Maruyama, H., Hirabayashi, Y., Shimada, S., Yoshida, A., Amano, T., Tominaga, A., Takatsu, K., & Ohta, N. (2003). Intraepithelial infiltration of eosinophils and their contribution to the elimination of adult intestinal nematode,

Strongyloides venezuelensis in mice. *Parasitology International,* Vol.52, No.1, (March), pp. 71-79, ISSN 1383-5769

Galioto, A.M., Hess, J.A., Nolan, T.J., Schad, G.A., Lee, J.J., & Abraham, D. (2006). Role of eosinophils and neutrophils in innate and adaptive protective immunity to larval *Strongyloides stercoralis* in mice. *Infection and Immunity,* Vol.74, No.10, (October), pp. 5730-5738, ISSN 1098-5522

Genta, R.M. (1989). Global prevalence of strongyloidiasis: critical review with epidemiologic insights into the prevention of disseminated disease. *Reviews of Infectious Diseases,* Vol.11, No.5, (September-October), pp. 755-767, ISSN 0162-0886

Genta, R.M. (1992). Dysregulation of strongyloidiasis: a new hypothesis. *Clinical Microbiology Reviews,* Vol.5, No.4, (October), pp. 345-355, ISSN 1098-6618

Grove, D.I. (1994). Strongyloidiasis: a conundrum for gastroenterologists. *Gut,* Vol.35, No.4, (April), pp. 437-440, ISSN 1468-3288

Grove, D.I. (1996). Human strongyloidiasis. *Advances in Parasitology,* Vol.38, pp. 251-309, ISBN 0-12-031738-9, London United Kingdom

Grove, D.I. (1989a). Clinical manifestations. In: Strongyloidiasis a major roundworm infection of man, D.I. Grove (Ed.), 155–174, Taylor and Francis, ISBN 0-85066-732-1, London, United Kingdom

Herbert, D.R., Lee, J.J., Lee, N.A., Nolan, T.J., Schad, G.A., & Abraham, D. (2000) Role of IL-5 in innate and adaptive immunity to larval *Strongyloides stercoralis* in mice. *Journal of Immunology,* Vol.165, No.8, (October), pp. 4544-4551, ISSN 1550-6606

Igra-Siegman, Y., Kapila, R., Sem, P., Kaminski, Z.C., & Louria, D.B. (1981). Syndrome of hyperinfection with *Strongyloides stercoralis. Reviews of Infectious Diseases,* Vol.3, No.3, (May-June), pp. 397-407, ISSN 0162-0886

Iriemenam, N.C., Sanyaolu, A.O., Oyibo, W.A., & Fagbenro-Beyioku, A.F. (2010). *Strongyloides stercoralis* and the immune response. *Parasitology International,* Vol.59, No.1, (March), pp. 9-14, ISSN 1383-5769

Keiser, P.B. & Nutman, T.B. (2004). *Strongyloides stercoralis* in the immunocompromised population. *Clinical Microbiology Reviews,* Vol.17, No.1, (January), pp. 208-217, ISSN 1098-6618

Kerepesi, L.A., Hess, J.A., Nolan, T.J., Schad, G.A., & Abraham, D. (2006). Complement component C3 is required for protective innate and adaptive immunity to larval *Strongyloides stercoralis* in mice. *The Journal of Immunology,* Vol. 176, No.7, (April), pp. 4315-4322, ISSN 1550-6606

Kimura, K., Song, C.H., Rastogi, A., Dranoff, G., Galli, S.J., & Lantz, C.S. (2006). Interleukin-3 and c-Kit/stem cell factor are required for normal eosinophil responses in mice infected with *Strongyloides venezuelensis. Laboratory Investigation,* Vol.86, No.10, (October), pp. 987-996, ISSN 1530-0307

Kinjo, T., Tsuhako, K., Nakazato, I., Ito, E., Sato, Y., Koyanagi, Y., & Iwamasa, T. (1998). Extensive intra-alveolar haemorrhage caused by disseminated strongyloidiasis. *International Journal for Parasitology,* Vol.28, No.2, (February), pp. 323-330, ISSN 1879-013

Kishimoto, K., Hokama, A., Hirata, T; Ihama, Y., Nakamoto, M., Kinjo, N., Kinjo, F., & Fujita, J. (2008). Endoscopic and histopathological study on the duodenum of *Strongyloides stercoralis* hyperinfection. *World Journal of Gastroenterology*, Vol.14, No.11, (March), pp. 1768-1773, ISSN 1007-9327

Klion, A.D. & Nutman, T.B. (2004). The role of eosinophils in host defense against helminth parasites. *Journal of Allergy and Clinical Immunology*, Vol.113, No.1, (January), pp. 30-37, ISSN 0091-6749

Krishnan, S., Barger, G., & Chandrasekar, P. (2006). Recurrent *Strongyloides stercoralis* hyperinfection syndrome case report and a brief review. *Infectious Diseases in Clinical Practice*, Vol.14, No.4, (July), pp. 240–243, ISSN 1056-9103

Kobayashi, T., Tsuchiya, K., Hara, T., Nakahata, T., Kurokawa, M., Ishiwata, K., Uchiyama, F., & Nawa, Y. (2008). Intestinal mast cell response and mucosal defence against *Strongyloides venezuelensis* in interleukin-3-hyporesponsive mice. *Parasite Immunology*, Vol.20, No.6, (June), pp. 279-284, ISSN 1365-3024

Lantz, C.S., Min, B., Tsai, M., Chatterjea, D., Dranoff, G., & Galli, S.J. (2008). IL-3 is required for increases in blood basophils in nematode infection in mice and can enhance IgE-dependent IL-4 production by basophils in vitro. *Laboratory Investigation*, Vol.88, No.11, (November), pp. 1134-1142, ISSN 1530-0307

Ligas, J.A., Kerepesi, L.A., Galioto, A.M., Lustigman, S., Nolan, T.J., Schad, G.A., & Abraham, D. (2003). Specificity and mechanism of immunoglobulin M (IgM)- and IgG-dependent protective immunity to larval *Strongyloides stercoralis* in mice. *Infection and Immunity*, Vol.71, No.12, (December), pp. 6835-6843, ISSN 1098-5522

Lindo, J.F., Dubon, J.M., Ager, A.L., de Gourville, E.M., Solo-Gabriele, H., Klaskala, W.I., Baum, M.K., & Palmer, C.J. (1998). Intestinal parasitic infections in human immunodeficiency virus (HIV)-positive and HIV-negative individuals in San Pedro Sula, Honduras. *American Journal of Tropical Medicine and Hygiene*. Vol.58, No.4, (April), pp. 431-435, ISSN 0002-9637

Link, K. & Orenstein, R. (1999). Bacterial complications of strongyloidiasis: *Streptococcus bovis meningitis*. *Southern Medical Journal*, Vol.72, No.7, (July), pp. 728-731, ISSN 0038-4348

Machado, E.R., Ueta, M.T., Lourenço, E.V., Anibal, F.F., Sorgi, C.A., Soares, E.G., Roque-Barreira, M.C., Medeiros, A.I., & Faccioli, L.H. (2005). Leukotrienes play a role in the control of parasite burden in murine strongyloidiasis. *Journal of Immunology*, Vol.175, No.6, (September), pp. 3892-3899, ISSN 1550-6606

Machado, E.R., Carlos, D., Lourenço, E.V., Sorgi, C.A., Silva, E.V., Ramos, S.G., Ueta, M.T., Aronoff, D.M., & Faccioli, L.H. (2009). Counterregulation of Th2 immunity by interleukin 12 reduces host defenses against *Strongyloides venezuelensis* infection. *Microbes and Infection*, Vol.11, No.5, (April), pp. 571-578, ISSN 1286-4579

Machado, E.R., Carlos, D., Sorgi, C.A., Ramos, S.G., Souza, D.I., Soares, E.G., Costa-Cruz, .JM., Ueta, M.T., Aronoff, D.M., & Faccioli, L.H. (2011). Dexamethasone effects in the *Strongyloides venezuelensis* infection in murine model. *American Journal of Tropical Medicine and Hygiene*, Vol.84, No.6, (June), pp. 957-966, ISSN 0002-9637

Mahmoud, A.A. (1996). Strongyloidiasis. *Clinical Infectious Diseases*, Vol.23, No.5, (November), pp. 949-952, ISSN 1537-6591

Maizels, R.M. & Yazdanbakhsh, M. (2003). Immune regulation by helminth parasites: cellular and molecular mechanisms. *Nature Reviews Immunology*, Vol.3, (September), pp. 733-744, ISSN 1474-1733

Marcos, L.A., Terashima, A., Dupont, H.L., & Gotuzzo, E. (2008). *Strongyloides* hyperinfection syndrome: an emerging global infectious disease. *Transaction of the Royal Society of Tropical Medicine and Hygiene*, Vol.102, No.4, (April), pp. 314-318, ISSN 0035-9203

Mir, A., Benahmed, D., Igual, R., Borrás, R., O'Connor, J.E., Moreno, M.J., & Rull, S. (2006). Eosinophil-selective mediators in human strongyloidiasis. *Parasite Immunology*, Vol.28, No.8, (August), pp. 397-400, ISSN 1365-3024

Montes, M., Sanchez, C., Verdonck, K., Lake, J.E., Gonzalez, E., Lopez, G., Terashima, A., Nolan, T., Lewis, D.E., Gotuzzo, E., White, & A.C.Jr. (2009). Regulatory T cell expansion in HTLV-1 and strongyloidiasis co-infection is associated with reduced IL-5 responses to *Strongyloides stercoralis* antigen. *PLoS Neglected Tropical Diseases*, Vol.9, No.6, (June), pp. e456, ISSN 1935-2735

Negrão-Corrêa, D., Pinho, V., Souza, D.G., Pereira, A.T., Fernandes, A., Scheuermann, K., Souza, A.L., & Teixeira, M.M. (2006). Expression of IL-4 receptor on non-bone marrow-derived cells is necessary for the timely elimination of *Strongyloides venezuelensis* in mice, but not for intestinal IL-4 production. *International Journal for Parasitology*, Vol.36, No.10-11, (September), pp. 1185-1195, ISSN 1879-0135

Olsen, A., van Lieshout, L., Marti, H., Polderman, T., Polman, K., Steinmann, P., Stothard, R., Thybo, S., Verweij, J.J., & Magnussen, P. (2009). Strongyloidiasis-the most neglected of the neglected tropical diseases? *Transaction of the Royal Society of Tropical Medicine and Hygiene*, Vol.103, No.10, (October), pp. 967-972, ISSN 0035-9203

Padigel, U.M., Lee, J.J., Nolan, T.J., Schad, G.A., & Abraham, D. (2006). Eosinophils can function as antigen-presenting cells to induce primary and secondary immune responses to *Strongyloides stercoralis*. *Infection and Immunity*, Vol.74, No.6, (June), pp. 3232-3238, ISSN 1098-5522

Pampiglione, S. & Ricciardi, M.L. (1972). Geographic distribution of *Strongyloides fuelleborni* in humans in tropical Africa. *Parasitologia*, Vol.14, pp. 329–338

Patel, N., Kreider, T., Urban JF Jr., & Gause, W.C. (2009). Characterisation of effector mechanisms at the host: parasite interface during the immune response to tissue-dwelling intestinal nematode parasites. *International Journal for Parasitology*, Vol.39, No.1, (January), pp. 13-21, ISSN 1879-0135

Paterson, S., Wilkes, C., Bleay, C., & Viney, M.E. (2008). Immunological responses elicited by different infection regimes with *Strongyloides ratti*. *PLoS One*, Vol.3, No.6, (June), pp. e2509, ISSN 1932-6203

Porto, A.F., Neva, F.A., Bittencourt, H., Lisboa, W., Thompson, R., Alcântara, L., & Carvalho, E.M. (2001). HTLV-1 decreases Th2 type of immune response in patients with strongyloidiasis. *Parasite Immunology*, Vol.23, No.9, (September), pp. 503-507, ISSN 1365-3024

Rajapurkar, M., Hegde, U., Rokhade, M., Gang, S., & Gohel, K. (2007). Respiratory hyperinfection with *Strongyloides stercoralis* in a patient with renal failure. *Nature Clinical Practice Nephrology*, Vol.3, No.10, (October), pp. 573-577, ISSN 1745-8331

Rivasi, F., Pampiglione, S., Boldorini, R., & Cardinale, L. (2006). Histopathology of gastric and duodenal *Strongyloides stercoralis* locations in fifteen immunocompromised subjects. *Archives of Pathology & Laboratory Medicine*, Vol.130, No.12, (December), pp. 1792-1798, ISSN 1543-2165

Rodriguez-Hernandez, M.J., Ruiz-Perez-Pipaon, M., Cañas, E., Bernal, C., & Gavilan, F. (2009). *Strongyloides stercoralis* hyperinfection transmitted by liver allograft in a transplant recipient. *American Journal of Transplantation*, Vol.9, No.11, (November), pp. 2637-2640, ISSN 1600-6143

Roxby, A.C., Gottlieb, G.S., & Limaye, A.P. (2009). Strongyloidiasis in transplant patients. *Clinical Infection Diseases*, Vol.49, No.9, (November), pp. 1411-1423, ISSN 1537-6591

Sathe, P.A. & Madiwale, C.V. (2006). Strongyloidiasis hyperinfection in a patient with membranoproliferative glomerulonephritis. *Journal of Postgraduate Medicine*, Vol.52, No.3, (July-September), pp. 221-222, ISSN 0022-3859

Schad, G.A. (1989). Morphology and life history of *Strongyloides stercoralis*. In: Strongyloidiasis a major roundworm infection of man, D.I. Grove (Ed.), 85-104, Taylor and Francis, ISBN 0-85066-732-1, London, United Kingdom

Schaeffer, M.W., Buell, J.F., Gupta, M., Conway, G.D., Akhter, S.A., & Wagoner, L.E. (2004). *Strongyloides* hyperinfection syndrome after heart transplantation: case report and review of the literature. *The Journal of Heart and Lung Transplantation*, Vol.23, No.7, (July), pp. 905–911, ISSN 1053-2498

Seet, R.C., Lau, L.G., & Tambyah, P.A. (2005). *Strongyloides* hyperinfection and hypogammaglobulinemia. *Clinical and Diagnostic Laboratory Immunology*, Vol.12, No.5, (May), pp. 680-682, ISSN 1098-6588

Shea-Donohue; T.B. & Urban, J.F.Jr. (2004). Gastrointestinal parasite and host interactions. *Current Opinion in Gastroenterology*, Vol.20, No.1 (January), pp. 3-9, ISSN 1531-7056

Siddiqui, A.A. & Berk, S.L. (2001). Diagnosis of *Strongyloides stercoralis* infection. *Clinical Infectious Diseases*, Vol.33, No.7, (October), pp. 1040-1047, ISSN 1537-6591

Siddiqui, A.A., Stanley, C.S., Skelly, P.J., & Berk, S.L. (2000). A cDNA encoding a nuclear hormone receptor of the steroid/thyroidhormone-receptor superfamily from the human parasitic nematode *Strongyloides stercoralis*. *Parasitology Research*, Vol.86, No.1, (January), pp. 24-29, ISSN 1432-1955

Speare, R. (1989). Identification of species of *Strongyloides*. In: Strongyloidiasis a major roundworm infection of man, D.I. Grove (Ed.), 11-84, Taylor and Francis, ISBN 0-85066-732-1, London, United Kingdom

Tefé-Silva, C., Souza, D.I., Ueta, M.T., Floriano, E.M., Faccioli, L.H., & Ramos, S.G. (2008). Interference of dexamethasone in the pulmonary cycle of *Strongyloides venezuelensis* in rats. *American Journal of Tropical Medicine and Hygiene*, Vol.79, No.4, (October), pp. 571-578, ISSN 0002-9637

Tefé-Silva, C., Beneli, C.T., Celes, M.R., Machado, E.R., Ueta, M.T., Sorgi, C.A., Floriano, E.M., Faccioli, L.H., & Ramos, S.G. (2012). Dexamethasone reduces bronchial wall remodeling during pulmonary migration of *Strongyloides venezuelensis* larvae in rats. *Parasitology International*, Accepted, ISSN 1383-5769

Trajman, A., MacDonald, T.T., & Elia, C.C. (1997). Intestinal immune cells in *Strongyloides stercoralis* infection. *Journal of Clinical Pathology*, Vol.50, No.12, (December), pp. 991-995, ISSN 1472-4146

Urban, J.F.Jr., Madden, K.B., Svetić, A., Cheever, A., Trotta, P.P., Gause, W.C., Katona, .IM., & Finkelman, F.D. (1992). The importance of Th2 cytokines in protective immunity to nematodes. *Immunology Reviews*, Vol.127, (June), pp. 205-220, ISSN 1600-065X

Vadlamudi, R.S., Chi, D.S., & Krishnaswamy, G. (2006). Intestinal strongyloidiasis and hyperinfection syndrome. *Clinical and Molecular Allergy*, Vol.4, No.8, (May), ISSN 1476-7961

Valar, C., Keitel, E., Dal Prá, R.L., Gnatta, D., Santos, A.F., Bianco, P.D., Sukiennik, T.C., Pegas, K.L., Bittar, A.E., Oliveira, K.T., & Garcia, V.D. (2007). Parasitic infection in renal transplant recipients. *Transplantation Proceedings*, Vol.39, No.2, (March), pp. 460–462, ISSN 0041-1345

Vilela, E.G., Clemente, W.T., Mira, R.R., Torres, H.O., Veloso, L.F., Fonseca, L.P, de Carvalho E Fonseca, L.R., Franca, M.C., & Lima, A.S. (2009). *Strongyloides stercoralis* hyperinfection syndrome after liver transplantation: case report and literature review. *Transplant Infectious Disease*, Vol.11, No.2, (April), pp. 132–136, ISSN 1399-3062

Viney, M.E. & Lok, J.B. (2007). *Strongyloides* spp. *WormBook*, Vol.23, No.2, (April), pp. 1-15, ISSN 1551-8507

Werneck-Silva, A.L., Alvares, E.P., Gama, P., Damiao, A.O., Osaki, L.H., Ogias, D., & Sipahi, A.M. (2006). Intestinal damage in strongyloidiasis: the imbalance between cell death and proliferation. *Digestive Diseases Sciences*, Vol.51, No.6, (June), pp. 1063-1069, ISSN 1573-2568

Wilkes, C.P., Bleay, C., Paterson, S., &Viney, M.E. (2007). The immune response during a *Strongyloides ratti* infection of rats. *Parasite Immunology*, Vol.29, No.7, (July), pp. 339-346, ISSN 1365-3024

Williams, J., Dralle, W., Berk, S.L., & Verghese, A. (1988). Diagnosis of pulmonary strongyloidiasis by bronchoalveolar lavage. *Chest*, Vol.94, No.3, (September), pp. 643-644, ISSN 1931-3543

Wirk, B., & Wingard, J.R. (2009). *Strongyloides stercoralis* hyperinfection in hematopoietic stem cell transplantation. *Transplant Infectious Disease*, Vol.11, No.2, (April), pp. 143-148, ISSN 1399-3062

Yassin, M.A., El Omri, H., Al-Hijji, I., Taha, R., Hassan, R., Aboudi, K.A., & El-Ayoubi, H. (2010). Fatal *Strongyloides stercoralis* hyper-infection in a patient with multiple myeloma. *The Brazilian Journal of Infectious Diseases*, Vol.14, No.5, (October), pp. 536-539, ISSN 1678-4391

Zumla, A.I. & James, D.G. (2002). Immunologic aspects of tropical lung disease. *Clinics in Chest Medicine*, Vol.23, No.2, (June), pp. 283-308, ISSN 1557-8216

15

Lymphatic Filariasis Transmission and Control: A Mathematical Modelling Approach

Asep K. Supriatna and N. Anggriani

Padjadjaran University
Indonesia

1. Introduction

Lymphatic filariasis has an effect on almost 120 million individuals all over the world. The disease may cause a chronic morbidity if the persons who are infected are left untreated. It is endemic in many parts of tropical countries. To prevent worldwide parasite transmission, the World Health Organization initiated the Global Programme to Eliminate Lymphatic Filariasis (GPELF) by eliminating filarial parasites from their human hosts (Molyneux & Zagaria, 2002). Various GPELF implementations are done in many participating countries. In 2004 alone there were more than thirty countries have started elimination program and this number is still rising. Various degrees of success have emerged as a result of the implementation of this program. Although it was reported that in some places the program has interrupted the transmission, in many other places the program could not stop the transmission of the disease (WHO, 2005). It has been argued that strategic choices and operational or biological factors contribute to the success or failure of the program. In general, it is difficult to evaluate the success or the failure of a health program, especially in the beginning of the program.

A mathematical model provides useful tools for planning and evaluation of control program in disease elimination (Goodman, 1994). In our earlier work (Supriatna *et al.*, 2009) we develop a mathematical model for the transmission of Lymphatic Filariasis disease in Jati Sampurna, Indonesia. In Indonesia, the disease is already alarming. For example, the incidence of filariasis in Jati Sampurna (a district in the West Java province) is more than 1%. Within less than five years since the date of the publication confirming that Jati Sampurna is an endemic area, almost all regions nearby Jati Sampurna, and other relatively far distance areas are affected by the disease, and some of them are also categorized as endemic areas. Other cases of filarial prevalence are reported outside Java island, such as in Alor islands (the province of Nusa Tenggara Timur). On Alor islands, both *B. timori* and *W. bancrofti* are circulated, with a prevalence of up to 20% (Supali *et al.*, 2002). Indonesia joined the GPELF since 2001 and implemented administration of a single dose regimen of diethylcarbamazine (DEC) and albendazole in endemic areas (Krentel *et al.*, 2006). Our previous model tries to capture the effectiveness of this scenario in the attempt of controlling the spread of the disease, inspired by the transmission of the disease in Jati Sampurna.

The model assumes that acute infected humans are infectious and treatment is given to a certain number of acute infected humans found from screening process. The screening is done every time a new chronic reported. The treated acute individuals are assumed to be remains susceptible to the disease. The model is analyzed and it is found a condition for the existence and stability of the endemic equilibrium. A well known rule of thumb in epidemiological model, that is, the endemic equilibrium exists and stable if the basic reproduction number is greater than one, is established. Moreover, it is also shown that if the level of screening is sufficiently large, current medical treatment strategy will be able to reduce the long-term level of incidences. However, in practice it is not realistic for the following reasons.

One important concept in mathematical epidemiology regarding transmission of a disease is the basic reproduction number. It measures the number of new infections caused by an infective during the life time of the infective. Although our previous model is able to gain some insights on how the provision of a medical treatment can reduce the level of disease incidence, however it is worth to note that the basic reproduction number does not depend on the level of the treatment. It means that the treatment, no matter how large it is, will not be able to annihilate the endemicity of the disease. This is some what surprising and unexpected, because normally, in many epidemiological models, any medical treatment should reduce the basic reproduction number.

Our earlier work shows that the medical treatment given in the model scenario cannot eliminate the disease, in terms of reducing the basic reproduction number. Our previous model has also ignored an important factor in the transmission stage, namely the time delay. The model has assumed that once an individual infected, he/she become infectious without any delay. Nonetheless, the reproduction number can be reduced by giving additional treatments, such as reducing the biting rate and mosquito's density. This suggests that there should be a combination of treatment to eliminate the disease. In this chapter we review our earlier model of the filariasis transmission and a new model based on the earlier work is developed and analysed. The chapter gives a step by step improvement of our previous model. We do not carry out a heavy mathematical analysis instead some simulations of the models are presented. Finally, some interpretations are derived from the results.

2. Mathematical model with no time delay in infection period

To formulate the model we use the assumptions that initially the human population is virgin, *i.e.* there is no infection, and the total population of human is constant. We assume that there is an invasion by few infective individuals of either human or mosquitoes. There is only one species of worm and one species of mosquito, and there is no vertical transmission of the disease, either in human or mosquitoes populations. The human population is divided into three subpopulations, susceptible S_H, infected-carrier A and infected-chronic K, with the total number of the population given by N_H. We assume that once a human individual is infected then without any delay the individual becomes infectious. However, we strictly assume that transmission to the mosquitoes is only from the acute population. All chronic individuals are isolated perfectly. This strict assumption will be relaxed in some simulation later on. The mosquitoes are divided in two subpopulations, susceptible S_V and infected I_V mosquitoes, with the total number N_V. Related parameters in the model are the human recruitment rate R_H, human death rate μ_H, successful rate of transmission from mosquitoes to susceptible human p_H, mosquitoes biting rate on human

b , symptomatic rate δ , mosquitoes recruitment rate R_V , mosquitoes death rate μ_V and successful rate of filarial transmission from human to susceptible mosquitoes p_V. If the medical treatment is quantified by n number of people screened by the health authority, for every single chronic found, with the successful probability of the treatment p_0, then the governing differential equations describing the mathematical model of the disease transmission are given by the following equations:

$$\frac{dS_H}{dt} = R_H - \frac{bp_H I_V S_H}{N_H} - \mu_H S_H + \frac{p_0 n \delta A^2}{N_H} , \tag{1}$$

$$\frac{dA}{dt} = \frac{bp_H I_V S_H}{N_H} - \mu_H A - \delta A - \frac{p_0 n \delta A^2}{N_H} , \tag{2}$$

$$\frac{dK}{dt} = \delta A - \mu_H K , \tag{3}$$

$$\frac{dS_V}{dt} = R_V - \frac{bp_V A S_V}{N_H} - \mu_V S_V , \tag{4}$$

$$\frac{dI_V}{dt} = \frac{bp_V A S_V}{N_H} - \mu_V I_V . \tag{5}$$

We can evaluate the effectiveness of the medical treatment n in managing the disease within the presumed policy, by inspecting its appearance in the endemic equilibrium and in the basic reproduction number. From the model, by assuming the host and vector populations are constant, so that $N_H = \frac{R_H}{\mu_H}$ and $N_V = \frac{R_V}{\mu_V}$, we found the endemic and non-endemic equilibria of the model related to the basic reproduction number

$$R_0 = \frac{\sqrt{b^2 R_H R_V \mu_H p_H p_V (\delta + \mu_H)}}{R_H \mu_V (\delta + \mu_H)} . \tag{6}$$

We also establish a theorem saying that "if $R_0 > 1$ then the endemic equilibrium of the system is locally asymptotically stable, otherwise it is unstable". The details of the derivation can be seen in Supriatna et al. (2009). In terms of controlling the disease it means that we should keep the basic reproduction number as low as possible so that it is lower than the unity by adjusting the level of the treatment n. The basic reproduction number is obtained using the next generation matrix (see Diekmann & Heesterbeek, 2000). It is worth to note that the basic reproduction number does not depend on the level of screening n, and hence, current presumed method of treatment does not annihilate the endemicity of the disease. This is partially because of the re-susceptibility of the treated population. However, our earlier work show that it indeed reduces the number of the acute population in the long-term as shown in the following section.

2.1 Numerical examples for the model with no delay time in infection period

To facilitate some interpretation regarding the results in our previous work, we present numerical examples using the parameters shown in Table 1. The simulation uses Powersim Constructor Ver. 2.5d with the program listing equivalent to basic model of equations (1) to (5) is provided in the Appendices. Powersim code for other models in the preceding section can be easily modified from this basic model. We give two examples: the first example assumes that a virgin population is invaded by acute infected human (via human immigration) and the second example assume that a virgin population is invaded by infected mosquitoes (e.g. a container un-intentionally transporting infected mosquitoes from an endemic area).

Parameter	Value	Parameter	Value
R_H	2,500	R_V	1,000,000
μ_H	1/70	μ_V	365 (1/30)
δ	0.25	b	250
p_H	0.01	p_V	0.1
n	0	p_0	0.75

Table 1. The main values of parameters used in the numerical examples

Figure 1 depicts the following scenario. Suppose that a population is initially virgin and stays at its equilibrium. We assume that it is then invaded by 10 acute infected human individual, with all the mosquitoes are also virgin. Using the parameter values given in Table 1, we obtain the value of the basic reproduction number is 3.02, which means that the disease will increase if there is no intervention. Figure 1 shows the dynamics when there is no treatment ($n=0$). The effect of the values of the parameters on the basic reproduction number is clear from equation (6). However its effect on the dynamics and the endemic equilibrium is not so obvious. Figure 2 shows the same dynamics as in Figure 1, with an addition that in the 25th year after the invasion of infective individuals there is a medical treatment with $n=200$. Figure 3 shows the same dynamics as in Figure 1, but here the treatment is carried out as early as the 5th year after the invasion with only 100 screening ($n=100$). These figures reveal that an early average treatment is better than a late huge treatment.

The scenario in Figures 1 to 3 assumes that the medical treatment given to the infected persons does not affect the transmission parameters given in Table 1 other than the screening parameter n. The screening parameter n does not appear in the basic reproduction number formula (6). Hence, this treatment does not affect the endemic status of the disease. In reality, there are some treatments that could alter the values of the disease transmission parameters. For example, if we assume that some portion of the population is treated by giving them some insect repellent, then the biting rate b could be altered. Let us assume that an effective insect repellent could decrease the biting rate to 50% of its current level. Figure 4 shows the dynamic when there exist this effective insect repellent, and used from the 5th year in the absence of the medical treatment ($n=0$) and Figure 5 shows the same scenario as in the previous figure but in the presence of the medical treatment with $n=100$ given by the same time as the insect repellent provision. Compared to the case when there is no insect repellent (Figure 1), the introduction of the insect repellent is significantly reduces the level of the disease outbreak (Figure 4) and in the same time reduces the endemic level of the disease (changing the value of the basic reproduction number from 3.02 to 1.51). Meanwhile, if we also apply the medical treatment with only average treatment ($n=100$), then the level of the outbreak is relatively the same, but apparently with a shorter period of the outbreak (Figure 5).

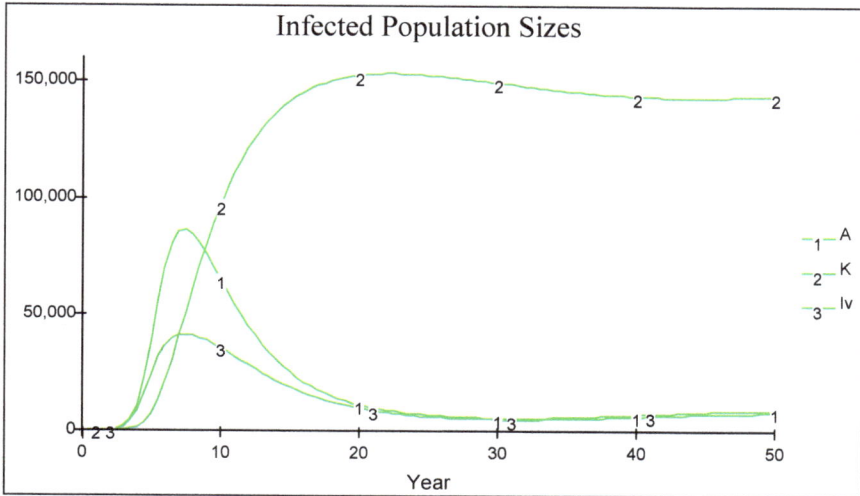

Fig. 1. The dynamics of infected population when there is no medical treatment after the invasion of 10 infected human.

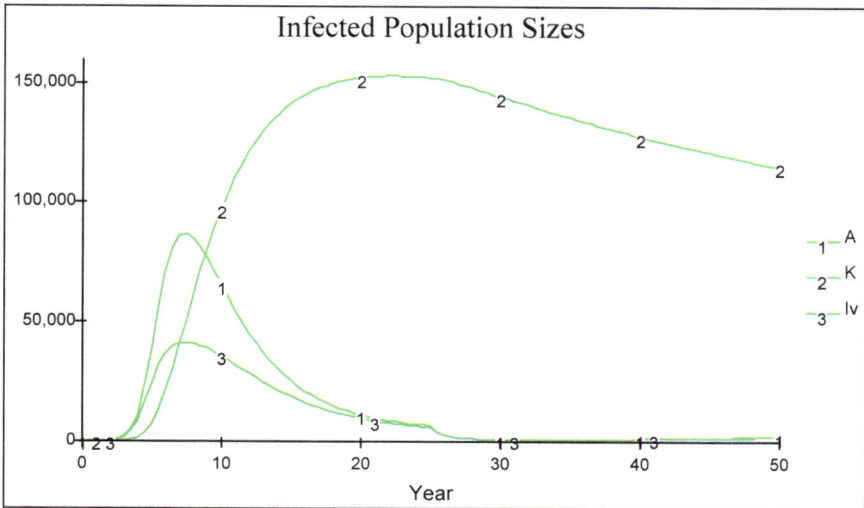

Fig. 2. The dynamics of infected population when there is a medical treatment in the 25th year with $n=200$.

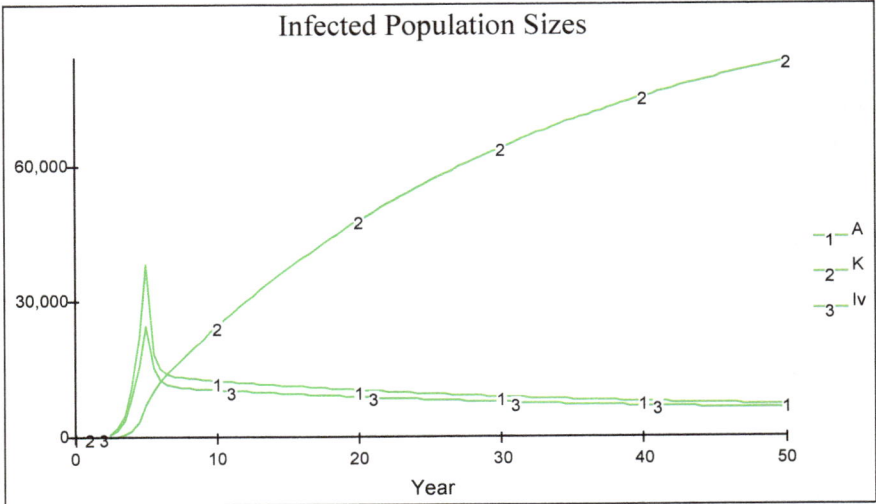

Fig. 3. The dynamics of infected population when there is a medical treatment in the 5th year with n=100.

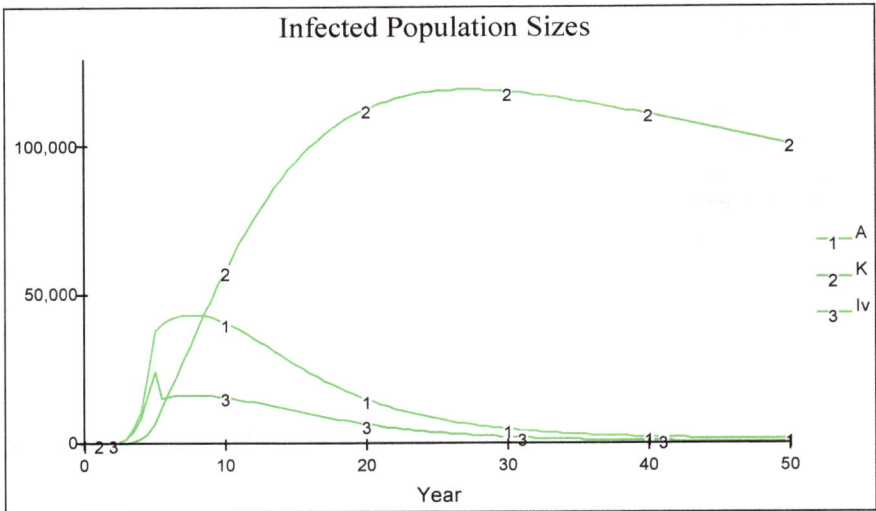

Fig. 4. The dynamics of infected population when there is an effective insect repellent which changes the biting rate to its 50% of the current level with no medical treatment in the 5th year after the disease invasion (n=0).

Other scenarios could also be considered. Some are already known to be ineffective if only applied solely, such as fogging (Soewono & Supriatna, 2002) and other still unexplored, such as newly developed method for shortening mosquitoes life expectancy (Turley et al., 2009). Supposed that with some ways we can reduce the mosquito life expectancy down to 50 % of the existing level (from 30 days as in Table 1 to 15 days). Figure 6 shows its

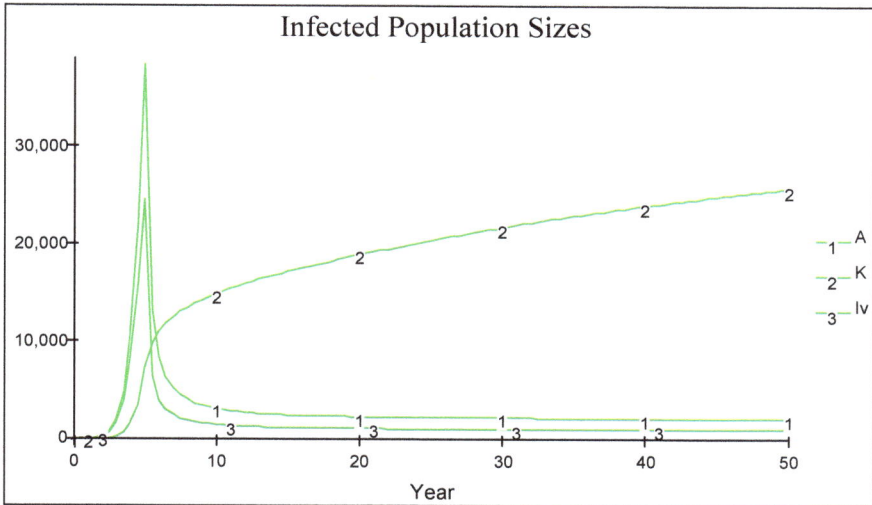

Fig. 5. The dynamics of infected population when there is an effective insect repellent which changes the biting rate to its 50% of the existing level combining with average medical treatment in the 5th year after the disease invasion (n=100).

dynamics which is the same as the dynamics in Figure 4. This is not surprising considering the form of the basic reproduction number (equation (6)), in which the decrease of biting rate acts the same as the decrease of the mosquitoes life expectancy (equivalently the increase of the mosquitoes mortality rate μ_V). If we decrease both values, i.e. the values of the biting rate and the life expectancy, then their effect in reducing the basic reproduction number doubled, such as shown by Figure 7, resulting in the value of the basic reproduction number to be less than one (only 0.755), which means the disappearance of the disease is guaranteed. Even in the absence of medical treatment, Figure 8 shows that if we do this strategy before one year has elapsed then the disease does not have any chance to grow. This suggests that preventive action is better than curative action.

In the previous example we assume that invasion is done by infected human. Next in the following example we assume that invasion is done by infected mosquitoes from an endemic area. Considering the short distance of the mosquito flight, we can assume that this invasion happens un-deliberately, for example via container and other transportation modes. However, considering the stability theorem of the endemic equilibrium point in our previous work (Supriatna et al., 2009), we expect that the long term behaviour of the disease transmission dynamics would be the same as in the first example. In other words, there is an independence of initial values, such as illustrated by Figure 9, in which we assume that there are 100 infected mosquitoes invades the virgin population as described in the first example (Figure 1).

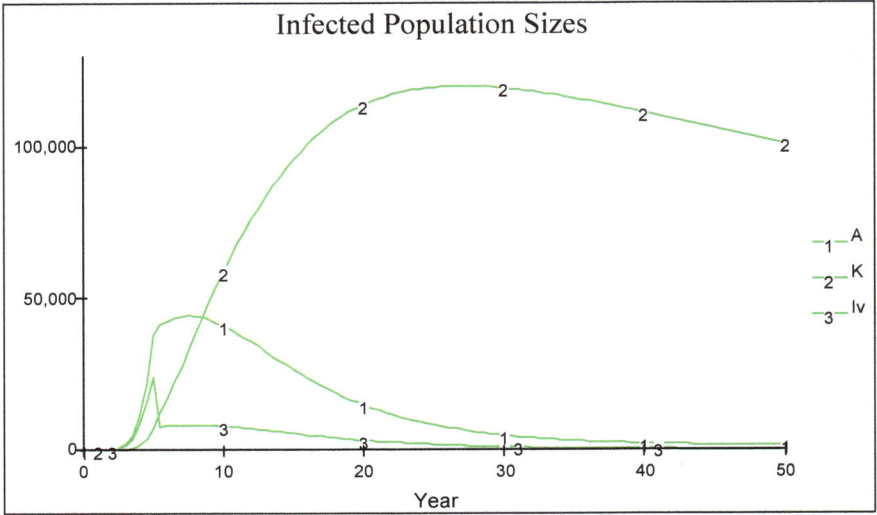

Fig. 6. The dynamics of infected population when there is an intervention which changes the mosquitoes life expectancy to its 50% of the current level with no medical treatment in the 5th year after the disease invasion ($n=0$).

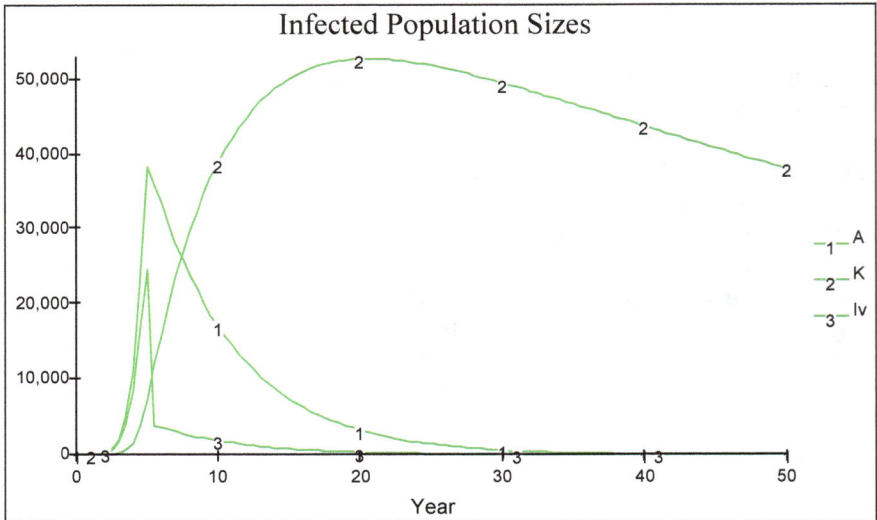

Fig. 7. The dynamics of infected population when there is an intervention which changes both the mosquitoes life expectancy and the biting rate to their 50% level with no medical treatment in the 5th year after the disease invasion ($n=0$).

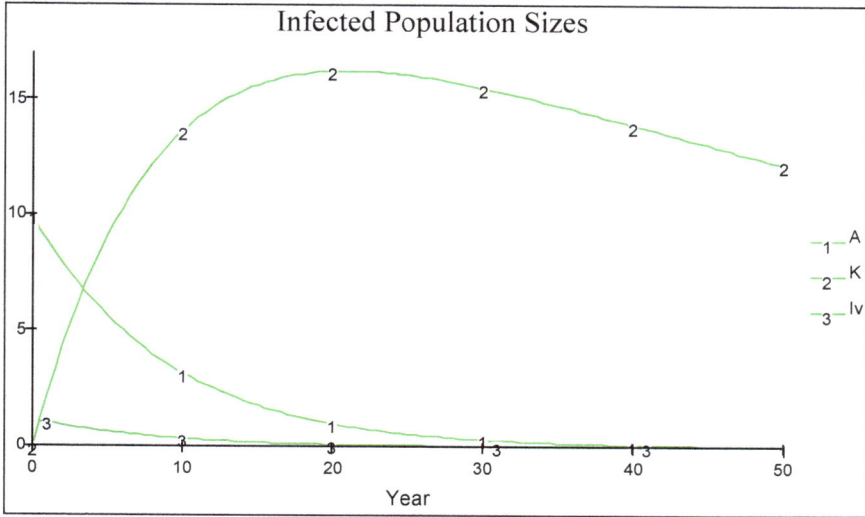

Fig. 8. The dynamics of infected population when there is an intervention which changes both the mosquitoes life expectancy and the biting rate to their 50% level done before one year after the disease invasion has elapsed ($n=0$).

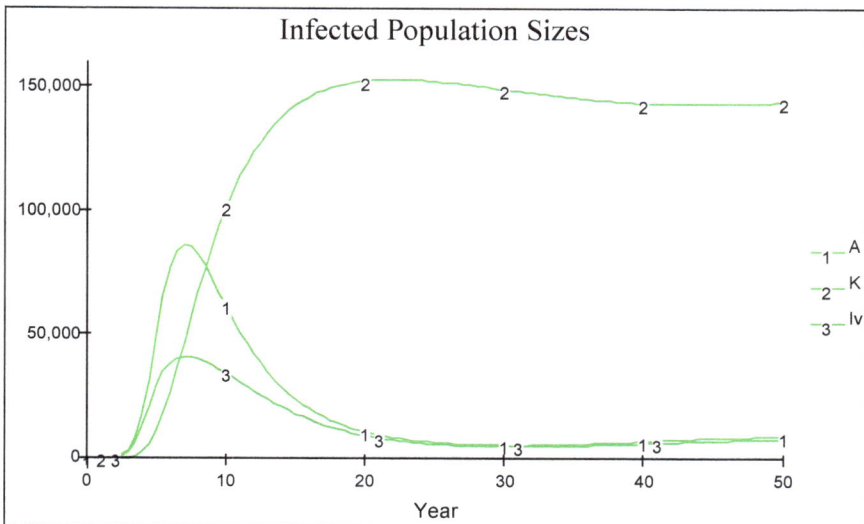

Fig. 9. The dynamics of infected population when there is no medical treatment after the invasion of 100 infected mosquitoes into a totally virgin population. The figure is similar to Figure 1 in which invasion is done by 10 infected human.

3. Mathematical model with delay time in infection period

In this section, we take a delay time into account and re-analysed the resulting model by introducing a new compartment to mimic the presence of the delay time. This is done by adding a sub acute or minor acute compartment A_m into the previous system. The sub acute population has a lower force of infection than the acute population considering their worm burden status, and it might be not infectious yet. This is reflected by a lower successful rate of filarial transmission p_{V2} from the sub acute to susceptible mosquito population, compared to the successful rate of filarial transmission from the acute population p_{V1}. In this case, we can consider the sub acute compartment consist of exposed or latent individuals. Individuals stay in sub acute compartment with the sojourn time $1/\gamma$ before they leave to the acute compartment. The system of equations takes form as the following,

$$\frac{dS_H}{dt} = R_H - \frac{bp_H I_V S_H}{N_H} - \mu_H S_H + \frac{p_0 n \delta A}{N_H}(A + A_m),$$ (7)

$$\frac{dA_m}{dt} = \frac{bp_H I_V S_H}{N_H} - \mu_H A_m - \gamma A_m - \frac{p_0 n \delta A A_m}{N_H},$$ (8)

$$\frac{dA}{dt} = \gamma A_m - \mu_H A - \frac{p_0 n \delta A^2}{N_H} - \delta A,$$ (9)

$$\frac{dS_V}{dt} = R_V - \frac{b(p_{V1}A + p_{V2}A_m)S_V}{N_H} - \mu_V S_V,$$ (10)

$$\frac{dI_V}{dt} = \frac{b(p_{V1}A + p_{V2}A_m)S_V}{N_H} - \mu_V I_V.$$ (11)

3.1 Numerical examples for the model with delay time in infection period

As in the previous section, we provide a simulation for the model of equations (7) to (11) to gain some insights. The parameters are the same as before unless it is stated explicitly.

Compared to Figure 1, in which there are 10 acute infected human initially, Figure 10 shows that the present of time delay, by assuming that the sojourn time in the sub acute compartment is 5 years (hence γ is 1/5) with the probability of transmission to the mosquitoes is only 10% of the probability of the acute compartment (hence p_{V2} is 0.01), has an effect on significantly delaying the accumulation of the chronic and reducing the number of acute human population. However, the total infectious ($A + A_m$) in Figure 10 is slightly greater than the total infectious (A) in Figure 1.

We can also simulate if in fact we were unable to perfectly isolate the chronic individuals, hence there is a transmission from a portion of them to the mosquitoes. We would expect the transmission rate from the chronic is far greater than the one from the acute population, say the transmission is more certain considering the worm burden carried by them. One of

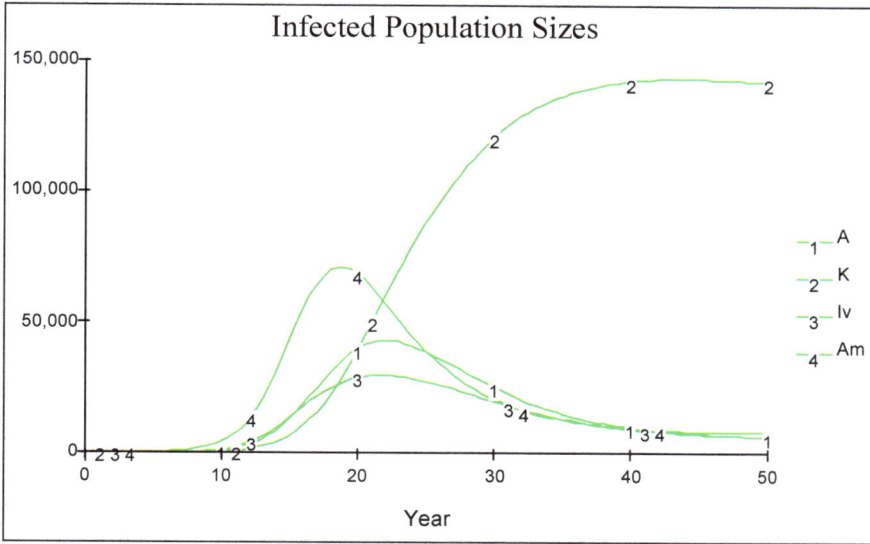

Fig. 10. The dynamics of infected population when there is no medical treatment after the invasion of infected human comprising of 10 acute individuals. Here we assume that there is no sub acute individual, initially.

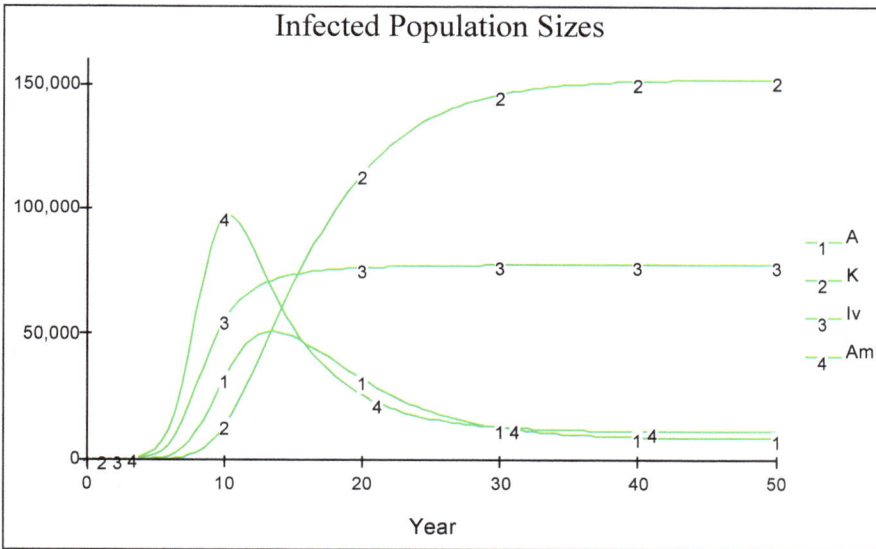

Fig. 11. The dynamics of infected population as with all parameters as in Figure 10, with an addition that infection also occurs from the chronic by assuming there is no perfect isolation.

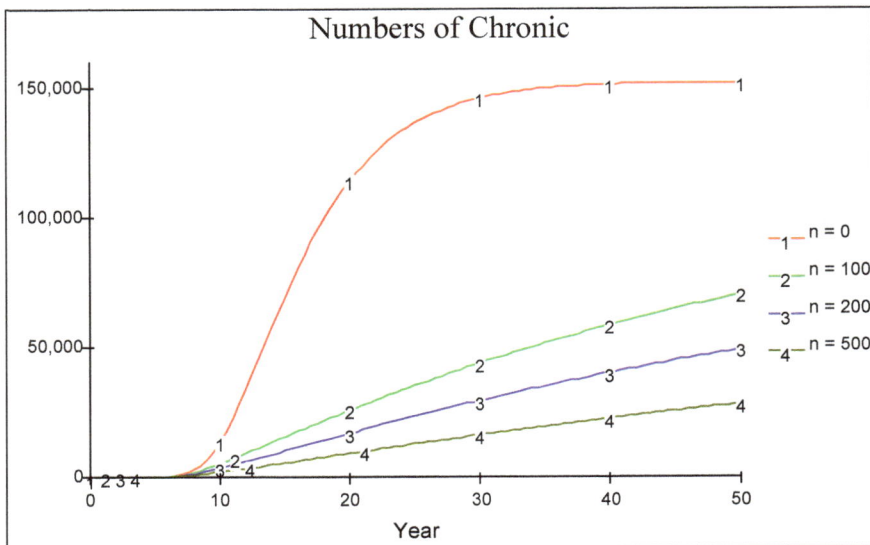

Fig. 12. The dynamics of chronic population when there is an early medical treatment with various values of n.

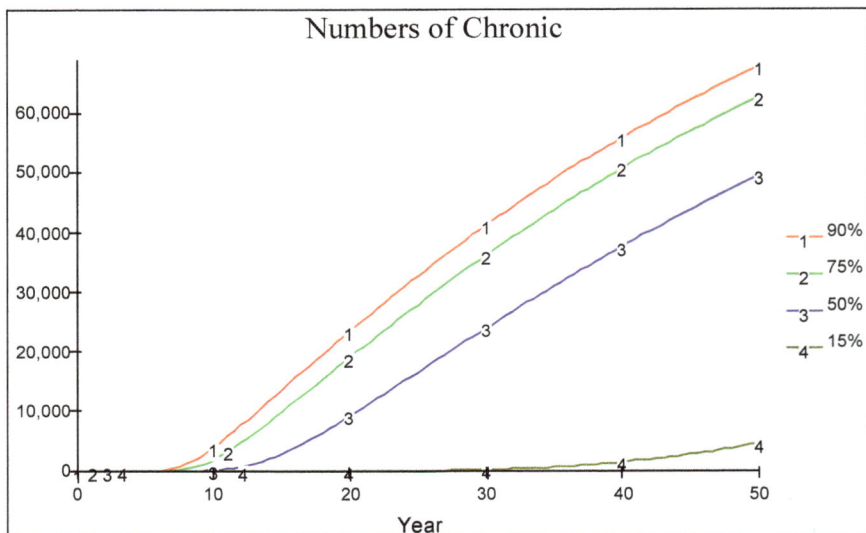

Fig. 13. The dynamics of chronic population when there is an early medical treatment with $n=100$ together with the various reduction of the biting rate up to a certain level.

the realisations is shown in Figure 11. The figure reveals that the peak of the outbreak is higher and reached earlier compared to that in Figure 10. Note that in the early years, there is an iceberg phenomenon, in which the number of chronic is far less than the number of acute. This indicates that early treatment is better than late treatment. Suppose that we administer a medical treatment as in the previous section, measured by the number of screening n. Figure 12 shows various regimes of treatment done continuously since the beginning of the course of the epidemic. Figure 13 shows that a low level of medical treatment combined with the high reduction of biting rate (e.g. up to 15% of the original biting rate) performs better than that resulting from high level of medical treatment with no reduction in biting rate.

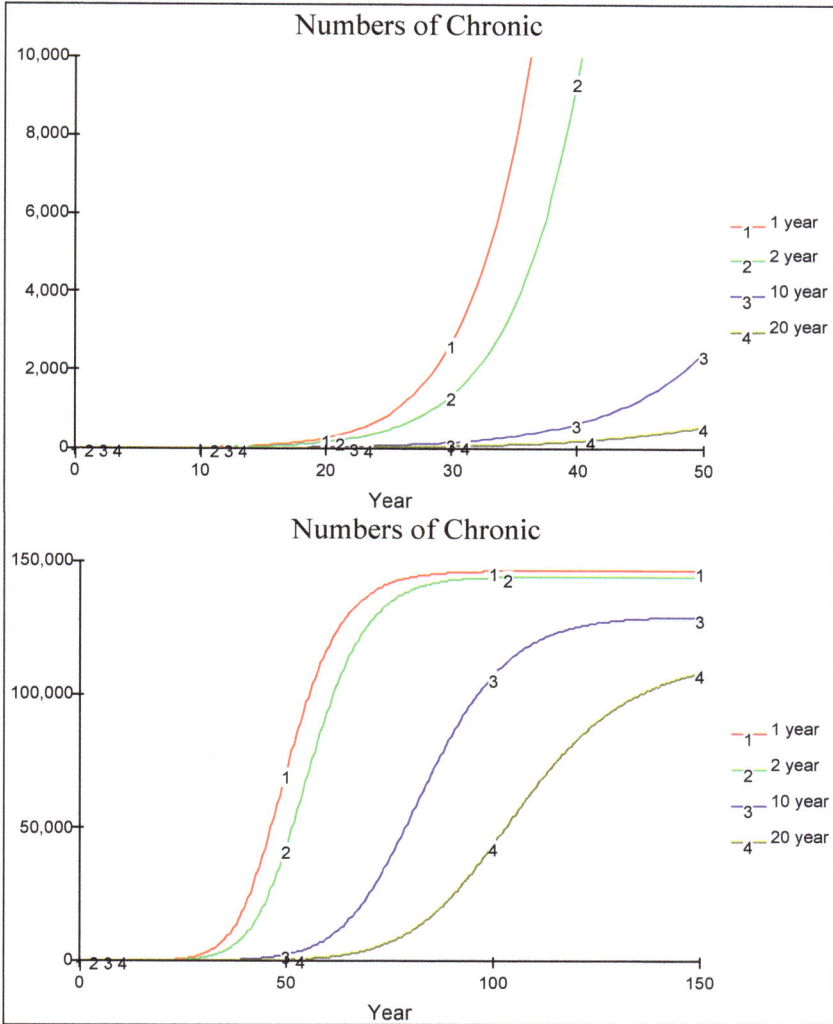

Fig. 14. The dynamics of chronic population when prophylaxis is given to the whole population with various effects to the sub acute sojourn time (equivalent to the reciprocal value of the recruitment rate from sub acute to acute population).

Suppose now that we have another scenario of treatment, that is giving prophylaxis to all the populations (set $n=0$, simply to evaluate the effectiveness of this prophylaxis). The prophylaxis works by inhibiting the growth of the worms inside human, say by delaying the recruitment into the acute population A from the sub acute population A_m. Technically this is done by varying the values of the transition rate γ (or equivalently the sub acute sojourn time $1/\gamma$) in the model. Figure 14 shows the effect of delay for various sojourn time due to the effect of the prophylaxis application. It seems that all the graphs increase exponentially (upper figure), but in fact at the end they end up to their stable equilibrium (lower figure) with different speed and different peak. This indicates that controlling the density of worm inside the body of infective human is effective in reducing the number of filarial infection. The model assumes that the delivery of prophylaxis has a result in a constant effect over time, which doesn't reflect the reality. To increase the realism, we should consider the decrease of prophylaxis effectiveness by modifying or refining the model. Nevertheless, we still can apply the current model by only believing the short-term prediction given by the model, say only in one to two years prediction and use it as guidance in a periodic delivery of a mass drug administration program.

The introduction of a single exposed compartment is not without a problem. Getz and Lloyd-Smith (2006) showed that a single exposed compartment will produce an exponentially-distributed sojourn time in the exposed stage. Referring to our delay model (equations (8) and (9)), this distribution has mean at $1/\gamma$ while its modus is at 0, which is a poor match to the real distribution of latent periods. Plant and Wilson (1986) pointed out that the drawback can be resolved by introducing a distributed delay or staging delay time approach comprising of k classes of sub acute or exposed individual. This approach gives a gamma-distributed total time of individuals staying in the exposed class with mean $1/\gamma$ and variance $1/(k\gamma^2)$. Note that a fixed time delay $1/\gamma$ is obtained whenever the number of delay stages k approaches the infinity.

In this part we use this approach (see also Getz and Lloyd-Smith (2006)) to our delay model by introducing multiple exposed compartments which is more appropriate to the disease like filariasis which has more than one different exposed stages. The general model is the same as equations (7) to (11) except that equations (8) and (9) are replaced by

$$\frac{dA_{m1}}{dt} = \frac{bp_H I_V S_H}{N_H} - k\gamma A_{m1} - \mu_H A_{m1} - \frac{p_0 n\delta A A_{m1}}{N_H}, \tag{12}$$

$$\frac{dA_{mi}}{dt} = k\gamma(A_{mi-1} - A_i) - \mu_H A_{mi} - \frac{p_0 n\delta A A_{mi}}{N_H}, \qquad i = 2,...,k, \tag{13}$$

$$\frac{dA}{dt} = k\gamma A_{mk} - \mu_H A - \frac{p_0 n\delta A^2}{N_H} - \delta A. \tag{14}$$

The system is much more complex since it consists of 15 differential equations compared to just 6 differential equations in the previous model. However, numerical example in Figure 15 shows that for $k = 10$ (and also for any $k > 1$), the simpler model of equations (7) to (11), qualitatively, is a good approximation of the more realistic model of the same equations but with equations (8) and (9) are replaced by equations (12) to (14). Initially, the prediction of simpler model ($K1$ in Figure 15) slightly overestimates, but then after a certain years it begins to underestimate, the "true" numbers of chronic individuals ($K10$ in Figure 15). However in the long-term both model produce the same equilibrium point (not shown in the Figure).

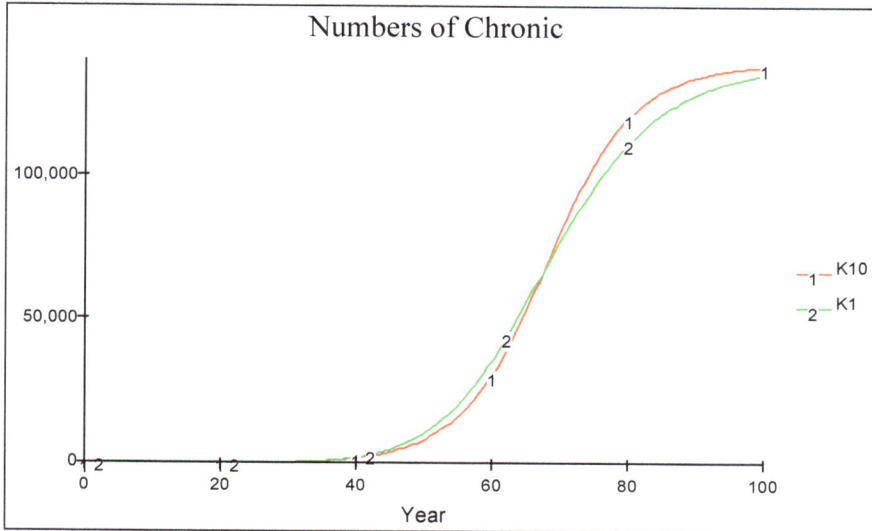

Fig. 15. The dynamics of chronic population predicted by the simple model of equations (7) to (11) and the more realistic staging delay time model of the same equations but with equations (8) and (9) are replaced by equations (12) to (14).

4. Conclusion

In this chapter we review a mathematical model of filarial transmission in human and in mosquitoes. Some simulations are carried out to obtain some insights regarding the transmission and possible actions to control the transmission. Some refinement of the model could be done in many directions to increase the realism of the model and to obtain a more accurate prediction. New directions may include the evolutionary, sosio-economics, and climatology aspects of the disease (Levin, 2002).

In the evolutionary issues of epidemiology, some agents of diseases may develop resistance to certain drug. It is worth to explore how this affects the transmission of the diseases. In many situations, especially in developing countries, there always competing interests related to limited resources and budget. There are many other important diseases, other than filariasis, needs for attention. Choosing the right priorities are among the concerns of health managers and authorities. In the absence of sufficient health budget it is important to address questions like the long term consequences when the treatment is terminated, either purportedly, e.g. because the budget is re-allocated to a higher priority health problem (to other endemic places of the same disease or to other disease problems) or inadvertently (due to the decreasing compliance of the program implementation). This is an example of sosio-economics issues in epidemiology (Supali *et al.*, in prep.). Climate change also regarded as a factor contributes to current emerging and re-emerging infectious diseases. For example, since the global temperature is rising then suitable habitat for mosquitoes becomes wider. It is reported that many parts in the globe of previously free from mosquito is now invaded by incoming mosquitoes. To obtain a better prediction of global filarial transmission, this climatology aspect also should be considered. We believe that there are many other venues are possible for future research in mathematical aspect of filariasis transmission.

5. Acknowledgment

Part of the research is funded by the Indonesian Government through the scheme of Penelitian Hibah Kompetensi 2012.

6. Appendices

6.1 Powersim diagram of the basic filariasis model

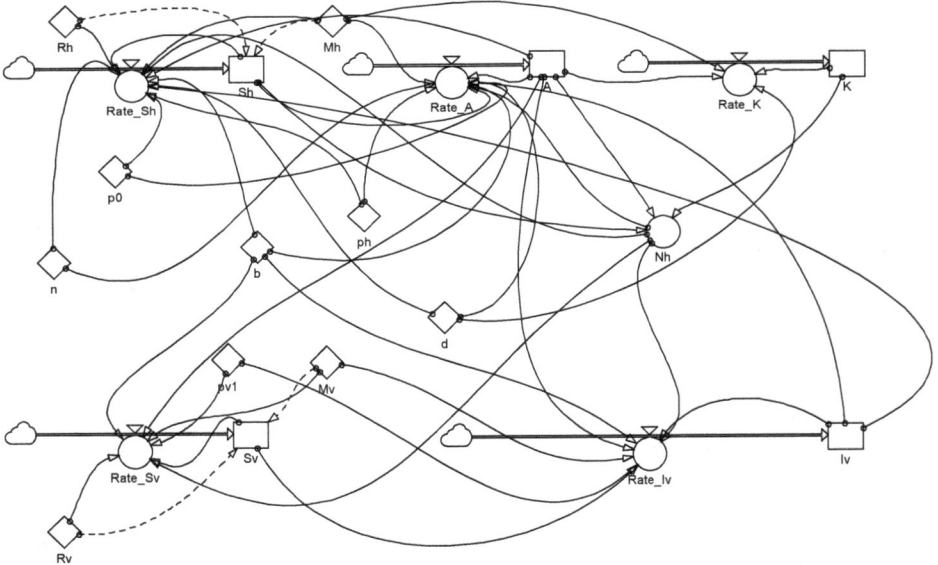

6.2 Powersim listing program of the basic filariasis model

```
init      A = 10
flow      A = +dt*Rate_A
init      Iv = 0
flow      Iv = +dt*Rate_Iv
init      K = 0
flow      K = +dt*Rate_K
init      Sh = Rh/Mh
flow      Sh = +dt*Rate_Sh
```

init   Sv = Rv/Mv
flow   Sv = +dt*Rate_Sv
aux   Rate_A = ((b*Iv*Sh*ph)/Nh)-Mh*A-((p0*n*A*d*A)/Nh)-d*A
aux   Rate_Iv = ((b*Sv*A*pv1)/Nh)-Mv*Iv
aux   Rate_K = d*A-Mh*K
aux   Rate_Sh = Rh-((b*Iv*Sh*ph)/Nh)-Mh*Sh+((p0*n*A*d*A)/Nh)
aux   Rate_Sv = Rv-((b*Sv*A*pv1)/Nh)-Mv*Sv
aux   Nh = Sh+A+K
const   b = 250
const   d = 0.25
const   Mh = 1/70
const   Mv = 365/30
const   n = 0
const   p0 = 0.75
const   ph = 0.01
const   pv1 = 0.1
const   Rh = 2500
const   Rv = 1000000

7. References

Diekmann, O. & Heesterbeek, J.A.P. (2000). *Mathematical Epidemiology of Infectious Diseases*, John Wiley & Son, ISBN 978-0471492412 , New York, USA

Getz, W.M. & Lloyd-Smith, J.O. (2006). Basic Method for Modeling the Invasion and Spread of Contagious Diseases, In: *Disease Evolution: Models, Concepts, and Data Analyses*, Z. Feng; U. Dieckmann & S. Levin (Eds.), 87-105, AMS, ISBN 0-8218-3753-2, USA

Goodman, B. (1994). Models Aid Understanding, Help Control Parasites [News]. *Science* 264: 1862-1863

Krentel, A.; Fischer, P.; Manoempil, P.; Supali, T.; Servais, G. & Ruckert, P. (2006). Using Knowledge, Attitudes and Practice (KAP) Surveys on Lymphatic Filariasis to Prepare a Health Promotion Campaign for Mass Drug Administration in Alor District, Indonesia. *Tropical Medicine and International Health*. 11: 1731–1740

Levin, S.A (2002). New Directions in the Mathematics of Infectious Disease. In: *Mathematical Approaches for Emerging and Reemerging Infectious Diseases: Models, Methods, and Theory*, Castillo-Chavez, C *et al.* (Eds.), 1-5, Springer, ISBN 0-387-95355-8, New-York, USA

Molyneux, D. & Zagaria, N. (2002). Lymphatic Filariasis Elimination: Progress in Global Programme Development. *Ann. Trop. Med. Parasitol.* 96 (Suppl 2): S15-40

Plant, R.E. & Wilson, L.T. (1986). Models for Age-Structured Population with Distributed Maturation Rates. *J. Math. Biol.* 23, 247-262.

Soewono, E. & Supriatna, A.K. (2002). A Two-Dimensional Model for the Transmission of Dengue Fever Disease. *Bulletin of Malaysian Mathematical Sciences Society* 24(1): 49-57

Supali, T.; Wibowo, H.; Ruuckert, P; Fischer K.; Ismid, I.S.; Purnomo; Djuardi, Y. & Fischer P. (2002). High prevalence of Brugia timori infection in the Highland of Alor Island, Indonesia. *Am. J. Trop. Med. Hyg.*, 66(5), 2002, pp. 560–565

Supali, T.; Tasman, H.; Supriatna, A.K.; Soewono, E. & Nuraini, N. Long Term Effects of Mass Drug Administration on Lymphatics Filariasis Transmision, In Prep.

Supriatna, A. K.; Serviana, H. & Soewono, E. (2009). A Mathematical Model to Investigate the Long-Term Effects of the Lymphatic Filariasis Medical Treatment in Jati Sampurna, West Java. *ITB Journal of Science* Vol: 41 Issue: 1 Pages/record No.: 1-14

Turley A.P.; Moreira, L.A.; O'Neill, S.L. & McGraw, E.A. (2009). Wolbachia Infection Reduces Blood-Feeding Success in the Dengue Fever Mosquito, Aedes aegypti. *PLOS Neglected Tropical Diseases*. 3(9): e516

World Health Organization (2005). Global Programme to Eliminate Lymphatic Filariasis - Progress Report For 2004. Wkly. *Epidemiol. Rec.* 80: 202-212

Permissions

The contributors of this book come from diverse backgrounds, making this book a truly international effort. This book will bring forth new frontiers with its revolutionizing research information and detailed analysis of the nascent developments around the world.

We would like to thank Prof. Alfonso J. Rodriguez-Morales, for lending his expertise to make the book truly unique. He has played a crucial role in the development of this book. Without his invaluable contribution this book wouldn't have been possible. He has made vital efforts to compile up to date information on the varied aspects of this subject to make this book a valuable addition to the collection of many professionals and students.

This book was conceptualized with the vision of imparting up-to-date information and advanced data in this field. To ensure the same, a matchless editorial board was set up. Every individual on the board went through rigorous rounds of assessment to prove their worth. After which they invested a large part of their time researching and compiling the most relevant data for our readers. Conferences and sessions were held from time to time between the editorial board and the contributing authors to present the data in the most comprehensible form. The editorial team has worked tirelessly to provide valuable and valid information to help people across the globe.

Every chapter published in this book has been scrutinized by our experts. Their significance has been extensively debated. The topics covered herein carry significant findings which will fuel the growth of the discipline. They may even be implemented as practical applications or may be referred to as a beginning point for another development. Chapters in this book were first published by InTech; hereby published with permission under the Creative Commons Attribution License or equivalent.

The editorial board has been involved in producing this book since its inception. They have spent rigorous hours researching and exploring the diverse topics which have resulted in the successful publishing of this book. They have passed on their knowledge of decades through this book. To expedite this challenging task, the publisher supported the team at every step. A small team of assistant editors was also appointed to further simplify the editing procedure and attain best results for the readers.

Our editorial team has been hand-picked from every corner of the world. Their multi-ethnicity adds dynamic inputs to the discussions which result in innovative outcomes. These outcomes are then further discussed with the researchers and contributors who give their valuable feedback and opinion regarding the same. The feedback is then collaborated with the researches and they are edited in a comprehensive manner to aid the understanding of the subject.

Apart from the editorial board, the designing team has also invested a significant amount of their time in understanding the subject and creating the most relevant covers. They scrutinized every image to scout for the most suitable representation of the subject and create an appropriate cover for the book.

The publishing team has been involved in this book since its early stages. They were actively engaged in every process, be it collecting the data, connecting with the contributors or procuring relevant information. The team has been an ardent support to the editorial, designing and production team. Their endless efforts to recruit the best for this project, has resulted in the accomplishment of this book. They are a veteran in the field of academics and their pool of knowledge is as vast as their experience in printing. Their expertise and guidance has proved useful at every step. Their uncompromising quality standards have made this book an exceptional effort. Their encouragement from time to time has been an inspiration for everyone.

The publisher and the editorial board hope that this book will prove to be a valuable piece of knowledge for researchers, students, practitioners and scholars across the globe.

List of Contributors

Ross Parker and Kevin Leary
Uniformed Services University of the Health Sciences, USA

Benjamin G. Koudou
Vector Group, Liverpool School of Tropical Medicine, Pembroke Place, Liverpool, UK, Centre Suisse de Recherches Scientifiques, Abidjan, University of Abobo-Adjame´, Abidjan, Côte d'Ivoire

Marcel Tanner and Juerg Utzinger
Department of Epidemiology and Public Health, Swiss Tropical and Public Health Institute, Basel,
University of Basel, Basel, Switzerland

A. Samie
Molecular Parasitology and Opportunistic Infection Program, Department of Microbiology, University of Venda, Private Bag X5050 Thohoyandou 0950, South Africa

A. ElBakri and Ra'ed AbuOdeh
Medical Laboratory Technology Department, College of Health Sciences,University of Sharjah, Sharjah, United Arab Emirates

Akila Fathallah Mili
Laboratory of Parasitology, Farhat Hached Hospital, Sousse, Laboratory of Parasitic Epidemiology and Ecology (LEEP) - LR00SP04, Institut Pasteur, Tunis, Tunisia

Fatma Saghrouni and Moncef BenSaid
Laboratory of Parasitology, Farhat Hached Hospital, Sousse, Institut Pasteur, Tunis, Tunisia

Zeineb BenSaid
Service of Dermatology, Farhat Hached Hospital, Sousse, Institut Pasteur, Tunis, Tunisia

Yusr Saadi- BenAoun and Ikram Guizani
Laboratory of Parasitic Epidemiology and Ecology (LEEP) - LR00SP04, Institut Pasteur, Tunis, Tunisia

Oscar Bruna-Romero and Dulcilene Mayrink de Oliveira
Department of Microbiology, Instituto de Ciências Biológicas, Universidade Federal de Minas Gerais – UFMG, Belo Horizonte-MG, Brazil

Valter Ferreira de Andrade-Neto
Department of Microbiology and Parasitology, Centro de Biociências, Universidade Federal do Rio Grande do Norte – UFRN, Natal-RN, Brazil

Consuelo Giménez Pardo and Lourdes Lledó García
Alcalá University, Spain

Andrés F. Flórez
German Cancer Research Center (DKFZ)/ Division Theoretical Systems Biology, Heidelberg, Germany, Universidad de Antioquia/Programa de Estudio y Control de Enfermedades Tropicales – PECET, Medellín, Columbia

Stanley Watowich
University of Texas Medical Branch/Department of Biochemistry and Molecular Biology and the Sealy Center for Structural Biology and Molecular Biophysics, Galveston, USA

Carlos Muskus
Universidad de Antioquia/Programa de Estudio y Control de Enfermedades Tropicales – PECET, Medellín, Columbia

Iván S. Marcipar
Laboratorio de Tecnología Inmunológica (LTI), Fac. Bioquímica y Cs. Biológicas, Universidad Nacional del Litoral, Argentina

Claudia M. Lagier
Instituto de Química Rosario (IQUIR-CONICET), División Química Analítica, Fac. Cs. Bioquímicas y Farmacéuticas, Universidad Nacional de Rosario, Argentina

Antoni Soriano Arandes and Frederic Gómez Bertomeu
University Hospital Joan XXIII of Tarragona, Spain

Josué de Moraes
Supervisão de Vigilância em Saúde, SUVIS Casa Verde, Secretaria de Saúde da Cidade de São Paulo, Rua Ferreira de Almeida, São Paulo, SP, Brazil

Aline S. de Aluja
Departamento de Patología, Facultad de Medicina Veterinaria y Zootecnia, Universidad Nacional Autónoma de México, Ciudad Universitaria, D. F., Mexico

Julio Morales Soto
Lab. MVZ. Aline S. de Aluja, Facultad de Medicina Veterinaria y Zootecnia, Universidad Nacional Autónoma de México, Ciudad Universitaria, D. F., Mexico

Edda Sciutto
Lab. de Inmunología, Instituto de Investigaciones Biomédicas, Universidad Nacional Autónoma de México, Ciudad Universitaria, D. F., Mexico

Louis-Albert Tchuem Tchuenté
University of Yaoundé I, Laboratory of Parasitology and Ecology, Centre for Schistosomiasis and Parasitology, Yaoundé, Cameroon

Adisak Bhumiratana
Department of Parasitology and Entomology, Faculty of Public Health, Mahidol University, Center for EcoHealth Disease Modeling and Intervention Development Research, Faculty of Public Health, Mahidol University, Environmental Pathogen Molecular Biology and Epidemiology Research Unit, Faculty of Veterinary Medicine, Mahanakorn University of Technology, Bangkok, Thailand

Apiradee Intarapuk and Danai Sangthong
Environmental Pathogen Molecular Biology and Epidemiology Research Unit, Faculty of Veterinary Medicine, Mahanakorn University of Technology, Bangkok, Thailand

Surachart Koyadun
Ministry of Public Health, Department of Disease Control, Office of Disease Prevention and Control 11 Nakhon Si Thammarat, Thailand

Prapassorn Pechgit
Department of Parasitology and Entomology, Faculty of Public Health, Mahidol University, Bangkok, Thailand

Jinrapa Pothikasikorn
Department of Microbiology, Faculty of Science, Mahidol University, Bangkok, Thailand

Eleuza R. Machado and Lúcia H. Faccioli
Department of Clinical Analyses, Toxicology and Bromatology Faculty of Pharmaceutics Sciences of Ribeirão Preto, University of São Paulo, Brazil

Cristiane Tefé-Silva and Simone G. Ramos
Department of Pathology, Faculty of Medicine of Ribeirão Preto, Brazil

Asep K. Supriatna and N. Anggriani
Padjadjaran University, Indonesia